HEAL CANCER: CHOOSE YOUR OWN
SURVIVAL PATH

HEAL CANCER: CHOOSE YOUR OWN SURVIVAL PATH

Dr Ruth Cilento, MB, BS, DBM, DAc

HILL OF CONTENT
Melbourne

First published in Australia 1993
by Hill of Content Publishing Company Pty Ltd
86 Bourke Street, Melbourne, Australia 3000

© Copyright Ruth Cilento 1993

Reprinted 1993

Typeset by Midland Typesetters, Maryborough, Victoria
Printed in Australia by Australian Print Group, Maryborough, Victoria

National Library of Australia
Cataloguing-in-Publication data

Cilento, Ruth, 1925–
 Heal cancer: choose your own survival path.

 Bibliography.
 Includes index.
 ISBN 0 85572 213 4.

 1. Cancer—Popular works. I. Title.

616.994

FOREWORD

Of all the diseases known to man, cancer is the most feared. Each year millions die of cancer of the lung, breast, intestines, prostate and dozens of other forms. Individuals who escape the tragedy of cancer are blessed, and families free of cancer have much to be grateful for.

Although medical science claims to be winning the war on cancer, the mortality statistics show otherwise. Even when cancer is discovered and treated early, many patients ultimately succumb to the disease. Despite the latest advances in treatment, the cure rate for certain forms of cancer remains abysmal.

Why is this so?

The crux of the matter is that the cause of cancer is still not well understood by medical scientists. Nor does medical science recognise the role of the hidden killer in the picture, the so-called 'cancer microbe'—the infectious agent that is always present and active in cancer. As the cancerous process continues, these microbes greatly increase in number and toxicity. Unrecognised by medical scientists, it is this hidden infectious process that causes the debilitation, weight loss, loss of appetite and deterioration that every dying cancer patient experiences. Our inability to cure cancer largely stems from the refusal to recognise the existence and importance of the cancer microbe.

For many years traditional medicine has used surgery, radiation and chemotherapy as the primary forms of treatment for cancer. For some patients this has proved successful. However, for all those who have died of cancer these forms of therapy must be considered a failure. Obviously, new forms of cancer therapy must be undertaken if we are to improve our ability to cure it.

The extreme resistance of orthodox medicine to alternative forms of cancer treatment is legendary. Any form of therapy that does not include surgery, radiation or chemotherapy is likely to encounter severe condemnation by the medical establishment.

The conventional approach to cancer treatment is directed at killing the cancer by surgery, radiation and chemotherapy. In this process the patient is expected to do little else but cooperate fully in the oncologist's treatment plan. If the treatment fails, the physician sadly declares that everything that could have been done was done. The cancer simply did not respond to the treatment.

It is a rare doctor who will challenge the system and dare to suggest that more can be done and should be done for the healing of cancer. It is a rare doctor who will encourage the patient to use the power of the mind and suggest meditation and affirmations in the fight against disease. Rarely do physicians suggest dietary changes, or the addition of supplements, vitamins and minerals as adjuncts for cancer treatment.

In this book, Ruth Cilento bravely presents unorthodox and controversial elements of cancer healing for your consideration.

In addition, Dr Cilento brings the reader a treasure trove of knowledge derived from the research of the great cancer pioneers who have studied the cancer microbe, and who have developed therapies to combat its harmful effects in the body. 'Wholistic' treatment methods for cancer are often criticised as being unscientific; however, in the light of cancer microbe research studies, the rationale for wholistic treatment begins to take on additional meaning and significance.

For many years I have studied the cancer microbe, not only in cancer but also in other immunologic diseases, including AIDS. I am often asked how the cancer microbe can be killed.

It took me many years to figure out that the cancer microbe is, in reality, inseparable from us. The cancer microbe resides in everyone, the healthy people and the sick. It is in us and of us and cannot be destroyed—only transformed.

People who have been cured of cancer are living in harmony with the cancer microbe.

Everything that happens to us serves as an opportunity for growth and transformation. Even a diagnosis of cancer can serve as a stimulus for positive change in our lives.

Each of us must pioneer our healing in the way that is best for us. Doctor Cilento has vast experience as a medical healer. I applaud her willingness to share her experiences with others in need of guidance and support in difficult circumstances.

I admire Dr Cilento's courage in presenting the controversial ideas contained in this book. It is my belief that cancer can eventually be conquered by opening our minds to new ideas about its origin and treatment. In this process we will undoubtedly discover new facets of our mind-body-spirit relationship which also connects us all to one another, to the planet and to the cosmos.

Alan Cantwell Jr, MD

Doctor Alan Cantwell MD is a dermatologist and cancer/AIDS researcher who has written over thirty published papers on cancer, AIDS, and other immune deficiency diseases. He is the author of *AIDS: The Mystery and the Solution*, *AIDS and the Doctors of Death*, and *The Cancer Microbe*. He lives and practices in Los Angeles.

ACKNOWLEDGEMENTS

It seems that this writing has gone on forever; at least so long has it been filling my wakeful nights that I have sometimes forgotten all the people who have made it possible for me.

My long-term secretary Fay Henley, who has now retired, was my constant helper when this book began, and has brought to it her skill at typing, setting out and interpreting my confused script to make legible copy. Nicholette Wray, my present secretary and office manager, also has these skills. She inherited these somewhat onerous tasks and is my helper and close friend in discussing material. Helen Fowler, our second in command, also helps mightily to bring order out of chaos in our busy office. Valerie Dommett, the indomitable worker, offered to put the second draft on her computer. I was hesitant about accepting this providential offer because Val also has a business and family to run, but the manuscript could never have been finished without her great help and encouragement. Thanks to Gwen Hussie for corrections at short notice. A special thanks also to those patients who read the manuscript. I am profoundly grateful to all these loyal and efficient people who have given me so much more help than the call of duty requires.

I have carefully acknowledged most of the material quoted here and there in the book, but in some instances I have found permission difficult to obtain because there has been no address or source to contact. In some cases, the words were written long ago and the author has died. I have tried to acknowledge the author and the source within my text, hoping that there will be tolerance in understanding that I have never willfully stolen someone's words but simply been enthralled by the concurrence with my own thoughts, and so shared that with the reader. If I have failed to acknowledge, for instance in the 'affirmations' at the bottom of the pages and in quotes from magazines, it is because I can't find the source. So I apologise here and now and ask forbearance. The list of authors and publishers in the Bibliography gives the source and the acknowledgement for some of the material not specifically mentioned.

The publisher Michelle Anderson and all the staff, and Helen Chamberlin, the editor, from the first day of contact have been enthusiastic, encouraging and efficient. I thank them.

I also wish to thank the readers for their advice and encouragement. My cousin, Wendy Porter, and her writer husband, James, who read the manuscript first were really instrumental in making me finish it when I had cold feet. Tom Walker, my mother's cousin, and his wife, Grace, added their approval after reading the tangled draft. Because writing is such a solitary occupation and I was so bound up in my own thoughts, the support and impressions of these kind people have been essential for me in gauging reader reaction.

We learn all through life so how could I possibly remember all my wonderful teachers and helpers through school, university and hospital years. Even those who put obstacles in the way taught me valuable lessons. But most of all I wish to acknowledge the part my patients and group members have played in teaching me, supporting my ideas, putting up with my scolding and believing in our ever-progressing knowledge and applying it with the amazing courage and resource that is the strength of the human spirit.

CONTENTS

Foreword v
Acknowledgements ix
Introduction 1

PART ONE: FINDING THE RIGHT PATH
1 Starting the search 7
  Making a more workable plan 11
  Looking for a like-minded colleague 11
  Why don't you teach other doctors? 12
  My parents, my helpers 14
  The Cilento Survival Plan 15

2 We Are Losing the Fight 16

PART TWO: STEPS ON THE ROAD TO RECOVERY
3 Healing the body 21
  Preliminaries 21
  Making the lifestyle changes 24

4 The trouble with statistics 31
  Results of treatment study 35
  How long have I got? 36

5 Lifestyle changes necessary for survival 41
  Build up the general health 41
  Build up the immune system 41
  Eliminate anything that causes cancer to grow faster 43
  Support the liver 45
  Look on Changes as a Challenge 46
  Establish peace of mind 46

6 Understanding the Survival Plan	47
Guidelines for the food plan	47
Special situations	48
The fluids	49
What's for breakfast?	51
7 The diet and supplements for cancer control	66
Food Plan	67
Why use supplements in such high doses?	75
How come I did all that and I still got cancer?	78
8 Clearing the Mind	81
Understanding the brain—a new science	81
We are born with life energy and survival emotions	83
Families that fight, families that fear	84
What is your attitude of mind about healing?	88
Life force	88
Relax for better health	89
Thinking in pictures: teach your body to do your mind's bidding	91
Affirmations	94
Open-eye meditation on colour	96
9 Reviving the spirit	98
Confidence and self-esteem	98
The spirit rules	101
Quality of Life Support Group	101

PART THREE: ON THE TRAIL OF DISCOVERY

10 Taking the road to America	107
Making a film of the blood	107
The Cancer Control Society annual convention	110
The Livingston Medical Clinic	115
Dr Issels, the vaccine and dead teeth	117
Is light important to health? Dr John Ott	121
Showing the film in Brisbane	122

PART FOUR: PHYSIOLOGICAL SIGNPOSTS

11 Why don't we all get cancer?	125

12	What is the immune system?	128
	Some good food sources of vitamins and minerals	133
13	What is a vaccine?	135
	Who can use a vaccine?	137
	More cells	138
14	Biological products in treatment	139
	Herbs for healing	145
	Is chemotherapy harmful to the immune system?	149
	What about radium?	150
	Who are the healers?	151

PART FIVE: THROUGH THE MAZE OF CANCEROUS CHANGES

15	What are stressed cells?	155
	Energy source	155
	Other factors influencing the pre-cancerous change	157
	The cell membrane	158
	Contact inhibition	159
	The ongoing work of Dr Caroline Mountford	160
	The discoveries of Udo Erasmus and Johanna Budwig	161
	Lecithin	164
	Adrenal overaction and stress	165
16	How do stressed cells become cancerous?	168
	Varmus, Bishop and retroviruses	168
	Other researchers	169
17	The role of pleomorphic organisms	173
18	Early vaccine makers	178
19	Why is there so much dissension in research?	182
	The cell discoveries of Emanuel Revici	183
20	Internal cell defence, peptides or antineoplastons	189
	Stanislaw Burzynski	189
	Stages in cancer formation	191

xiv *Heal Cancer*

21 The cell diagram ... 193
    The initiating and precipitating stages of cancer formation ... 193
    The changes making a normal cell into a stressed cell ... 194

PART SIX: SIDETRACKED

22 No vaccine available ... 199
    Who will make a vaccine? ... 200
    Taking the road to Japan ... 203
    Who was Dr Kiichiro Hasumi? ... 206
    Learning in Japan ... 212

23 Obtaining autovaccines ... 215
    Permits to import biological products ... 215

24 More pioneers with vaccines ... 221
    The candida spore controversy ... 232
    We are on the brink ... 234

PART SEVEN: GOING IN THE RIGHT DIRECTION

25 Recovery, remission or recurrence ... 239

26 Case 1: Bruce Huxley—Chrondro-Fibrosarcoma ... 240
    Causative factors ... 240
    Healing reactions ... 243
    The effects of vibrations, light and x-rays ... 245

27 Case 2: Ian Whitmee—Bladder cancer ... 247
    The Gerson Therapy ... 248
    All clear ... 250
    Infections or recurrence? ... 250
    Lessons to learn ... 252
    The blessings of our society ... 253

28 Case 3: Belinda—Bowel cancer ... 255
    The Stress Background ... 258
    The Gerson therapy doesn't suit everyone ... 262

29 Case 4: Robert Neville—Melanoma ... 264
    Hard decisions about lifestyle ... 265
    Relieving stress ... 267
    Assessing treatment choices for melanoma ... 268
    Interferon and chemotherapy ... 268

	Skin treatments	269
	Petty Spurge	270
30	Case 5: Gwen Clark—Skin cancer	272
31	Case 6: Lesley—Breast cancer	274
	Factors in recovery	276
	Benign cystic hyperplasia or chronic mastitis	277
32	Case 7: Althea—Breast cancer	281
	Cancer markers	281
	The natural history of untreated breast cancer	283
	Why do people refuse treatment?	283
	Childhood illness	284
	Overcoming destructive patterns	287
	Making the choice to die	289
	Living and dying	291
33	Case 8: Geraldine—Breast cancer	300
	Iscador	301
	No permit allowed	303
	Comparing Althea and Geraldine	304
	Ernesto Contreras in Tijuana	305
	Geraldine has radium	309
	Geraldine, the surgeon and Iscador	310
	Geraldine, the Bhagwan and energy levels	311
	Geraldine and the Gerson program	312
	More self-awareness, magnetic therapy and crystals	312
	Dolphins	313
	Vis medicatrix naturae, the healing force	314
34	Case 9: Megan McNichol—Melanoma	319
	The Livingston Medical Clinic	321
	Lifestyle changes	322
	Purified Protein Derivative Tests and BCG	323
	Removing the last lump	324
	Healing attitudes	325
	Cancer formation and spread	326
	Urea and Dr Danopoulos	328
	Setbacks to cancer recovery	330
	Avoiding destructive treatments	331

35	Case 10: Nancy—Rectal cancer	332
	High cholesterol: which type?	334
	Domestic brawling	337
36	Case 11: Tom—Melanoma	339
	Causative factors	340
	Candida	341
	Extra benefits of the survival plan	348
37	Case 12: Philip Lindsay—Bowel cancer	350
	Immunoglobulins	351
	Tuberculin, PPD or Mantoux test	352
	Sweet tooth	353
	Herpes and mouth ulcers	356
	The herpes family	357

APPENDIXES

1	What form of vitamin C will I take?	369
2	Cilento Survival Plan shopping guide, menus and recipes	371
3	Why we need vitamin supplements, by Lady Phyllis Cilento	378
4	Correct breathing for physical and mental health	383
5	Description of the cancer organism—Gaston Naessens	385
6	Healing institutions	390

BIBLIOGRAPHY 392
INDEX 400

very good results, ones which, I hope, will have lessons for all who read the case histories in the last section.

In the appendices are notes on further reading, and addresses of other clinics.

There is a great gap in our treatment of cancer. The person seems to lose identity as the case is diagnosed. It is a sad enough outlook for anyone without the added psychological burden of feeling relegated to a different status and often put down, just because your illness is considered incurable by most people, even doctors.

It need not be this way. I encourage my patients to take an active interest in their treatment and their healing processes. Many make a strong commitment to change and recover. Even those who know they cannot turn the disease round altogether rally remarkably in body, mind and spirit. The gift of hope is the greatest lifter of the human spirit and, with it, the immune system's defence system. There is no such thing as 'false hope'. When there is no hope, there is no hope for the person to recover or even to feel better. It is so much better to recover that free feeling of being in charge of one's life, of taking responsibility, of being able to make informed decisions, and of remaining a valued member of the family, even if working capacity has gone.

About 14 per cent of my terminally ill patients survive the five-year period which is supposed to indicate sustained remission or 'cure'. At least 65 per cent will have a temporary remission, will feel better, will have more energy, will sleep better, eat better and have better general health. The program can slow the cancer up tremendously, not only by following physiological principles of nutrition with the food and the supplements, but also by clearing the mind to work on healing with meditation, relaxation and prayer.

It is not an easy road. There may be some rocky patches along the way but, with guidance in the right direction, many come through. Those who don't have a gentle passing, usually without pain, and with the peace and dignity that they deserve.

Maybe if you read this book you will be able to help yourself or others along the road to a healthier life.

Ruth Cilento
1993

Part One

FINDING THE RIGHT PATH

1 STARTING THE SEARCH

I was my mother's apprentice but, I admit, not a really dedicated one for many years. Her constant discussion of new research findings and her continual reports of the success of nutritional treatment in her own patients became not only commonplace and unheeded but rather tedious to me. I thought all that information had gone in one ear and out the other until she first became ill at the age of eighty-four and allowed me to help her in her practice. I found that what she had been telling me was undoubtedly true. So I went through a baptism by fire for the next ten months. I studied the literature and research night and day so that I could look after her patients while she was away recovering.

After many years in general practice I studied child psychiatry in the State Health Department, working first in the Welfare and Guidance Section and later in the adult psychiatric clinic. From 1970 to 1976 I was also in charge of a busy alcoholism clinic at a leading hospital in Brisbane.

At the psychiatric and alcoholism clinics I had considered nutrition only in passing with my patients. Now, applying my sounder knowledge in conjunction with the stress control methods I had always used, I found that people responded better and became well much faster.

In my previous work there had been little opportunity to see people suffering from cancer. Then, in the first three months that Mother was away, I saw sixteen people with the disease—each one different. It was as though they had been sent especially to teach me and stimulate my study of this horrible illness. They were all classed medically as 'terminally ill'; that is, in the 'nothing-more-can-be-done' category. Yet all improved and felt better with modified nutrition, and many could go off their pain medication. I was amazed.

That was the beginning of the stream of people who have come for advice and support ever since.

In adopting and adapting my mother's simple anti-cancer diet I knew, through the research of many reputable scientists, that I was following physiological principles in giving the beleaguered immune system all the nutrients it needed to pick up strength to defend the body. That was the first rule I learned: always go back to the basic physiology of how cells work, then find out why they go wrong, in order to understand what must be changed to help the body right itself again.

As I carefully noted and recorded the progress of patients on Mother's original diet and my anti-stress program (which I have constantly been revising and improving), this great and profoundly simple truth emerged:

The right food and the right environment (physical and mental) keep cells normal.

Even when some cancerous changes have already occurred, much can be done to reverse the sick state of the body to stop cancer progressing in it. Moreover, if the sick chemistry is *not* reversed, it is most unlikely that the patient will *ever* recover from the cancer, no matter how much surgery, radiation or chemotherapy is given. Although the older textbooks considered that cancer was incurable once it had moved from its original site, either locally or by way of the blood or lymph circulation systems, this view is modifying under the impact of newer therapies.

Throughout the history of man *herbs* have been used as medicine. They are still used successfully by those versed in their value. Then there was *surgery*, which is becoming more and more technically efficient. 'If surgery doesn't fix it, nothing will', was the belief last century. Next came *radiation* therapy. It has now been recognised that it has good and bad outcomes, but radiation therapy is still used to treat the local area where the cancer is seen by the eye or by scans, X-rays and Nuclear Magnetic Imaging. Lastly, with *chemotherapy* which is carried everywhere by the blood, the medical world came closer to recognising that cancer is not a series of lumps to be cut out, but a state of the whole body.

Researchers over the last 150 years have recognised that cancer occurs only in tissue that has cells with a nucleus. It progresses:

- firstly from nuclear changes,
- secondly to affect the whole cell, the cell tissues,
- thirdly the chemistry of the organs it is in,
- then finally the whole body chemistry.

Emmanuel Revici*, among many others, has demonstrated these facts.

> Although generally considered as a unity, the differences between an early intraepithelial cancer (cancer in situ) and terminal cancer are so great as to oblige us to recognise that they are of the utmost importance in the pathogenesis (development) of this complex disease. While the factors responsible for the transformation of cancer from a clinically innocuous cell disturbance to a lethal disease are usually considered as secondary characters, my research has emphasised the roles of these manifestations and the factors which intervene to bring them about. I have tried to correlate each of the successive clinical phases in the evolution of cancer with the intervention of different processes, and thus determine their part . . .

Clinically these *stages* are now measured carefully by our tests of the cells and the body chemistry and by the signs, appearance and symptoms of the patient. 'Staging' of the cancer now precedes the doctor's pronouncement of its 'curability'.

Every school of therapy has its own attitudes or protocol for what is proper treatment. There is no *one* treatment that is infallible and there is no *one* substance that can cure cancer.

The factor that most therapists have disregarded until very recently is the spirit. The spirit is the essence of the person, and the mind and the body are its tools. All need to be in order to effect a turning-round of the situation. Unfortunately, by the time patients come to me they have often reached the stage when it is impossible to turn the chemistry round. Then no amount of surgery, radiation or chemotherapy can do anything but make the patient feel worse.

---

* This is from his book *The Control of Cancer with Lipids*, Institute of Applied Biology, New York, 1955.

Say: *I have the freedom to dream.*

However, instead of recognising that they have come to this stage, anxious, fearful or angry people sometimes rush around from one therapy to another looking for an elusive 'cure'. The patient may be worn out by this stressful waste of energy and emotion while the cancer progresses, causing more and more discomfort.

I used to have only one consultation with a person with cancer, lasting from an hour to an hour and a half. Everything I wanted to say had to be fitted into this time because I was seeing the person only once, with no follow-up. It didn't work very well. I was frustrated at not giving them all the information I thought they needed, and they were bewildered because I wished them to change their lifestyle for reasons that I had no time to explain. At that time I was working in my mother's rooms, driving 240 kilometres down from the country, where I had my angora goat stud and my alternative energy village, to see patients for just three days a week.

Because some people felt better and some began to recover, more and more people came and the number of patients soon became too many. Sadly, I had to leave my interests in the country and move back to Brisbane in 1983. At first I saw people in my house until I converted the ground floor garages into consulting rooms. Though there was less travelling, living and working on the same premises is always stressful.

The number of patients still increased and the time was inadequate, so in February 1985 I started the Nutrition and Stress Control Centre at Kelvin Grove, where I could teach terminally ill people and their helpers proper cooking methods, meditation, organic gardening, home nursing, diet, nutrition, the rudiments of the physiology of cancer and how to deal with it. It was in the patients' changing attitudes and enthusiasm that I was to find the most encouragement.

The five staff members at the Centre worked with me as a team. The results were very good, and it was all most rewarding, except financially. I went broke and had to give the lovely old house back to the bank. This was because we often had only three patients for the two-week course, and I had no time to see enough other paying patients to make ends meet. I paid the staff well, and many patients who learnt at that course still survive, but I went deeply into debt.

Making a more workable plan

When Mother died in 1987 she left me some money so I could build onto my consulting rooms at home. In that way I could start a smaller but more concentrated course to give information to the ever-increasing number of people who wanted it.

So, in 1988, by pruning out much of the part people can read in books, I reorganised my two-week program for new patients into one full, seven-hour day each fortnight. I was thus able to interview, assess and advise more new patients.

This one-day program has worked well enough; while I was grossly overloaded with patients it was the only way to fit them in, I thought, but I felt dissatisfied with the results. It was a very long and tiring day for me, too. I found that the patients had much less energy and had lost concentration after the good organic lunch we provided, so that much of what I told them about the food plan, stress control, goals and change had lost its punch, if they remembered it at all. The result was that, after each intake of new patients, there was a constant barrage of phone calls to verify or discuss points that they had missed and were now reading in their notes. Daytime consultations were being disrupted to such an extent that I had to put all phone queries off till the evenings, which made night seem very long. 'Burn out' was fast approaching. I was so cranky that one of my secretaries left.

I decided to review and reorganise the practice, perhaps with a helper, and more time to write and think.

Looking for a like-minded colleague

There are many 'natural' therapies, some of which I have researched. I have investigated and used the most promising ones which have proved successful elsewhere, but I cannot comment on those I have not had the opportunity to study or which are prohibited in Australia.

We are lucky here. In spite of the recently implemented, restrictive Therapeutic Goods Act, Australian citizens are mostly allowed to use whatever method they choose for themselves so long as the

Say: *I have the power to make my dreams come true.*

choice does not involve importing or selling prohibited substances or trying to treat other people.

Fear and ignorance of what cancer *is* puts most patients under the power and complete control of their doctors. The choices the doctors are obliged to make depend on the training they have had, whether as general practitioners, physicians, surgeons, haematologists, radiotherapists or whatever. This puts a heavy load of responsibility on the doctors—it can very often mean the difference between life or death for the patients.

How can my colleagues achieve a comprehensive assessment and treatment when our teaching in medical school and thereafter almost entirely leaves out the fundamental nutrition necessary for healing the body, and gives no instruction at all in building up the factors necessary for healing the mind and spirit?

In the last ten years, since I have been combing and sifting the research literature and learning from hundreds of cancer patients, I have noticed many young medicos becoming more enquiring and educating themselves in these matters at the risk, of course, of attracting the wrath and opprobium of their peers ('peer sneer', I call it). Many more than in 1982 are referring their terminally ill patients to me for nutritional advice and stress control, or for help through the process of dying, which Dr Elizabeth Kubler-Ross (an authority on research into dying) calls the 'final stage of growth'.

One of the reasons I am writing this book is to help those therapists who want to give their patients a better chance of recovery and a better quality of life to sort out which of the various nutritional and psychological therapies will help each type and stage of cancer, and why it does so. It is only by experience and reading research that I am learning all the time. Very few of my colleagues are really on the same track in cancer treatments.

Why don't you teach other doctors?

Many patients ask me why I don't find other doctors as assistants. I have tried to do that several times. To help people who are desperately ill needs commitment; it is not just a job. Once I advertised for an assistant with a view to partnership.

Of the doctors who applied, one was a young graduate who had no experience of general medicine and wanted a stepping stone to go on to what he thought would be a 'real' specialty, dermatology. This has an advantage in that no-one dies and responsibility is minimal. A doctor coming into my situation can expect that at least half the patients will die and that he or she must face death with all the patients. Not many choose to do that.

Another applicant was a retired anaesthetist who did not value nutrition, was drug oriented and knew nothing about how the mind works. He thought a few afternoons chatting with patients would be comfortable between his games of golf!

One man came from Victoria and wanted to relocate in a warmer climate because his children had asthma. He doubted that he could make enough to live on with what patients paid in my practice. He learned at the outset that the salary he had been expecting was more than I ever received. He knew little about cancer and almost nothing about vitamin therapy.

Many well-meaning doctors phone or write for information when patients show them the Survival Plan, the hourly schedule and the supplement list: 'Send me all the information you can, they ask. Books by well-known researchers are most helpful here. I normally recommend *Cancer and its Nutritional Therapies* by Richard Passwater[1], *Getting Well Again* by Carl O. Simonton and Stephanie Matthews Simonton[2], and *You Can Conquer Cancer* by Ian Gawler[3]. There are dozens of other books too[4]. It is no wonder that many doctors graduate with no knowledge of treating cancer at home. In medical school we learn so much about illness but so little about lifestyle for health. Nutrition and stress control are not exact scientific subjects, they are part of our very being. With chemotherapy and radiation the protocol can be written out in precise detail in text books—the exact dose and how to give it. Patients accept the things

---

[1] Keats Publishing Co., Connecticut, 1978
[2] Bantam Books, New York, 1978
[3] Hill of Content, Melbourne, 1984
[4] For example: *Anatomy of an Illness* Norman Cousins, Bantam Books, New York, 1979; *Cancer and its Nutritional Therapies*, Richard Passwater, Pivot, Keats Publishing Co., Connecticut, 1978.

Say: *My dreams are so fragile but so strong.*

that are done to them because they are given by the doctor in charge, but the doctor may not know how to advise about what and how to eat or how to overcome fear and anxiety. Many doctors are making themselves conversant with these matters by reading and listening to their patients.

Many doctors find it easier to believe the propaganda of governments—all over the world—that great strides are being made against cancer, that new 'breakthroughs' are being followed up and that a cancer cure is imminent. Then it is all being taken care of by somebody else—the GP, the surgeon, the oncologist, the radiotherapist. I would so much like to run courses for doctors on how to manage the treatment of cancer in the home.

My parents, my helpers

My parents set the stage for me. They were pioneers in their field. Vitally interested in the development of our enquiring minds, they taught my five brothers and sisters and me by example, not by pressure. We had a childhood unusually free from restrictions. We were led into independence in so many ways.

My parents were both doctors with active, intelligent, enquiring minds. In treating people, my mother followed her own favourite slogan, as she often states in her books: 'Leave no stone unturned'. She continually fossicked for the truth to present to people in an easily understood form. 'You need to go over what you have to say in writing many times to cut out all the blemishes. You need to hone it down and polish it up till your meaning stands out clearly', she told me.

My mother gave all six of us the freedom she had as a child. We were never pampered or cajoled or ridiculed, but were encouraged to be self-reliant, to have a go and to try making and doing things ourselves. Father taught me to satisfy my investigative urge by reading. He gave me the run of his extensive library when I was eleven years old—except for some books by Havelock Ellis, which I found hidden under the window seat when I was twelve. He told me that if I wanted to succeed at something, I should gather all the information I could about it, sift it, test it and verify it. When I was satisfied I knew enough, I was then to put it into practice in a way that could not cause harm but would benefit others. So that is what I have always aimed to do in everything.

I believe my final introduction into the work with cancer was made possible by leaving the exacting full-time management of the alcoholism clinic in Brisbane to take my angora goat herd up to Stanthorpe, where I built the 'sun-powered Eukey complex'. It was there that I learned to have the courage to put into practice what I had researched, planned and found would really work.

The Cilento Survival Plan

Originally, when I was working with my mother, she called her programs of nutrition for various ills the 'Cilento Way'. This became even more firmly established after the *Courier Mail* newspaper published a collection of her newspaper articles under that name. I naturally continued calling the diets the 'Cilento Way' even though, year by year in my treatment of cancer, I have revised the original food plan to encompass many more of the physiological principles necessary for survival.

So I have now called what has evolved the 'Cilento Survival Plan'. This gives guidance for people of all different metabolic types. We are all aware that one person may fatten on the same amount and type of food that would cause another to lose weight.

At first the Survival Plan consisted of 75 per cent raw food. The main idea of this was to replenish the natural and easily assimilable minerals and vitamins that are so depleted for so long in people with cancer. This was fine for the first three to six weeks of detoxification, but it caused many people to lose too much weight because they were too full of raw foods to take the more calorific cooked ones.

We all need five to eight glasses of fluid a day. So I found that a more acceptable way for all concerned of gaining these essential natural medicines was to take them as the essence or juice of the raw foods. *This is why the juices are so very important a part of the Cilento Survival Plan.* Read about them in 'Healing the body', pages 21-30.

2 WE ARE LOSING THE FIGHT

Unfortunately, all through history, knowledge has not been used as it should be. Time and time again, the old human frailities of greed, pride, jealousy and power interfere with the good that knowledge can bring. Vital discoveries have been suppressed, researchers ridiculed, fortunes made and lost in legal costs, violence, destruction and even murders have been committed in the name of science and the protection of the public, and especially in the name of the fight against cancer.

In the last thirty years it has become obvious, in spite of widespread cover-up attempts, that the survival rate for people with cancer has not improved and that cancer is increasing in the Western World at a steady and alarming rate.

In mid-April 1987, the US Government's General Accounting Office of Statistics reported to Congress that, although:

Progress has been made, it is not as great as that reported by the National Cancer Institute (NCI) monitor of the 'Conquest of Cancer' program begun during the Richard Nixon era.'

Jan McLean reports in *The Australian Doctor* on 8 August 1986:

'We are not winning the battle against cancer, according to Professor Martin Tattersall of the Ludwig Institute of Cancer Research in Sydney. 'In spite of intensive research and a range of new treatments, the prognosis for most cancers hasn't really changed over the past 30 years,' he said.

Professor Tattersall supports the view, expressed by Dr John Bailar of the Harvard School of Public Health and Dr Elaine Smith of the University of Iowa Medical Centre in a *New England Journal of Medicine* report (8 May 1986), that anti-cancer efforts should concentrate on prevention rather than on new methods of treatment.

The main conclusion we draw is that some 35 years of intense effort focused largely on improving treatment must be judged a qualified failure, the US researchers wrote.

For Americans, the risk of dying from cancer has increased over the last three decades, they point out. In 1950, 170 in every 100 000 people in the US died of cancer. In 1982, after the figures were adjusted to reflect the ageing population, there were 185 deaths in 100 000—an 8 per cent increase.

Improved five years survival rates may give the impression that progress is being made against the disease. But if cancer is diagnosed earlier, for instance, the patients will survive longer from the time of diagnosis, even if they are still dying at the same age as before. Both earlier diagnosis and improved screening techniques may give a false picture.

Australian cancer statistics, recorded since 1954, also reveal little change in the overall incidence of cancer and associated mortality.

Say: *Dreams light up my brilliant goals.*

Part Two

STEPS ON THE ROAD TO RECOVERY

3 HEALING THE BODY

The means of destruction are approaching perfection with frightful rapidity.

Baron Antoine Henri Jomine, 1838.

Preliminaries

The decision to make the lifestyle changes necessary to implement the Cilento Survival Plan is a full commitment. Before I accept a person with cancer as a patient, he or she reads the contact notes, which go with a questionnaire we send out in order to understand the statement of policy it contains. *I am not intimating that the cancer will be cured;* no-one can give guarantees about that. The policy states clearly that by following the Survival Plan the person hopes to build up natural immunity and, with it, natural healing power. The following contact notes, which we usually send to each enquirer, spell out the policy.

Nutrition and Stress Control Centre contact notes

Thank you for your enquiry about the assessment and program at the Centre. It is the only one of its kind in Australia and aims to help you change your life for the better and, if possible, to halt or slow down your illness by using your own healing power.

Each person is unique and responds differently to our program. The response depends largely on your motivation to get well, your attitude to change and how depleted you are due to disease and its treatment. If you are presently taking chemotherapy or radiation, you may still benefit from our program, because it is supportive, helpful and informative and will not interfere in any way with the treatment you are now using. We aim to teach you how to improve, not deplete, your immune system. WE DO NOT CLAIM TO CURE YOUR DISEASE, but by changing your lifestyle, you may stimulate your own immune system to do that.

At the Centre, we provide a supportive setting where we will teach you how to manage stress, how to understand the illness and how it came about, and what you may do to help prevent further deterioration. In order to ensure the success of this program, the following information should be understood and agreed upon by you, our welcome guest.

Statement of policy

The Nutrition and Stress Control Centre is an adjunctive medical clinic only. Each person is expected to be under the care of his/her own physician at home and there should be on-going communication with your own doctor. We are a medical, dietary assessment and teaching establishment, providing prescribed medication, immunology and appropriate tuition in relaxation techniques, physiology, hygiene, causes and treatments of deteriorating illnesses. We aim, through private consultations, groups and lectures, to teach you to live a healthier, happier life by using the appropriate nutrition and supplements for your condition and by using techniques of relaxation to reduce fear, pain and other negative emotions.

For those filling out the questionnaire, who, for geographic reasons, can only have a consultation by telephone, this policy still stands. For those who are able to come to the centre personally it must be understood that prospective patients should be ambulatory and are expected to be able to hear, to understand English, to see and to be able to manage their personal needs. Exceptions may be made if, by prior arrangement, a companion accompanies the disabled person.

If someone becomes incapacitated during a visit, or if physical status becomes unmanageable, decision as to further participation is at the discretion of our doctor.

Helpers

Once participants are established on the program, they take their new-found knowledge, plus supplies, to be administered at home. This is very difficult unless others in the household understand what they are trying to do. Participants are encouraged to bring a spouse, relative or helper with them so that the program will be fully understood and much more easily carried out.

Program arrangements

The questionnaire is to be filled out carefully and returned by post before your appointment. It saves a great deal of time and helps doctor to assess your condition and the environmental and physical stresses being encountered. For those attending the centre, tests done on the first day will reveal the capacity of the immune system. In all cases, it will need to be stimulated into action against the cancer by the Cilento Survival Plan, which doctor will arrange. Participation in the full program includes:

- *Individual consultation with assessment of causes of the disease and nutritional, physical, work and emotional stresses compounding the problem.*
- *Lectures and discussion on diet, vitamin and mineral therapy.*
- *Pathology tests—such as full blood count, multiple biochemical analysis, Erythrocyte Sedimentation Rate or others.*
- *Tests for immune competence (Purified Protein Derivative) and yeast overload (Candida sensitivity).*
- *Discussion of books useful in cooking, nutrition, raising self-esteem and controlling stress.*
- *Lectures and participation in meditation, biofeedback, visual imagery and other techniques.*
- *Discussion of the physiology and control of cancer.*
- *Reprocessing of negative attitudes to dispel anger, fear and harmful habits of reacting.*
- *Discussion of blood and yeast sensitivity test results.*
- *Dicussion of goal-making for future lifestyle.*
- *Microscopic darkfield blood examination and discussion if time permits. (This is not a Hemaview screening.)*
- *Discussion of changes necessary for each person to avoid stress overload.*
- *Provision of the dietary, vitamin, mineral and injectable supplements for raising immune system status.*

Say: *We can bring beauty, love and joy to our environment.*

- Discussion on following the plan at home, making the diary, keeping appointments and participating in the free Friday Support Group.

It is then a matter of taking the steps necessary to reverse the factors that have caused the cancer, as much as it is possible, by helping your body chemistry, your mind and your motivation to recover.

Because fear and other emotional stresses have such a debilitating effect on the body's defences, special attention is given to helping the patient understand and eliminate negative influences. This may be facilitated by consultation and discussion and with lectures, videos, tapes, music, relaxation and visual imagery, both individually and in groups.

There are discussions and demonstrations, if time permits, about the various methods of administration and use of vaccines and immune system stimulation—the dietary program—the elimination of toxins—the control of pain—family help and involvement—what to do in a crisis—the use and abuse of vitamin and mineral supplements—and many other subjects that patients may need to have clarified.

If it is appropriate for your illness, doctor will arrange for further appointments to discuss the use of autogenous vaccines.

Attitudes

Success in treating your disease depends on taking responsibility for your own recovery and maintaining a determined, positive attitude and confident spirit. As you are sharing communal rooms, we encourage you to enjoy this time with a sense of companionship and consideration. You will help others and yourself by your cheerful smile, patience and friendliness. Love, laughter, harmony and understanding are the keynotes to the song of life!

On-going contact *with Doctor by progress consultations or by telephone is recommended most strongly, not only for the patient's benefit, but to help in our continuing research.*

Making the lifestyle changes

The Cilento Survival Plan helps the patient to make any necessary changes in lifestyle and gives support in carrying them out. With new-found knowledge, the patient takes responsibility for his or her decisions and, with the help of family and friends, follows the chosen plan as closely as possible.

There may be a psychological disadvantage in some patients from the start. Most therapists working with this disease have noticed the preponderance of personality types dedicated to nurturing others and feeling guilty or ashamed if they spend time taking care of their own needs. The classic work of Lawrence Le Shan* is perhaps the best-known research study of this.

Of course, this does not mean that all people who develop cancer are like this. Consider a two-year-old child who develops acute leaukaemia or an X-ray technician who develops cancer of the thyroid from prolonged exposure in his or her work. There are always many factors which can be implicated in tipping the balance of the body and mind towards ill health.

Positive attitudes of those around the sick person are of the utmost importance in assisting healing.

How do you interact with someone who has terminal cancer?

Here is a very brief questionnaire. Do you:
- Avoid him/her?
- Ignore the condition and go on as usual?
- Be solemnly sad and forget to smile?
- Anxiously expect the sick person to die anytime?
- Say it will all be fixed by the doctor?
- Tell the sick one to ask forgiveness for sins?
- Bargain: if only you get better I will always . . .?
- Deny that it is true?
- Feel angry or resentful?
- Tend to be over-sympathetic?
- Blame and criticise the patient, the doctor, the hospital or others?
- Be jolly and matter-of-fact?
- Tell the sick one to make a will?
- Look at the sick one's lifestyle or your own and try to change it?

---

* *You can Fight for Your Life*, Lawrence Le Shan, Jove Publishing, USA, 1978.

Say: *I believe in miracles, they are all around me.*

- Live with the sick one and help run the household?
- Other attitudes?

These are just a few of the many ways in which people react. What is your way? It depends on your past experience, your personality and your occupation, among other things. For instance, a doctor or nurse, a chaplain, a priest or other spiritual leader and a busy mother of four small children would probably all react quite differently.

The people who are afflicted also have many different views of the disease. The interaction of the helper's and the sufferer's views can make a very great difference to the outcome. There have been several large studies designed to assess the effects a patient's attitudes have on healing and one is currently being undertaken at Sydney University. A survey still being completed by the University of Pennsylvania Cancer Centre includes a series of questions which aim to discover which attitudes are more conducive to a good quality of life for those who are terminally ill.

It will be some time before this large survey, which covers many hospitals and clinics in all parts of America, is completed, but when it is, it will be found that some attitudes are related to further ill health because they result in handing the responsibility for recovery over to someone else. In the meanwhile, the attitudes below are, in my experience, some of the pre-requisites for healing.

- To have the desire, commitment and the goal to live.
- To have a strong belief in the group, the doctor, the therapist or whoever is the adviser and mentor.
- To have faith in the treatment itself and an intelligent interest in how it is carried out.
- To have perseverance and determination.
- To have a commitment to do everything necessary to reach the goal, even if it involves some sacrifice of comfort.
- To have peace of mind and to release fear and anger. This encompasses a feeling of self-worth and faith in God. It is a realisation that we are all part of the universal energy, source, light—or whatever your belief is.

If there are negative influences at work which interfere with these attitudes, either the influences must be removed or the patient must be removed from them. It is well nigh impossible for a patient with cancer to recover in a ward where everyone around is dying, in pain or surrounded by weeping relatives. The nursing staff do their best to make the wards more conducive to healing, but with overcrowded hospitals and overworked staff, the situation is sometimes impossible.

In any sort of unpleasant situation, the patient is desperate for some relief, for something to hang onto, for hope. Two of the best books you can give someone in hospital with cancer are *You Can Conquer Cancer* and *Peace of Mind*, both by Ian Gawler*, a veterinary surgeon who recovered from terminal bone cancer. Others that give hope and inspiration are listed on page 392-9.

All these books emphasise, from the writers' own experience, that if people take responsibility for themselves and do something to help, they can lift themselves out of depression, fear, anger and despair.

A positive attitude can stimulate the immune system to function again.

If change is needed, it may come slowly with the pain of self-searching, it may come fast in a crisis, or it may be a gradual, painless easing into a new lifestyle.

As well as the support and understanding of family and friends, a definite plan of action and a mentor or caring instructor to show the way and explain the reason why are needed. This is where my work comes in.

Assessment and Evaluation

It is certainly *not* possible to motivate everybody. That is why the Pennsylvania University survey, when it is evaluated, may help in weeding out those who will have no chance of recovery judging by their psychological attitudes. Dozens of sick people phone each week, most of them terminally ill. I speak to them all, or to a family

---

* *You Can Conquer Cancer*, Hill of Content, Melbourne, 1984; *Peace of Mind*, Hill of Content, Melbourne, 1987.

Say: *God makes miracles every day.*

member, but few want to make the commitment to do anything themselves. Many want advice over the phone, which is illegal for someone who is not already a consulting patient. Apart from that, it is most unwise as many misinterpretations can occur on the phone and there may be unwanted results.

Of those who do decide to come to the course, some renegue at the last minute because the family does not approve of diet, supplements or meditation. Some think that their other doctors will be angry; some think it is 'just a diet' and costs too much when they can get one from a naturopath or a health column in the local paper; there are all sorts of 'reasons'. Sometimes the family is desperate to make the commitment but the patient does not want to. Sometimes the patient is so ill or depressed that it is even more stressful and difficult trying to stick to a program. Sometimes the patient cannot read or is mentally backward.

If the Cilento Survival Plan was a routine part of all cancer treatment programs, undertaken as soon as the diagnosis of cancer was made, then many, many more people would survive cancer. As I stated in the introduction, there is nothing 'alternative' about the Plan. It is based on sound physiology and each part of it has been authentically researched and used effectively. It has taken many years of research into literally hundreds of different journals, scientific papers, books, letters, laboratories, clinic procedures and interviews for me to dig out the information required to make my decisions in individual assessments and treatments.

The Survival Plan is versatile; it must change to fit individual needs, even though the physiological principles are still the same. It is useless for me to prescribe liver for someone who gags at the very thought of it, for instance. For those who are in the midst of radium treatment or chemotherapy, the nutrients must be given in such a way that they can be assimilated, and so on.

Most surgeons, radiologists and oncologists are now giving some instructions to the patient or to nursing staff about short-term care over food, sleep and elimination. Unfortunately, once their treatment area is finished, no follow-up advice is given because most of these specialists are not conversant with continuing care at home. We are not taught much of any practical importance in medical school about nutrition, vitamins, minerals, anti-oxidants, detoxification, relaxation and meditation techniques or even simple home nursing.

Most patients don't even know how to use a thermometer! Whose responsibility is it to teach the patient? Nobody's, it seems.

Luckily there are many dedicated nurses who give wonderful service in training patients to manage dressings, hygiene, mouth toilets, lifting, turning, massaging and other essentials for sick people. But nurses, too, learn practically nothing about nutrition and stress control, which are essential parts of gaining and maintaining health.

Most patients come to me already diagnosed. I want to see the surgeon's and the pathologist's reports before I prescribe anything. I want to know what medication the GP and the physician have given, what the surgeon diagnosed and what prognosis was given. The questionnaire prospective patients fill in for me (and the computer) is ten pages long, but it saves much time and missed information.

General hospitals have been notoriously slow in sending results but most patients have a copy of their X-ray findings. I have tests for blood cells, immune system and cancer markers (see page 23), done every eight weeks or so, in any case, to monitor progress.

Patients have already been to a GP and a surgeon and had treatment of various types that seemed appropriate to their doctors. Many hundreds of patients come to me for advice, not because they are terminally ill, but because they have had the diagnosis and the surgery 'to get it all', but have a strong inner feeling that this is not enough. They feel that no-one, however good a surgeon, can 'get it all' because it is more serious than the manifestation of lumps that have been removed. They come to gain more information so that they can work out a plan for the future.

I don't only see the successes. I also see the people who don't know where else to go. Many have had a prognosis of 'terminally ill'. Some doctors are even so brash as to give a prognosis of the time of survival. This is unwise, even from a textbook. If the doctor is respected and believed, the prognosis can become a 'bone pointing' or self-fulfilling prophecy and the patient obediently dies at the stated time. Then there is the patient who defies the doctor's prognosis of 'two months to live' and displays himself twenty years later to

Say: *Strangers are friends I haven't yet met.*

prove the doctor wrong. If only the medical world could realise that everything works together for good in those who love God or the universal laws of nature, or whatever you like to call it!

I am in no way denigrating the great progress that is being made in cancer treatment on physiological lines. Such tremendous strides have been made in some ways—in diagnosis, in surgical techniques, in the provision of exceptional care in nursing, in the provision of social service funds by governments, religious and private agencies, and in drug therapies that do no damage. Nevertheless for all the great good, there are also horrendously bad things happening. Medicine is drawing further and further away from practical physiological means of helping people to heal. In fact, reading the journals constantly as I do, I see much evidence that doctors, researchers, scientists, technicians and others believe that *they* are doing the healing themselves. It is easy to make this assumption, especially if prestige, self-esteem, self-respect and economic livelihood depend on that attitude, yet we are all merely facilitators— we contribute by helping the life force of the sick person to heal from within.

4 THE TROUBLE WITH STATISTICS

It has been said by many that statistics are inexact and that they can be made to say anything a manipulator chooses. Smarting under this criticism, statisticians have tried hard to make statistics into a foolproof science, but I have learnt that, unless they are used by an expert, they prove nothing.

Cancer Facts and Fallacies seminar and its sequels

In May 1983, I organised a free seminar called 'Cancer Facts and Fallacies', at The Relaxation Centre of Queensland in Brisbane. About ninety people attended. Apart from my own presentation of what I saw as the facts, three of my patients gave accounts of their experiences, followed by open discussion. In the afternoon, I had asked three leading members of the medical profession—an experienced radiologist, a senior surgeon and a leading oncologist—to give their views. It was an eager and interested audience. In the panel question-time at the end of the seminar there were some heated discussions.

The oncologist came in for some unanswerable queries and a heavy barrage of unhappy blame and criticism about chemotherapy in general and his views in particular. This was most evident after his statements denigrating the use of meditation, stress control, vitamin and mineral supplements, diet and nutrition. To save him walking out, I suggested that we should conduct a study together on the effects of these basic modalities of treatment with his patients who were taking chemotherapy. He readily agreed in the face of the unpleasant situation, perhaps hoping that I would not follow up the suggestion, which had been unanimously applauded by the audience. The question about research into nutrition and vitamins had been put to them spontaneously and without any instigation from me, by an assertive young man whose wife had recently died of cancer.

There were three important sequels to this seminar. Firstly, I had spoken in the seminar about the value of a caring support group. Eight people waited after the speakers left, eager to find out when and where the first support group in Queensland was to be. 'Right here, next Friday afternoon between 2 and 5 p.m.,' I said glibly, though I had not yet asked if we could use that venue. They agreed, so that is where we held the meetings of the 'Quality of Life Group' for the next twenty months. They are still free for people with cancer and their families, and still at the same time, but the venue has changed four times in the last eight years.

The second event which concerned me a little was my receipt of a letter from the Australian Medical Association (A.M.A). I had been a member since 1950 and my parents had been life-long members and also distinguished physicians in Australia. I think this made a difference to the way the letter was worded. The Secretary was inviting me to answer serious questions that had been raised by the ethical committee, as to why I had publicly advertised myself as a medical lecturer and why I had set myself up as a specialist.

To be charged with unethical conduct is not just a reprimand from the A.M.A. Several years ago legislation was passed by the Government requiring all misdemeanours to be reported to the Medical Registration Board, which had the power to deregister doctors at its own discretion. There was no court of appeal to either organisation at that time and no *habeas corpus*. If a complaint was made to the A.M.A. by one of its anonymous informants, a 'please explain' was sure to be forthcoming.

I suppose that the complaint came from the oncologist I had chosen to lecture at the seminar since his therapy was the most questioned by the audience. There was a good reason for thinking so. The Australian oncologist, Dr Helen Manion, had warned me about his attack on her through the A.M.A. when, two years previously, she and her psychologist husband, Gerard, spoke at a seminar held on cancer at the University of Queensland under the auspices of the Relaxation Centre of Queensland Committee.

They said that doctors who pronounced a survival time for fearful and trusting cancer patients unknowingly gave a death sentence, in the same way that Aboriginal tribal elders can cause people to die by 'pointing the bone'. Their presentation at this congress and their paper, published in the *Australian Medical Journal*, was based on some of the same principles as the work of Dr Ainslie Meares, a Melbourne psychiatrist who had given up his speciality to devote himself to teaching meditation techniques to desperately ill people.

Dr Manion had worked for years at the huge Sloan Kettering cancer research hospital in New York and knew the terrible hazards of using chemotherapy without concomitant psychological support. In fact she had been so saddened and frustrated by the suffering of patients and the failure of methods used then, that she gave up her higher degree in oncology. Back in Australia, she and Gerard developed a Cancer Care Program, incorporating meditation with visualisation, relief of stress and many forward-looking techniques that have helped hundreds of people to withstand the psychological effects of illness.

After her lectures, the A.M.A. threatened Helen with the loss of her practising licence. A complaint had been made in quite abusive terms by a certain oncologist. So when I visited her in early 1983 with a patient who needed their program, she had warned me to beware of this complaining person. I thanked her for her advice but, after much thought, I decided that a man who felt so threatened should have the chance to present his side of the question by participating in my seminar. I thought that this might also save me from his sniping from behind. That is why he spoke at my seminar and why the A.M.A. representative was more cautious in his polite but pointed letter to me.

I answered the letter by pointing out, also most politely, that there was no question of advertising (which is prohibited by the by-laws of the A.M.A.) as the information about the Cancer Facts and Fallacies' Seminar appeared in a private newsletter in the same way as 'notice of events would be circulated in a private golf club. Secondly I wrote, 'My presentation was on nutrition and stress control, in which subjects I *do* consider myself a specialist. Unfortunately, I have been informed by the Dean of the Medical Faculty that these are not medical specialities. I hope that in the future they will become so and be as much part of general medical practice as efficient

Say: *Work is worship.*

book keeping and faithful history taking'. I also invited A.M.A. members to our cancer support group where they could learn relaxation techniques. That was a bit cheeky. I had a letter back stating briefly that my comments had been noted. Nobody came and nothing more happened.

The last outcome of the seminar was the follow-up study I was to organise with the oncologist. We had several lengthy and amicable discussions but could not find any common ground on how to go about substantiating the hypothesis: 'That supportive nutrition and stress control improve the outcome of cancer treatment with chemotherapy.' Neither of us knew enough about statistical analysis at that time.

I found a retired hospital matron, Pat Truesdale, who was finishing her PhD thesis and was well versed in statistical methods. She agreed to come to some of our discussions and help us work out a format. Pat explained to us that such a hypothesis was impossible to prove or disprove. We would have to make each part much more specific. What did nutrition mean? Were we including supplements? If so, which ones? For how long? In what type of cancer? Over what survival time? At what stage of illness? . . . and so on and so on, the list of variables was endless. Then there was the *validation* of each question asked so that the sense of it could be completely understood by each participant. Apart from all that, we could not decide on who would foot the bill for running a study that could take from two to five years, or who should be employed. Should we apply for a university grant or funding from some of the drug or vitamin manufacturers?

It was all too much. Finally, by the end of 1983, the oncologist put a stop to our problems by stating categorically that he could not agree to having his patients participating in any study where Vitamin C was used at more than the Recommended Daily Allowance of 30 mg. We were both relieved. We had made an honest attempt which taught us both some very important lessons about the enormity of statistical problems, about our ignorance of each other's specialities and about the great diversity of each other's opinions, which we both grew to respect with more tolerance.

Results of treatment study

In 1989 there was enough data in enough case histories covering five to six years to take out some results of treatment. I had a little Apple computer which I had not learned how to use, and my secretary at that time was also computer illiterate. However, when I talked to her about what I planned to discover, a friend who has some experience volunteered to help me.

I was grossly overworked. I didn't take the time to work out a list of valid questions from the study. We were quickly reintroduced to all the problems I had found in 1983, but by this time Pat was too busy working with a melanoma project to approach. Also I heard from the University that statisticians were charging a huge hourly rate that I could not afford. My friend undertook a tremendous effort in helping me. Just putting the data in to a useable form was difficult enough for her because the computer was so small it could not deal with more than four variables at a time. Luckily she could work only part time or it would have driven her crazy— poor lady! After four months, all the 'bytes' had been used up without finishing the questions, so we decided to ask the computer some questions with what she had put on it anyway.

Of 182 adult terminally ill patients randomly selected (every third chart) from those seen between January 1985 and December 1986, the answer came out: none had survived five years. This was absolutely wrong, since I could think of more than a dozen who were alive and well and still keeping in contact!

We went through the masses of data step by step. All it proved was that all but forty-two of the sample could be discounted for various reasons. This left us with a sample that was too small to be statistically valid and was no longer random. The dozen or so I remembered with my own brain computer would have been eliminated from the sample even if they had been chosen originally, because their data was incomplete. We abandoned the study because we realised I would need a bigger computer, a statistician and the money to provide these.

Say: *Dreams are the substance of future success.*

How long have I got?

By working through eighty-six histories of people who came to the two-week course from those two years at Kelvin Grove, we found twelve who were still alive five years later. That is nearly 14 per cent. The *how, why* and *what* are the important questions, however. *The percentage of survivors means very little on its own.*

Hundreds of people phone for information about the program, what it entails, how long it is, and what it costs. Many ask the questions, 'What is your success rate?' and 'How long have I got?' To answer these unanswerable questions, a large number of doctors and other health workers make up little stories that possibly make the doctor and the patient feel better but are openly untrue. This is probably not done dishonestly; perhaps the doctor or health worker believes what is written in some of the medical books, most of which are confusing. Many a humane doctor will try to work out an 'informed guess' from his or her own personal experience, too. In making such an assessment the adviser must take into account the following factors:

- **What type of cancer is it?**
  This is really a dozen questions in one. There are dozens of types of cancer. Each type has its own characteristics, mode of spread, rate of growth and susceptibility to various forms of treatment.
- **What stage of invasion has the cancer reached?**
- **When was it first diagnosed and how?**

Case comment: Bill Jackson

I think of Bill Jackson (he wants me to use his proper name). He is a Vietnam veteran who had radiation treatment to a left apical cancer of the lung, a very aggressive and spreading type. *He was told that he had six to eighteen months to live*—a prognosis from the text books. He undertook our program strictly and seriously. The tumour of the lung disappeared and never recurred. After two years with our program he thought he was cured. He was congratulating himself by playing golf again with his mates when he had a fit. X-ray showed a haemorrhage into a large secondary tumour in the brain that had been there all along. His oncologist had never X-rayed his head.

Now another year has passed and he is still fighting on, improving his lifestyle all the time. He has moved to a better home where he can tend a garden and plant trees. He has found that entertaining old folk on a Sunday with his beautiful singing voice has given him more peace of mind than worrying about how long he will survive. 'Most of the oldies I sing to will probably go before I do,' he told the support group. His good humour, self-sufficiency and banter help to give heart to our other exceptional survivors.

- **What is the state of the nutrition?**
Some people are already so debilitated when they seek treatment that their chances of survival are lessened. Some actually starve to death because food cannot pass an inoperable tumour. Hyperalimentation (feeding by intravenous drip) may make a great difference. Best of all, and this is proved by our experience, the food plan in this book picks people up dramatically once it becomes established. Usually, patients begin to feel better within about six weeks. Their tests improve, pain subsides and their state of mind and generally better health make life worth living again. **Many people outlive the textbook prognosis two, three or four times over; some remain in remission.**

If every cancer therapist used this program as soon as the cancer was diagnosed, the other modalities of treatment such as surgery, radiation and chemotherapy would have much better results too. This is not hospital fare, this plan is fresh, unrefined, unadulterated food and the natural vitamins and mineral supplements that the body uses as medicine for recuperation of body and mind in any illness.

- **What are the environmental factors?**
People who have been taking immuno-suppressive drugs for other illnesses and are still taking them have a very hard battle recovering from cancer. The classic case history from the literature is the person in dialysis for kidney failure who had a kidney transplant. Unfortunately the donated kidney had a tiny cancer in it which, under the influence of the transplant anti-rejection drugs, grew and became invasive in the recipient's body. The transplant was

Say: | *We are each needed to make a better world.*

removed, the immuno-suppressive drugs ceased and the cancers, which had spread to other parts of the body, disappeared.

So many hidden factors must be considered that it is obviously impossible for anyone to give a prognosis for 'how long have I got?' The answer is 'Only God knows'. On the other hand, the old adage, 'God helps those who help themselves', fits the situation entirely.

The most important way of helping the body and mind to become more viable is to provide the best of all possible nutrition and raw products.

Cancer cannot grow in a completely healthy environment. The body and mind can become strong in spite of it. The plan is to *stop the cancer reaching any lethal place.* Stop it in its tracks and *give the healthy immune system a chance to destroy it with the natural defence substances we can all make.*

Case comment: Bernard

Sometimes thoughtless words from a doctor can have a profound effect on prognosis—particularly when considering some meddlesome counter-productive protocols. Take the case of Bernard.

This intelligent, strong-spirited man is now eighty-two years old. He came to me in December 1988 with stomach cancer diagnosed by biopsy and considered inoperable. Bernard had been an engineer in Indonesia. He was imprisoned in a concentration camp with many of his compatriots in 1942 during the Japanese invasion. He weathered this period of great privation and stayed in the country after World War II to work, marry and raise a family of four children. They moved to Australia, then called the 'lucky country', in 1970 to give the children a better chance in life.

Bernard suffered from a chronic back injury which gave him great pain so, in 1983, he had an operation on the spine in an attempt to fix it. Unfortunately, while he was still in hospital a grave infection with an antibiotic-resistant germ, commonly known as 'golden staph', invaded the new bone. Many different antibiotics were tried, unsuccessfully, to bring it under control. After nine months of great pain and discomfort his body defences finally won but several

INTRODUCTION

In recording these results of therapy undergone by my cancer patients, especially those who were terminally ill and have now recovered, I wish to make one thing crystal clear. There is nothing 'alternative' about their therapy. In every case it follows sound physiological and psychological principles, basically aimed at restoring the person to the state of healthy equilibrium, called 'homeostasis', which does not allow cancer cells to grow.

You see, we all have cancer cells in us, just as we have germs, fungi, yeasts and viruses that we carry about for all of our lives. They are the hangers-on and we are the hosts, but the intruders can only subversively change our cells to do their bidding, to multiply and take over, if we let them. If conditions are not to their liking, most of them will die off, but those that remain will be controlled quite easily by our strengthened defence systems. So our job—our lifetime commitment—is to keep the chemistry of the body in perfect working order so that it cannot be influenced by these rotten apples in its midst.

Since 1983 more than two thousand people with cancer have had reason to ask for my help with their nutrition and stress control. The majority have been classed as 'terminally ill'; that is, they have the disease in such a severe form that no further surgery, radiation or chemotherapy will help them. Many come to me as a last resort, a final try to find some quantity and quality of life in a desperate situation.

There are a few who have taken responsibility for their own health at an early stage of the condition and who take a lively and intelligent interest in everything their doctors have been doing. They find it easier than others to put fear behind them and begin a change in their lifestyle from the first diagnosis.

Cancer is the ultimatum for profound change, says Dr Carl Simonton, an American Doctor of Radiotherapy. This is a great truth. Unless the body can regain its capacity to fight the illness by changing back to its proper state of biochemical balance, as it was before it developed cancer, then the cancer cells will progress inexorably until the end, no matter what procedures have been undertaken.

On a one-to-one basis there is a limited number of people I can help to make these changes. Although personal contact is the best way, writing down the instructions in book form will reach more and help further. Even though each person is different, the basic guidelines can be discussed so that, with a big step in the right direction, people may continue on the path of change themselves.

Being a practical person, I have kept theory to a minimum, though some physiology is necessary for people to understand the reasons for the changes they make, otherwise they let them slip or omit what is not to their liking. There is a plethora of books about cancer; many contradict each other and some are on the wrong track and cause much confusion. The guidelines I am mapping out are founded on physiological facts that have been researched by scientists and recorded in reputable journals over the last hundred years or longer. It is not just my opinion or funny idea. The diet is balanced, the recipes are tried and true. The stress control techniques are the most useful to most people. We still use them in the clinic with many patients.

I assess the supplements individually for each patient's type of cancer, body metabolism and state of health. The supplements discussed here are general aids and may be taken without fear of toxicity since they are naturally-occurring substances and are taken in the right proportion for stimulating the immune system, restoring the liver and balancing the electrolytes.

Digging the information out of the hundreds of journals, books and seminars is a lifetime job. It has taken me to the USA and Mexico four times, and to Japan and Kenya, to see for myself. I study research literature constantly to discover more.

I have tried to describe briefly where I went and what I learned here and there, especially from the experiences of the therapies used at other centres. Then, with my patients' help, we have put into practice the fruits of those experiences and come up with some vertebrae had been partly destroyed and distorted so that he is left with a severe and permanently fixed kyphosis or bent back.

The abnormal pressures from this bony deformity on the abdominal viscera soon caused a large hiatus hernia—a condition in which part of the stomach is pushed up through the diaphragm into the chest. This compressed the lungs, which are now also ailing. Then cancer developed in the herniated part of the stomach.

When I first saw Bernard he was grossly anaemic after his exploratory operation on the abdomen, but ready to fight in spite of the 'hopeless' prognosis. The surgeon said that there was 'nothing he could do' and that Bernard would be dead within six or twelve months.

His wife, Willy, was so incensed at this prediction that she helped him to embrace the whole program I gave them, taking all the foods, supplements and even the raw liver juice with care and dedication. His spirits, his general health and his blood tests steadily improved. The cancer markers and pain regressed quite quickly. For more than two years Bernard felt very well and convinced himself that the cancer had gone completely. I didn't care whether it had all gone or not, he was keeping it under control and that was all that mattered. I told him, 'Your healthy body has shrunk the cancer to a very small size, probably only the size of the top of a pencil now'. He said, 'I don't believe I have cancer at all. There is nothing there.' He told me that repeatedly.

You see, Bernard is a winner. He liked to tease his surgeons with the incorrectness of their prognosis. He was determined to show those doctors and surgeons that he had won outright, that he no longer had cancer and that our diet, the supplements and his wife's care had won. To do this he was willing, against my advice, to undergo the tests that his G.P. and surgeon devised. He was also lured into the limelight by being the subject of a clinico-pathological conference arranged by his hospital doctors to demonstrate his recovery to their colleagues.

The endoscopy (tubal examination of the stomach) was done with great difficulty because of his bent, bony frame. The X-rays showed nothing but a huge hiatus hernia. The endoscopy showed a flat

Say: | *I take time to listen to others.*

plaque. The case was classified as an '*indolent cancer*', which means that the cancer was *not growing*. (The expectation had been that, with its original invasiveness, it would have already taken over the whole body and caused his death.) Was that the end of the story? Triumph?

Unfortunately not. As you would have guessed, the stirring up of the condition, the stress of going into hospital again, that invasive cutting of the quiescent little flat tumour to take bits of it for testing and the chemicals and drugs given during the anaesthetic and operation have all caused a downturn in Bernard's immune system. He has not regained his health since the ordeal. He is unwell. He has lost his appetite; his food goes down with difficulty and his cancer markers have begun to rise.

This means that the condition of the cancer has changed from 'indolent' to 'active', maybe not as active as it had been originally, but progressive none-the-less. And there is pain again. So there can be pain killers, so there can be constipation—all the earlier problems that put the body into the struggling mode again. He is fighting gamely, but that certain lethargy has crept in; a case of 'losing heart' and 'having no stomach' any more. Keep on keeping on, Bernard! You will soon have grandchildren to see!

5 LIFESTYLE CHANGES NECESSARY FOR SURVIVAL

Please read the foodplan and supplements of the Cilento Survival Plan in conjunction with this next section.

The lifestyle changes should:

Build up the general health

Establish optimum nutrition to withstand infections and replace what is deficient. Almost all cancer patients are deficient in vitamins A, C and E, potassium and magnesium. Often zinc, vitamins B6 and B12, and essential fatty acids are very low too. These can be replenished by the right food and by supplements, if necessary, and will be discussed as we go through the program in detail.

Build up the immune system

To do this, the food must contain all the substances necessary for making good white cells (our defenders) and you should eliminate anything from the food or the environment that will overtax the liver (which makes white cells) or any other organ of the body, so weakening it. For example:

- Don't eat hydrogenated oils. Cooked and preserved oils, in fried foods, especially in deep fried take-aways where oil has been heated many times, may form carcinogenic substances.
- Avoid hard animal fats: no lard, suet, dripping or pastry made from them. Hard animal fats like lard collect all the nasties the animal can't eliminate easily, such as antibiotics and pesticides. Our own fat contains dieldrin and other insecticides.
- Eliminate margarine. Use butter mixture (recipe later).
- Use only cold-pressed oils. The liver has to detoxify any medication you may be taking, whatever it is, so any drugs you take over

a *long period* may cause damage. These must not be ceased without medical advice since they may be lifesaving, but take only what is absolutely necessary. Ask your doctor.

- Eliminate those sugars that feed the cancer. Our normal cells live on oxygen in a process called 'aerobic metabolism', whereas cancer cells live on sugars and alcohols that they make from sugars. This is called 'anaerobic metabolism' So refined sugar must not be used—no glucose, sugar, whether raw or refined, no maltose, glucodin, dextrose, or other refined sugars. In nature, sugars occur in fruits and root vegetables, with many other natural substance such as fibre and pectin. These combinations are food for the body cells. Refine them, that is alter the combination, and they are food for the cancer cells.

  Sugar, particularly refined cane sugar, can upset the absorption of the B group of vitamins too. It is only natural if it has its fibre with it, so use the sugar in fruit for sweetness.

  Avoid *white flour*, too. It is changed to sugars by digestion. Instead, use unrefined grains and starches, such as arrowroot, rice, tapioca, corn, sago and pea flour.

- Reduce salt. You need potassium and sodium in a certain ratio, so cut out the sodium to restore the proper balance and the right electrical charge on the cell membrane (see diagram of cell changes on the colour pages).

- Avoid red muscle meat, such as beef, mutton and pork, which contain substances which may encourage cancer cell growth. Use liver, kidney, fish and seafood from the deep sea, instead.

- Tobacco has more poisons than nicotine. *Stop smoking*. Don't just cut down, stop! Otherwise you are not really committed to healing yourself.

- Use no alcohol. The cancer lives on alcohols that it makes from sugars. It has a fermentive, anaerobic metabolism, which was discovered by Professor Otto Warburg in 1936. It is best not to drink *any* alcohol, because your liver needs all the help it can get to make tumour necrosing factor and so on. Don't give it alcohol to detoxify too. This is your choice.

- Keep out of air-conditioning if you can. Don't go into air-conditioned places, especially where there is smoking. You will be breathing a soup of other people's germs to add to the poisons in tobacco.

- Artificial colours, flavours and preservatives are almost all manmade chemicals that may affect us adversely and must be detoxified in the liver. The long-term effects of many on humans are not known and some are carcinogenic to rats.

Eliminate anything that causes cancer to grow faster

This applies to the environment, as well as to food. Go through your cupboards and garden shed if you have cancer in the family. Dispose of all chemicals, oils, sprays, insecticides, hydrocarbons, weedicides, thinners, paints, welding chemicals and fungicides. If you have to use something chemical, use gloves, use it in the open air and wash with soap afterwards.

Commonly used household poisons which should be banned include mineral oils that give rats cancer, such as baby oil and commonly available medicinal oils for constipation. Detergents, too, whether they are biodegradable or not, are damaging to us in many ways. Castile soap, plain Lux or Sunlight are satisfactory substitutes. All hair shampoos, gel or liquid, contain detergents, hair conditioners and dyes are also chemicals. Use harmless anti fungal powder in armpits and toes instead of deodorants*.

All artificial colours, flavouring and preservatives should be avoided. They are present in aerosol sprays, air fresheners and pest strips and factory-made and processed foods such as coloured jellies, sweets, cake mixes, sauces, mayonnaise, canned foods, breakfast foods, desserts and biscuits. Make up these foods yourself if you can, with pure ingredients.

Refined flour, especially from wheat, is now suspect too, since eight chemicals, some of which remain in the flour, are used to process it. Organically grown grains would be best, if available. Next best is unrefined grains. Try wheat, rye, oats, millet, corn, buckwheat, or other types.

---

* *Consumer Beware* by Beatrice Trum Hunter, Touchstone, 1972; and *Be Kitchen Wise*, Beatrice Trum Hunter, Unwin Paperbacks, Sydney, 1986; give alternatives to use in place of dangerous household stubstances.

Say: | *My strength is quietness, calm and trust.*

Control biological poisons

Bacterial, viral and fungal elements that prevent healing (such as bad teeth, warts, herpes and candida) need to be controlled.

Dehydration and debility (see page 292)

When a patient is extremely debilitated from lack of food or loss of fluid, the situation is quite different. The body cells are dangerously depleted and need fluids, salt and glucose desperately in this instance; for example before or after an operation, having chemotherapy or during blood loss and attacks of vomiting and diarrhoea. Then these electrolytes are given by intravenous drip or retention enema by the doctor and they may well be *lifesaving*.

The natural sweetener, honey, may be used very sparingly (one teaspoon a day) if you must, for those with a 'sweet tooth' but it is really better to forego sweet things 'cold turkey'. You will very quickly lose the craving for them. Some people who experience sugar cravings are low in the amino acid, glutamine. This is part of a protein molecule and could come back into the diet in skim milk, yoghurt, cottage cheese, liver, kidney and legumes.

Salt comes into the category of substances that feed cancer in quite a different way. In the discussion on the changes in cell metabolism which allow cancer to grow, we will see that sodium (ordinary salt is sodium chloride) is an element that should be found *outside* the cell in the fluids of the body, while potassium is *inside* the cell. In people with cancer many cells have lost the capacity to keep sodium outside and it enters the cell, bringing water molecules with it to disrupt the working balance. This happens particularly if there is an overload of sodium ions in the body.

The dietary program aims to push up the intake and balance of potassium so that it goes back into the cells. To achieve this, sodium must be cut down to a minimum. Enough sodium for good health occurs naturally in the fruits and vegetables. Adding salt to food is a habit that has been learned, often in childhood by imitating parents. It may also have been necessary for people who perspired freely, so losing salt in the sweat. For instance, salt tablets are taken to prevent dehydration, cramps, thirst and nausea, as wheat humpers, fruit pickers and some sports people will know very well. However, people with cancer should not be doing that sort of activity anyway—

so, cut out salt. If you must have something to shake on your food, use potassium salt, which can be bought from the chemists without a prescription. But use it sparingly—it does not taste the same and is actually potassium chloride, not sodium chloride.

Red muscle meat has a time-honoured place in the Australian diet because it was a very nutritious protein source in the days when there were not many choices. Now we have lavish choices but not all of them are nutritive. Unfortunately, red muscle meat has a protein in its composition that *may* either act as a growth activator for cancer or depress the defence peptides (see page 189) in our cells. There are hundreds of different amino-acid combinations making up the many and various proteins in food. This one is *probably* not good for people with cancer (see page 386: the cancer organism can be grown on beef broth). In this instance the problem does not lie in what the animals have been fed. It is inherent in the red muscle itself. Rabbit and kangaroo muscle do not seem to have this property.

Support the liver

Eliminate substances that put too much strain on the liver. The liver has hundreds of functions to perform. It is the 'kitchen' of the body. Among its many uses are the following:

- It makes all the steroid hormones from cholesterol.
- It takes raw products from food and processes them into substances we can use.
- It stores glucose as glycogen.
- It makes bile to help digest fat.
- It detoxifies many poisons that come into the body.
- It breaks down many waste products ready for excretion.

It is now common knowledge that pesticides such as DDT, which is used for lice, ticks and worms, and the insecticides, weedicides and fungicides that are used on farms and in the home are dangerous substances if used constantly.

In animals raised for food, the pesticides for lice and ticks, the vermifuges for worms and the growth-enhancing substances we give

Say: *In stillness each day I attune to divine direction.*

them collect in the fat of the animal. Human breast milk in Eastern Australia now contains DDT and radioactive substances, since these are cumulative and indestructible in the environment. Like domestic animals, we too collect and retain chemicals from the insecticides, weedicides and fungicides which contaminate our vegetable food. For this reason, we should use organically grown food if possible.

It is the liver which monitors all these. Later we will discuss it more thoroughly but, for the moment, remember that these nasties are contained in the *hard animal fat*. If you eat that fat, you just contaminate yourself further and give your liver more to do in trying to detoxify it and put it into your bile for excretion or your fat for storage if it cannot be excreted.

Caffeine stimulants in tea, coffee and cola also put a heavy strain on the liver when taken by mouth.

Tap water should be mentioned too. Use rain water or distilled water if you can. Tank water from a clean iron roof and a clean tank may also be suitable if there is no aerial spraying of crops in your area.

Our town water supplies must be processed with chlorine to destroy bacteria which used to take a lethal toll in the past, especially of children through summer diarrhoea. Chlorine is the antiseptic that keeps town water clear of the germs that cause typhoid, cholera, enteritis and many other dangerous diseases. Chlorine also destroys fungi and algae. Though it is easily boiled out of water, dissolved chemicals used in flocculating dirt and pesticide pollutants picked up from soil are still there. Some water purifiers are helpful, especially the reverse-osmosis types.

Look on changes as a challenge

Don't fight changes, go with them. Don't forget that we are what we *think* too. Know you are meeting the challenge and winning. Clean out negative thoughts with meditation, relaxation and/or prayer. Say the affirmation, 'I enjoy only the foods that are good to my body and mind'. Repeat it often and you will soon find it is true.

Establish peace of mind

Develop faith in yourself, belief in your healing power and the strong desire to live life to the full. These decisions may make you one of the *exceptional survivors*.

6 UNDERSTANDING THE SURVIVAL PLAN

Guidelines for the food plan

Please turn to the diet itself on pages 66-77 and read in conjunction with these notes. Now we will go through the food plan, meal by meal to give some brief guidelines. You can then use your imagination and my anti-cancer cookbook* to make innovations that suit your taste.

Remember, there is nothing here that will 'make you lose weight'. This is not a diet for putting on or taking off weight. It says *what to eat, not how much.* If you want to put on weight, eat more of the grains, soup, root vegetables and calorific fruits such as bananas. If you want to lose weight, put in a bigger proportion of raw salads.

Basically, this food plan has no cooked fat, no fried foods, no sugar, no salt, no red meat and no chemicals.

This is a diet you and your family could stay on for ever—it is a way of life which helps your body to build up the immune system to fight off infections and cancer, get rid of toxic material you have stored over the years and keep your systems functioning as well as possible. This is how it helps you to fight cancer: by putting the body back into the fit state it was or should have been in before you got cancer.

If you have never been really well, this is your chance to put your health in order. It will also help to give you a better outlook on life. We are not a lot of little unconnected separated bits. Body, mind and spirit work together. Inner spirit and faith in yourself

---

* *Anti cancer Cookbook* by Ruth Cilento 1989 available from 1 Trackson Street, Alderly, Brisbane 4051.

are the motivators of the mind. The mind wants to know so it can tell the body what to do. The body, given the learning experience, will fulfil, or try to fulfil, what the mind and the spirit direct it to do.

There is nothing difficult about this diet, but some people may take longer to establish themselves happily on it than others. Take one part at a time if you are finding it heavy going and try starting with taking the juices or changing one meal at a time. Fix the breakfasts you like first, then dinners, and so on.

Special situations (see also page 28 and page 292)

- For those who have no appetite the Vitamin B12 and Lysine will be helpful. It is no use making large meals; the patient may take just two or three mouthfuls and not manage any more. This is disappointing and frustrating for the cook as well as the patient. Try small, very small, meals often. Most freshly prepared foods will keep two days in the refrigerator and may be re-presented in a different form, but not recooked. For instance, rice can be reheated or made into rice salad the second day.
- For those who have some obstruction in the gullet from cancer of the oesophagus, or as an aftermath of surgery or radiation to the head or neck, most food is best taken as a puree. The blender and the juicer will both be used. For scarring, a rubber bougie may need to be passed daily to keep the tightening area open. Usually there is a nursing and/or medical team at the hospital where the treatment was carried out who instruct and monitor the patient's proficiency in this.

  Radium to the head and neck causes drying up of the salivary glands and loss of taste, usually only for a time. Artificial saliva, like artificial tears, may be taken before a meal or with it. Sips of water, or juice, between mouthfuls may help. Acidy fruits such as pineapple, kiwi fruit and passionfruit should not be taken, since they cause unpleasant stinging.

  Vitamin E is most valuable to stop scars becoming hard, fibrosed and constricting and should be taken daily for an indefinite period.
- For those with cancer of the stomach many little meals, often, made in the blender as purees, can prevent the severe and lethal malnutrition that accompanies this cancer.

  The stomach cancer patient must have weekly B12 injections,

Understanding the Survival Plan 49

too, since the stomach does not absorb this vitamin; in fact full nutrition is only possible with 1000 mgm of B12 intramuscularly every week. This is because the stomach wall is not making the intrinsic factor which allows this most important vitamin to be absorbed. The usual hospital fare is completely inadequate and contains so many chemicals, in the food preservatives, flavouring and colouring, that the patient should go on to home-made egg flips as soon as possible.

Eggflip, a highly nutritious and easily absorbed drink, can be made in the blender with skim milk powder ('Carnation' is free of preservative) mixed with rain water, a whole free-range egg (washed of course), shell and all; one ripe banana or rolled oats, soaked and blended with 2 teaspoons of honey. Pure vanilla essence or a few fennel seeds can be added, too, for flavour. Blend it well. It may be kept in the refrigerator for two days.

The body needs proteins, essential fatty acids, unrefined carbohydrates, vitamins, minerals, fibre and fluid. As much as possible is provided by food, but for those depleted by their illness, lack of appetite or poor absorption, supplements of these substances will be needed for healing. These will be discussed as we proceed through the food plan.

The fluids

Start the day with them. You normally need six to eight glasses of fluid a day. Select your fluids from:

Water: rain, tank, distilled, or from a purifier.

Juices: from fruits and vegetables, freshly made, not frozen. Always drink fresh juice within one hour of making it, because when oxidised (from standing in the air), they are less effective.

Herb teas: (made with pure water) dandelion, red clover, pau d'arco, (taheebo), chapparel, lemongrass, dried or fresh herbs (not grown in Europe—remember Chernobyl).

Skim milk: made with pure water and preservative-free skim milk powder (such as Carnation brand in Australia).

Say: | *I am stable and steady in the face of challenge.*

Some minerals in which people with cancer are deficient can best be taken with the first drink of the day; for example, *potassium* and *magnesium*, the most important. Potassium is contained, in this order of strength, in orange juice, tomato juice, skim milk, bananas, potatoes, oats, pears, peaches, apricots and all root vegetables. (This is not an exhaustive list, see the table on page 133).

Most people like orange or other citrus juice as a starter to the day, but other fruit juice is nutritious, too, for those who cannot take citrus.

Magnesium is most economically taken as Epsom salts (which is magnesium sulphate), but in this form it should only be taken in doses of a ¼ to ½ teaspoon, since it may have a laxative effect and be wasted. If the body just throws it out unabsorbed in a loose motion, too much is taken, so use your discretion. This small dose may be added to the orange juice without changing its taste.

Since magnesium is the 'metabolic manager' inside each cell, it causes energy from food to be delivered to the cell in the form of a substance called Adenosine Triphosphate (ATP). It also takes part in hundreds of other transactions. Dr Joan Caddell, working as a voluntary medical worker among starving African children, found that only those given a magnesium supplement were able to absorb the relief food and recover.

Tablets such as magnesium orotate or magnesium aspartate may be given, but it is better to put magnesium into the body in the foods that are rich in it, such as legumes (peas and beans), wheatgerm, potato, oatmeal, spinach, skim milk and brown rice (see the table on page 133).

The juices are the most important part of any anti-cancer diet. There are five juices in this program and they are crucial to success. They contain many vitamins and minerals but, most importantly, they contain **abscisic acid**. *This is a substance that stops cancer cells growing.* It does *not* kill them, but it has the property of destroying the growth hormone that they make. In botany abscisic acid is called 'dormin'. It is responsible for stopping the growth of fruit so that it will start to ripen and of leaves so that they will fall.

Abscisic acid is strongest in wheatgrass, green vegetables, mangoes and all fresh and raw juices of vegetables and fruit (see the table on page 69).

What's for breakfast?

Some people are not in the habit of eating breakfast, yet it should be the most important meal of the day. At this time the whole body, including the digestive processes, has not only been rested but also depleted of nutrients for up to twelve hours.

In one part of the world an Eskimo (Inuit) may have raw seal oil and raw fish oil for breakfast while an Indian villager would be having rice with curried vegetables and a Masai tribesman ox blood mixed with milk. All these people could be much healthier with this fare than the businesswoman who hurries off to the office after a cup of sugared coffee and a slice of white toast with margarine.

There is no one way that is absolutely right for everyone because there are at least four different types of metabolism in western races and many more in our mixed-up inheritance. The heating grain foods might suit a cool, slow or 'yin' type of person, while a hot, active 'yang' type could prefer the proteins of meat, eggs or fish for breakfast.

Habits that preclude the eating of certain foods at certain times or make it taboo to combine one food with another may have grown up in a race of people over thousands of years. The origin of habit probably came from a necessity lost in time. To some people the eating of pig products is a serious sin, while to millions of others it is their staple protein.

Approved habits vary culturally from two meals a day to constant nibbling, snacking or 'grazing', as it is now called. (Remember, however, that grazing animals have several long periods of rest to digest!)

The breakfast foods discussed below are those most commonly available in most parts of the world. *Try to include something from each group* because they are nutritious and protective. The amounts and proportions of each are variable and depend on your taste, your appetite and your early eating habits.

Say: *In stillness ideas start to flow.*

Muesli or mash

To save time each morning, it is wise to make up enough muesli or mash dry ingredients for a week and store them in a glass jar with a screw top. This can be kept in a cool dark place or in the fridge, and the moist ingredients can be added when you scoop out the amount you are having in the morning for breakfast. This can be a tasty breakfast if you use your imagination when adding other ingredients, such as chopped, pureed or mashed fruit. Each muesli ingredient is there for a purpose.

Grains are responsible for some of the commonest allergies, to the grains themselves, to the way the grain is grown (with poor, non-organic fertilisers that make magnesium and other minerals insoluble and so unavailable to the plant), or it may be to the way the grain is stored, milled and processed.

There are usually eight artificially made chemicals used in the production of grains like wheat, from the time the pre-emergence spray is applied to the pre-fertilised ground to the time the flour sits on the shelves in the supermarkets, where the chemical preservatives in each bag allow it to stay sterile and unchanged for many years longer than it ever did in all our history. Even mice won't eat it.

Some of the peoples of the world amongst whom cancer was unknown throughout the ages have included grain as a staple part of their diet: the Incas with maize, the Celts and Scots with oats, the Hunzakuts with wheat, and the Aztecs with millet. In Japan and China rice has been cultivated since before written history. In the stratified layers of human debris dating from 5000 BC in the Tehuacan caves of Mexico, corn that could seed itself is to be found—ancestor to the hundreds of varieties since cultivated that cannot seed themselves and must be planted by people. Wheat and flax were bartering entities, staple crops and an important part of the economy in ancient Egypt. Wheat granaries, made of adobe mud brick dating back to 6000 BC, are still extant and look just as they were depicted on the ancient papyrus.

The grains were no problem then; many civilisations survived on them. It is *what we do to grain* that can make it a problem today.

Biodynamic grain—grown with humus and mulch instead of chemicals—is costly and difficult to find. Use it if you can but if, like most of us, you are reliant on the supermarket or health food shops, choose carefully. Do not use refined grain if you can avoid it.

Dolomite contains two important ingredients in the proper proportions for use in the body: calcium and magnesium. I test the serum calcium level with each patient at the first appointment, if possible, and before each two-monthly checkup, to see that calcium is not raised. (If it is, we leave out the dolomite.) One teaspoon or two tablets is sufficient for most people, though it is poorly absorbed.

Brewer's yeast, as you will see by the food table on page 133, has all the B group vitamins and many other useful minerals and vitamins. Some people who have the yeast infection *Candida* are sensitive to a number of other yeasts and may not be able to take brewer's yeast while having treatment for Candida. Others may wish to take it as two tablets, instead of in powder form if the taste is disagreeable to them. (The best way of testing Candida overload is by a simple skin test, measurable in twenty minutes. Husband and wife should both be treated if tests are positive.)

Natural unsweetened yoghurt*, made from the action of the acidophillus bacillus of milk, is the best way of taking that most useful of all our bacteria. We have many different types of bacteria in our bodies, particularly in the parts that are in contact with the external world such as skin, mouth, nose, gut, vagina and lungs. The proportion of different bacteria (germs) is called our 'flora'. We have wonderful defences against the disease-causing germs in the bowel. Some natural inhabitants of the gut, Lactobacillus acidophillus and Lactobacillus bifidis, keep the other bacteria, yeasts and fungi in order, so that they do not harm us. There is more about this in the case studies on page 343.

The main thing to know is that these 'germs', which make yoghurt, are protective. If you do not like yoghurt, use the bacillus itself

---

* You can make your own yoghurt from skim milk (there is a recipe in the *Cilento Anti-Cancer Cookbook*, Creed and Lang, Warwick, 1988) or buy a natural, locally made one with no preservatives or sugar.

Say: | *I share my faith with others.* |

as ⅛ teaspoon of the live organisms in a capsule or tablet, one with each meal. It does not taste and can be taken with food, but *not cooked*. Lactobacillus acidophillus, bifidus or bulgaricus are all suitable.

Since there is one teaspoon of honey allowed per day, you may like to use it on your breakfast, however fresh fruit juices are better and are necessary for those who cannot take milk products.

Some things that can be added to the dry muesli or mash ingredients are:

- Sesame seeds, sunflower seeds, millet, rye, linseed, buckwheat. All these can be ground up into a coarse powder by your blender or grinder and a small amount of the mixture can be added to the mash.
- Fresh raw fruits of all sorts may be used and fruit, stewed slowly without sugar, is also tasty. Prunes, plums, peaches, apples and pears are most suitable. Do not forget that this breakfast is mostly raw, as is 75 per cent of the whole eating plan. If you have something cooked, it should make up only 25 per cent of that meal.
- Raisins, sultanas and dried apricots should be washed thoroughly until the water runs clear, since they often have glycerine and metabisulphite on them to keep them moist and to stop mould. Put the washed fruit in some pure water in a stainless steel saucepan and bring to the boil. Strain and discard the water and put the fruit in the fridge for later use. This can then be added to the dry ingredients in *small* amounts only, or used in biscuit making and flavouring. Raisins and sultanas contain much natural sugar that is concentrated in the drying process. Dates and figs have too much sugar and often contain mould. Walnuts, pecans and peanuts have too much oil and may also harbour carcinogenic moulds such as aflatoxin.

People who have had bowel cancer, have a colostomy, diverticulitis, gall bladder trouble or any cancers of the gastro-intestinal tract should be very wary of nuts, seeds and dried fruit since they easily grow fungi when caught up in the bowel and may then promote irritation and diarrhoea.

The cold-pressed vegetable oils

The extraction of oils from seeds, grains and beans has become mechanised and modernised in the last fifty years. This is to produce more oil which will stay saleable on the shelf longer. To achieve this, the oil is extracted with super-heated steam and chemicals, so what emerges is actually cooked oil.

Unfortunately this process changes one of the components of the oil which is very important for our immune systems. The 'gamma linolenic' form of essential fatty acid is changed into the 'translinolenic' form, which cannot be used by the immune system in making the prostaglandin PGEI, necessary for maturing the white cells*.

We cannot function without the *essential fatty acids*, but we cannot make them in the body and so they must be taken in our food. Some people who have been taking a completely fat-free diet for years (Health Revolution and Pritikin) in an effort to reverse heart disease, diabetes or obesity, have discovered that, even though they have overcome the disease, they become weak and listless after a time, usually after their own fat stores have been used up. Because all fats except for a little butter, are eliminated in our program, we must add the right amount of the right essential fatty acid (EFA) to make our immune system efficient.

The oil that contains the most gamma linolenic EFA. is cold-pressed linseed (flax) oil. You will notice it must be *cold pressed*; that is, extracted in the old way without heat or chemicals. (It is *not* the same as the linseed oil in paint.) You would have to take twice as much safflower oil, or four times as much olive oil to gain the same effect, but then you would need to take a great deal more Vitamin E because you have put the fat intake out of balance again. The polyunsaturated oils inhibit the absorption of this vitamin and actually exacerbate heart problems. So get cold-pressed linseed oil, if you possibly can. You will need less of it than of other cold-pressed oils. 'Melrose' brand, made in Canada, is the very best.

To take the *one full tablespoon* of linseed oil needed daily, you may have to divide it up into two teaspoons in your breakfast juice

---

* Read the excellent book by Udo Erasmus, *Fats and Oils* (Alive Books, Vancouver, 1986), which describes the metabolism of these so well. It is based on the work of Dr Johanna Budwig, discussed later.

Say: *I walk on the bright side of life.*

or cereal, and two in your salad dressing, or soup. It must *not* be cooked or it is no longer cold pressed.

Some people who have never eaten cereal for breakfast find the muesli mash unpleasant. Others get tired of it, and leave out important ingredients. Rather than do that and put the food intake out of balance, try having the mash blended up, all ingredients together, as a drink. Lace it with fruit juice if you like it sweeter, or with more yoghurt if you like it sour.

Other breakfast suggestions

- Fresh fruit salad with the lecithin and skim milk yoghurt instead of cream on top.
- Cooked grains are a staple breakfast for some people, especially in cold countries. To some, no breakfast is satisfying without rolled oats. So cooked rolled oats porridge with or without stewed fruit (no sugar), is permissible as long as the raw fruits and vegetables are taken later in the day.
- Boiled rice, bread, chappatis and croissants are commonly eaten for breakfast and are acceptable if made without violating the general guidelines first described. But if you have these, you must add the other ingredients of the mash—butter, yoghurt, dolomite, and cold-pressed oil—somewhere along the line, either in food, powders or capsules.

Humans are omnivorous. Different tribes and races through human history have flourished in thousands of different ecological systems in different parts of the world. There never was any 'typical' race. Different peoples have always adapted to the foods available in their particular environment. In our drug/chemical-dependent society, cancer is now epidemic. Now, with medicinal help, even the most unfit can survive to pass on their genes, but at a price. The price is often ill health of various kinds, especially susceptibility to allergic disorders, so some people are allergic to some grains.

The safest way to use grain is to grind it yourself, but this is not possible for most of us. Second best is to buy rolled or flaked grain such as rolled oats, barley, wheat, rye, linseed and rice. Do not put these together at first. Use each singly as the basis of the raw muesli, washed well or soaked overnight and cooked as a porridge the next day. In this way, many an allergy will be discovered.

Ordinary rolled oats are the best for their potassium content. If there is no allergic reaction, combine several together.

If you want to be really sure that the grain you use is safe, you can sprout it and eat the sprouts raw or make suncooked bread, 'Essene bread' from the sprouted grain.

Wheatgerm and oat bran are in vogue now. I find both of these brans are irritating to the bowel and gas producing. Again it is not that they are unhealthy themselves, it is the concentration of chemicals they contain. Wheatgerm does *not* go rancid in three hours or three days as some books suggest; it lasts for 5 or 6 months in a cool environment. However it often contains residues of chemicals used in wheat growing.

The vexed question, then, is what to use for bread. It is best to make your own bread with freshly ground unrefined flour, preferably biodynamically grown.

The *worst* grain product to use is white flour, especially in sweetened forms such as buns, biscuits, cakes, doughnuts and pizzas. It is second best to buy bread made of 100 per cent wholemeal flour with no artificial colouring, flavouring or preservatives, no sugar and no oil. Some salt and some mould inhibitor is just about universal in all commercially made bread. If you have only one or two slices a day of that, you will not be doing yourself much harm, as long as you have the detoxifiers: fibre and Vitamin C. Any grain can be used, not just wheat. For those who have sensitivity to gluten—the glutinous or sticky part of the flour—use rice, corn, millet or buckwheat, which do not contain it. Use flat bread without yeast if there is an allergy to yeast or candida.

More about juices

Juices can be made from most fresh, raw vegetables and fruit. All juicing machines of the trituration, grinding and pressing varieties are very expensive. In Australia, for instance, the Norwalk juicer costs thirty times the price of the electric centrifugal juicer—and it is very much slower in operation. Certainly the Norwalk is the

Say: *I meet all tasks with cheerful confidence.*

best but, if the others were of no use, no-one would be getting better. In fact they *are* recovering, using juice from the centrifugal type. Theoretically centrifugal juicers, by breaking up the cells of the plant very fast, cause more oxidation which *may* oxidise some of the vitamins faster than the Norwalk. To overcome this problem, please *drink the juice within an hour*. You can judge for yourself the time it takes for squeezed orange juice to acquire a stale flavour; that is the time it takes to oxidise.

Various clinicians have advocated various juices and carrot, apple and beetroot are the all-time favourites in western countries. However, the qualities of the vegetables, their biochemical composition, taste and fluid content depend on how and where they are grown. Vegetables and herbs should be grown 'organically', without man-made pesticides, weedicides, and other chemical pollutants. They should be harvested as close as possible to the time they are to be used. All is not lost if the crop is too large. An overabundance, if snap frozen without chemical preservatives, can be stored without much change in its vitamin content if it is used within a month. Once thawed, the vegetables must be used immediately, not kept for another day. Vitamin C deteriorates first, so juice from prefrozen produce must not be relied upon to supply this. Fresh, unfrozen vegetables will keep in the fridge for days, weeks or months, depending on the type of vegetable or fruit. Pumpkins and potatoes, for instance, keep fresh for months in the crisper.

All vegetables and fruit should be *washed thoroughly* before being juiced. Organically grown produce needs to be washed, but it needs less attention than produce from the greengrocer which is always more or less polluted with chemical pesticides, weedicides, insecticides, colour 'improvers', ripening aids, antifungals, mould inhibitors and sheen producers. These may be surface chemicals, in which case scrubbing with simple soap in a tub of water and rinsing in pure water is the easiest remedy. Some surface pollutants are removed more easily—for example, from leafy greens—by adding acetic acid to the water. It is available from grocers in the form of the cheapest, white, non-brewed vinegar. Add one tablespoon to a 9-litre bucket of water. Since acetic acid is a cleaner and *not* to be taken by mouth, it must be rinsed off in pure water. If in doubt, *peel it*.

Common questions about juices

1 *Why can't I just eat the fruits and vegetables without juicing them?*

There are several reasons. Firstly, the amount of actual solid food you would need would be impossible to eat in one day. In the five juices in the Cilento Survival Plan for instance, there could be about eight carrots, four green apples, one kilo of grapes, two big oranges, two chokos, half a bunch of celery, half a kilo of green beans and half a kilo of leaves of cabbage, kale, silverbeet or other greens. There would be no room to eat any of the other necessary foods.

Secondly, the very purpose of removing the solids and releasing the chemicals from the fibre is to enable the body to assimilate the vital elements of the fruit and vegetables quickly, without any hinderance to the digestion and without destroying any of the plant enzymes and vital healing compounds that we can use. Plant pulp and fibre take hours to digest, while juices may take only twenty minutes, leaving the stomach empty for more solid food. (The pulp and fibre can be used in soups, fed to the chooks or made into compost for the garden. Don't just throw it away.)

2 *How much juice should I take?*

You may think the answer should be: 'as much as you can'. However, some guidelines are necessary. Most people need six to eight 275-ml glasses of fluid a day. The Cilento Survival Plan advises five or six glasses of juice a day, which gives 1500 ml.

In the detoxification plan (washing out of toxics) which I sometimes use as a preliminary to starting the Cilento Survival Plan, more fluid can be taken, since very little solid food is used for 72 hours.

In the Gerson diet 3000 ml of juices are taken daily. These include, three carrot juices containing fresh, unfrozen, raw young calf's liver. These are crucial to the success of that program.

3 *What fruits and vegetables can I combine?*

In spite of the many books giving advice on this subject, there are *no* hard and fast rules. There are at least ten different patterns of human metabolism that have been categorised not only in Ayuvedic and Traditional Chinese medicine, but also by recent computer

Say: | *I am strong in body, mind and spirit.*

studies of optimal eating habits in humans. The confusion arises because some nutritionists, who have had success in treating one sort of person with one disease, have generalised from specific cases and published their generalisations. The copycats have kept on reproducing these supposed 'facts'. I have found by clinical experience and my own research that people find their own best combinations.

As long as the important healing substances are contained in the produce and can be assimilated by the patient, it does not matter what is put with what. Each person can exercise his or her imagination; everyone is different.

Most clinicians have their own favourite formulae for juices which they advise their patients to take; carrot, greens, beetroot and its tops, grape juice and apple juice are the most commonly advocated. Go by your own tastes and use your imagination when making combinations. You *may* combine fruits and vegetables very successfully, if that is what suits you, but start with caution combining only two, such as apple and carrot. Then try apple and celery, or apple and broccoli, or some other green. As long as there is no adverse reaction, such as excessive wind or nausea, you may add a third vegetable, and so on. So that you can keep a track of any side effects and remember your favourite combinations, it is a good idea to note your experiments in your logbook.

A few rules about juices

There are a few rules that I advise: for example, do not put too many of the same botanical family together in a juice. For instance, members of the cabbage family are cabbage, kale, broccoli, brussel sprouts and cauliflower; members of the beet family are silver beet, rhubarb and beetroot; and members of the nightshade family are tomato, tamarillo (tree tomato), eggplant (aubergine), red and green capsicum, bell pepper, pepito, chilli and potato. Too much gas or flatulence can result from having too many from one family.

Below are some general characteristics of the commonest varieties of juices.

Green vegetation contains *chlorophyll* and its chemical components can be used by a host of land and sea creatures for conversion by digestion and assimilation into their own tissue. Humans are no exception; vegetation is no less a food for us than it is for a grasshopper or a goat, although we may use it in different ways. The huge variety of plant tissues containing thousands of combinations of the 264 elements of the earth are an integral part of the food chain of all creatures of land, water and sky. It is the means by which solar energy is used to release oxygen for life forms.

Another vegetable that is reported to be very beneficial is green asparagus. Bernie Lutz, an independent biochemistry researcher in Pittsburg, has been using it for years as an adjunct in the successful treatment of squamous cell cancers of the bladder, lung and skin. One report of his is published in *Cancer Journal News*, Vol. 14, No. 4, December 1979. In it he suggests that asparagus could be eaten raw, but preferably cooked to make it softer. Asparagus may be tough and stringy, though. It is best to make a puree in a blender, store it in the refrigerator and take four tablespoons twice daily. Improvement should be noted within two to four weeks, according to Dr Lutz.

I suggest that you take asparagus as a juice. Don't forget that large amounts of vegetable fibre may collect like wet cotton wool and, even if pureed, can block up the small lumen of the bowel, where a bypass operation has been performed to give food passageway through or past a cancerous growth. For this reason I advocate that only *juices* be taken of asparagus, mango, pineapple, celery and other very fibrous substances by people who have had such surgery or who have any potentially obstructive condition of the gastrointestinal tract.

As they ripen, all fresh and raw fruits and vegetables develop *abscisic acid* (dormin). This is a substance akin to the caratinoid family of substances which inhibit the growth hormone in plants, so allowing leaves to stop growing, age and fall, and allowing fruits to stop growing so that they will ripen. Abscisic acid does not inhibit *normal* human cell growth but it plays a very important part indeed in healing for people with cancer. It serves the same principal as in plants, inhibiting the growth hormone that cancer cells make, so slowing down their rapid and abnormal reproduction. Taken

Say: *The spirit of God is always with me.*

consistently in enough quantity, abscisic acid has allowed many people to slow up the growth so much that the immune system can destroy the cancer.

This is why fresh and raw vegetable and fruit juices are part of the nutritional program of most enlightened cancer clinics in the world, such successful program as those of the following:

- Dr Ernesto Contreras in Tijuana, Mexico;
- Dr Alex Forbes in Bristol, England;
- Dr Yolande Friare in Tijuana, Mexico;
- The Gerson Hospital in Tijuana, Mexico;
- Dr Josef Issels in Germany;
- Livingston Medical Clinic in San Diego, USA;
- Dr Moerman in Holland;
- Dr Hans Neiper in Hanover, Germany;
- The Centers that follow Ann Wigmore's teaching in Boston and San Diego, USA, Mudgereeba, and my own Nutrition and Stress Control Centre in Australia.

These are the ones I know best. No doubt there are hundreds of others with similar good results.

Foods containing abscisic acid

Abscisic acid is contained in the following:

- *All fruits*, especially mangoes, grapes, avocadoes, pears, oranges (with the white underpeel and pulp), apples and strawberries.
- *All fruit blossoms and leaves* used as tea (such as peach flowers, strawberry leaves, cherry flowers, apple blossoms and fresh herb teas) and mature leafy green vegetables.
- *All vegetables*, especially lima beans, potatoes, peas, yams, sweet potatoes, asparagus, tomatoes, onions, spinach and root vegetables, (especially carrots).
- *All nuts and seeds.*

Foods containing caratinoids

Most red, orange, deep yellow and deep green fruits and vegetables contain caratinoids. These all have strong anti-cancer properties but *beta carotene* is the best and most easily assimilated. It is strongest in carrots, mangoes, pink and orange coloured sweet potatoes, pumpkins, cantaloupes (rock melons), tomatoes, tamarillos, papaws, silverbeet and wheatgrass.

Beta carotene may be changed in the liver to Vitamin A or retinol (It is *not* Vitamin A, but its *precursor*.) If the liver cannot convert it because of disease, or if there is too much retinol stored in the liver already, then there is no conversion to Vitamin A. Hydrochloric acid made by the stomach is necessary for the conversion process. If people are taking more carotene than the body needs at the time it is stored in the skin where it shows, particularly in the hands and feet, as an orange colour. This substance is also in the blood where it is called 'Caratenaemia'.

Some doctors who are ignorant of the healing properties of carotene become worried by the orange colour, thinking it is Vitamin A (retinol), which can be toxic in malnourished people. Giving hydrochloric acid to those with Caratenaemia may cause it to be rapidly used or excreted.

Remember that, although daily doses greater than 100 000 units of retinol may give symptoms of overdosage in some rare cases, *carotene is non-toxic*. The orange colour fades from the skin within a few weeks if the substance containing it is replaced by other vegetables and fruit in the juice.

Other important ingredients of juices are the electrolytic elements potassium, magnesium, calcium, sodium and the trace minerals, especially selenium and germanium. Potassium is found in celery, spinach, potatoes and carrots, especially; calcium and magnesium is present in greens and grains; and sodium is found in celery, cucumber and the melon family.

Some of the vegetables and fruit obtainable for juicing in season in Australia are the following:

Vegetables

Artichoke (Jerusalem)
Artichoke (Green)
Asparagus
Aubergine (eggplant)

Bean sprouts
Beetroot and tops
Brussel sprouts
Broccoli

Say: *I give no one the power to hurt me.*

Cabbage
Capsicum, red and green; Bell pepper
Carrot
Cauliflower
Celery
Choko
Coconut
Cress
Cucumber
Dandelion
Endive
Fennel
Garlic
Kale
Kelp
Kohlrabi
Leek
Lettuce
Lettuce (Cos-Romaine)
Mint
Mustard Greens
Nasturtium leaves
Nettle and Dandelion
Okra
Onion
Parsley
Parsnip
Pepper (*not* hot ones)
Potato
Pumpkin (some types are too hard)
Radish
Rhubarb
Seaweed
Silverbeet
Sorrel (buckwheat)
Spinach (English or New Zealand)
Stringbean
Swede turnip
Sweet potato and greens
Tomato
Turnip (white)
Watercress
Zucchini

Fruits

Abiu
Apple
Apricot
Berries
Cherry
Citrus fruit (not skins)
Custard apple
Fig
Five corner
Grape
Grapefruit
Guava
Lemon
Lichi
Mandarin
Mango
Melon
Nectarine
Orange
Passionfruit
Papaw (Papaya)
Peach
Pear
Pepito
Persimmon
Plum
Pomegranate
Prickly pear (Sabe)
Sapote
Tamarillo

Understanding the Survival Plan

Bananas and avocadoes are too squashy and quinces are too dry and hard, while some pumpkins are too unproductive of juice to be worthwhile. These can be used in other ways.

Too much cabbage, silverbeet or green capsicum sometimes causes gas in those who are so toxic that their digestive enzymes are not working very well.

In the Survival Plan there are five juices of fresh and raw fruit and vegetables (about 140-280 ml, depending on the capacity of the person). There is no set time to take these, although it is best to space them out over the waking hours. In the diet plan I have put them in the time slot where we usually have a drink: on rising, at mid-morning, mid-afternoon, as an aperitif before dinner, and at supper-time. There is no hard and fast rule.

Take them when it suits you, but *it is preferable not to take a drink with a meal*, especially if you have limited stomach capacity. Juices are best absorbed and assimilated on an empty stomach, too. For those with intestinal cancer, see the notes on page 48 for special instructions.

When preparing fruit juices, cut apples in quarters to make sure there is no mould in the core. Do not use over-ripe banana and cut out any little blemishes in the skin of fruits. These are often patches of bacterial or fungal growth.

Say: *I am part of the miracle of life.*

7 THE DIET AND SUPPLEMENTS FOR CANCER CONTROL

This is the condensed plan as described in detail previously under Guidelines for The Food Plan Section 6. See also special sections pages 48 and 292.

Please note that there is nothing 'alternative' in this program. It is all sound, basic physiology which everyone can and should use as soon as cancer has been diagnosed. The rest of the family can use it too, though they do not need to take the juices and supplements or avoid the red meats, salt and additives.

> The basis of treatment is to build up the body's immunity so that effective antibodies against the growth of cancer cells can be formed. It is important to cut out any allergy makers (allergens) from other sources to give the body its best chance of combatting the major allergen (cancer). For this reason, it is necessary to:
>
> - **Remove all chemicals, insecticides, herbicides. sprays, oils, paints, etc, from your household.**
>
>   Do not use:
>
> - **tobacco**
> - **red meats**
> - **alcohol**
> - **canned foods**
> - **refined grains**
> - **coffee and tea**
> - **salt**
> - **processed food including white flour**
> - **cooked oils and fats**

- **sugar and foods containing it**
- **commercial preservatives**
- **perfumes, deodorants, aerosol sprays**
- **hair dyes, chemical cosmetics**
- **artificial flavourings and colourings**

No deodorants, aerosol sprays and chemical cosmetics should be used. It is wise to keep the skin absolutely clean since it can eliminate much waste material daily if the pores are clean. Showering or bathing at least once daily with unscented soap such as 'Sunlight' or Castile soap is desirable. Use hot or cold baths as directed. 'Mycil' antifungal powder under the arms and toes is allowed; also UV cream for sun protection. The Body Shop, Nutrimetics, Grace, 'Innoxa' and 'Blackmores' are just some firms which make natural, chemical-free skin moisturisers and other suitable products.

Food plan

Potassium and Magnesium

Cancer depletes potassium and magnesium. Those used to large amounts of salt *may* want to substitute Pressor K (available from chemists) which is potassium instead of sodium salt, but only use a small amount. Potassium is plentiful in vegetables and fruit (see list on page 133) especially root vegetables, oats, apples, apricots and bananas.

For magnesium, take pure water, warm or cold, containing ¼ teaspoon of Epsom salts (magnesium sulphate both magnesium and sulphur are protective). This is not enough to be a laxative. Epsom salts may also be added to juice or herb tea. Otherwise you can take one magnesium orotate tablet twice daily.

Abscisic Acid

Abscisic acid (dormin) is contained in all the raw fresh juice. It destroys the growth hormone made by some cancer cells.

Say: *God's way is the positive way.*

It occurs in all seeds, fruits and fresh vegetables. Your juices are thus the *most important* part of your diet. Never leave them out.

The five juices

You may take juices at any time throughout the day. I have put them in this order because these are the times most people take a drink anyway. They make up five or more of the six to eight glasses of fluid you need daily. The first is taken first thing in the morning and consists of a 200-275 ml glass of freshly squeezed, unstrained juice of two whole oranges or other fruit.

Breakfast

1 Fresh fruit.
2 Cereal mash or muesli containing many cancer-preventing ingredients. This cereal mixture is *raw* and may be taken in three ways: as a muesli; on top of cooked oatmeal porridge; or made up in a blender, for those who cannot eat solids, as a 'smoothie' or 'fortified milk' drink.

   To make the mash or muesli, mix the dried ingredients (you can make up enough for a week) in the following proportions:

   - wheatgerm, 1 tablespoon
   - Unprocessed bran of wheat, oats, rice or rye (delete if bowels are loose), 1 teaspoon
   - Lecithin granules, soya, 1 tablespoon
   - Dolomite Powder *or* two Dolomite tablets (delete if calcium is raised), 1 teaspoon

For each meal, add: **Natural yoghurt**, 1-2 tablespoons *or* 1/8 teaspoon of acidophillus powder as ordered (unsweetened, low-fat). **Skim milk** made of 'Carnation' powder which contains no preservative, or fresh fruit juice if you are allergic to milk. **Cold-pressed linseed or cold-pressed safflower oil**, 2 teaspoons.

   This can be sweetened with 1 teaspoon of honey if

allowed, or with fruit juice. Chopped fresh fruit makes it tasty too. Add raisins and/or washed apricots, if liked.

3 Egg. If you still have room and if your doctor advises, have a free-range egg, cooked with a runny yolk (not fried), with vegetable leftovers.
4 One slice of wholemeal toast and butter mixture (see recipe on page 72).

Mid-morning

1 Second juice: Drink 200–275 ml of raw vegetable and fruit juice (for example, four carrots and one Granny Smith apple), or 115 ml of 'fortified milk', which is the blended breakfast mixture plus pure water.
2 Choose bread, fruit, home-made biscuits, dried fruit preparation, sandwiches, wholemeal biscuits such as Ry-Vita, Vita-Weat, Crusket, with cottage cheese, onion, tomato, etc, but *no white flour*.

Green Juice

Drink the third fruit juice at anytime—200–275 ml of fruit and vegetable juice. Include one or more greens in the following 'green juice':

Juice together enough to make 200–275 ml of juice of any of the following: beetroot and tops, celery, parsley, lettuce, spinach, one of the cabbage family (cauliflower, brussel sprouts, broccoli), choko, green beans, any green herbs or greens from the vegetable list, *plus* pineapple, grapes, apple or other sweet fruit, if liked.

Start with the fruit juice plus a little of one green per day, and experiment to suit your taste, adding only one more green at a time to discover what suits you. *Do not* put too many together at first, or you will not be able to identify the culprit if the juice disagrees with you. Keep a food diary to record your favourites.

Say: | *It takes courage to say no.*

Lunch

Use foods in this order:

1. *Proteins.* Choose from free-range eggs, fish, cottage cheese, legumes or unrefined grains.
2. *Salad.* Any vegetables, five or more, raw and fresh, such as carrot, ¼ avocado, lettuce, onion, tomato, sweet corn, cucumber, celery, red capsicum (see vegetable list for juices).
3. ½ cup mung bean sprouts, ten raw almonds *or* five raw and fresh walnuts or pecans *or* six raw macadamias. These all contain laetrile. *Do not eat alfalfa sprouts* since they contain far too much growth hormone and your abscisic acid is wasted in destroying it.
4. Mayonnaise made with cold-pressed linseed oil or cold-pressed safflower oil, for linolenic essential fatty acid, with egg yolk and plain yoghurt,
   or
5. Dressing. Cold-pressed linseed oil, ½ in half with apple juice, cider vinegar or lemon juice, and with garlic and fresh herbs according to your tastes.
6. All-vegetable soup (see recipes on page 372). Make several different ones each week. They will keep for two or three days in the fridge. It is very boring to put everything in together each time.
7. One to three slices of wholemeal bread or roll (with no artificial colouring or flavouring) with one to three walnut-sized pieces of butter mixture. Do *not* eat bread first and then not have room for salad and soup.
8. A piece of fruit if desired.
9. Skim milk, fruit juice or herb tea if still thirsty.

Mid-afternoon

As for mid-morning, along with the fourth juice.

Fourth juice

50–250 g raw calf's liver juiced with four carrots **if directed by doctor**. *The liver must be young, not frozen, and eaten only within three days of slaughter. Don't forget to strain it.* (No, it doesn't taste horrible!)
or

take three dried liver tablets daily with carrot juice. Only *fresh, young, raw* and unfrozen liver contains the substances that are so important for the manufacture of tumor-necrosis factor, peptides and macrophages. Liver cooked, dried, frozen or made into tablets is good food but it does not contain these essentials. If you are strongly averse to eating liver or if the very thought of it makes you gag, then forget the liver, just continue with a fruit and vegetable juice for this one but add a freeze-dried liver tablet.

Fifth juice

200-275 ml fruit and vegetable juice.

Dinner

1. Many small portions are best to tempt your appetite. Choose dishes made from liver, kidney, fresh fish, legumes and unrefined grains, eggs, cottage cheese, fresh breast of free-range turkey*.

2. Three to six cooked vegetables—at least one green leafy vegetable and one red or yellow. You may dry bake, steam, casserole or cook in any way except fried or microwaved. Low heat and long cooking is best for grains, beans, potatoes and other starchy vegetables.

3. Any fresh or stewed fruit. Skim milk and its products, yoghurt, arrowroot, sago and tapioca.

A good routine is salad first, then all-vegetable soup, a cooked vegetable and protein dish, then fruit—cooked or raw—with or without skim milk yoghurt or skim milk home-made ice-cream. Frozen fruit put through the blender makes a good ice-cream with yoghurt. You can also add fruit puree as a sweetener for pancakes and cakes. Stewed fruit, fruit juice

---

* Chicken is not allowed. Jelly from veal bones and sharks' fins is allowed. These special proteins can be added to soups instead of chicken stock.

Say: | *I am brave enough to speak up.*

and dried (washed) fruit are also good sweeteners. Add vegetables such as tomatoes, turnips and onions pureed as sauces raw or cooked.

You may have anything in this diet, but nothing not in it. All fruits and vegetables, fresh and preferably organically grown, are suitable. There is ample protein of the right kind on this plan. *It is not a diet for gaining or losing weight*—that depends entirely on the amount you eat. Little meals often are best. If you can't eat a big salad at lunch, have two small ones, one at lunch and one at dinner, or have them as snacks between meals. (See notes on page 00 for special types of cancer problems.)

Recipes for Juices

(Have 200–275 ml per serve.)
- Apple and carrot juice. Use Granny Smith Apples, wash well, do not peel. Cut into pieces. Cut tops off carrots, but do not peel. Scrub with a soft nailbrush. Make juice half and half.
- Wheatgrass juice. This may be taken daily but start slowly, with only 50 ml; you may work up to 200 ml if tolerated.
- Liver juice. (Beginners should start with only 50g). 250g fresh raw calf's liver and 250g fresh carrots. Wash carrots well and cut into strips. Cut liver into strips. Feed equal amounts of liver and carrot through juicer together. Strain through a nylon mesh (stocking is good) and drink juice immediately!

   Have some sliced apple, orange or lemon ready to cleanse the mouth.

To make butter mixture

Beat ½lb softened butter with ¾ cup of cold-pressed linseed or cold-pressed safflower oil.

Herb teas

Use red clover, chaperal, dandelion, peppermint, basil, lemon grass, chamomile, valerian, horsetail, corn silk, lemon balm or other herbs. Preferably use fresh herbs—you can grow them in pots.

Wash everything well to remove ingrained dirt and chemicals. Use a tablespoon of white vinegar or a teaspoon of bicarbonate of soda to wash vegetables and fruit in a bucket of water.

Always use fresh, live unadulterated foods

- Cooked lamb or calf liver should be taken twice a week to gain all the right nutriments; kidney once a week; and fish or other deep-sea seafood twice a week or more (seafood should be unsalted, bought raw and fresh and cooked at home). Some bought, frozen seafood is dipped in anti-mould preservative so is unsuitable. Use fresh fish and cook it yourself or buy it just cooked from the trawler. If you catch your own, you may snap freeze it.
- You may have Ryvita or Vita-weat biscuits, dried fruit leather, flat bread, rice cakes, or other breads or biscuits with no sugar or white flour. Use unrefined grains.
- Bread and cereals should be 100 per cent wholemeal of wheat, rye, oats, corn, etc, *not* white bread coloured with dye or caramel. It should contain a minimal amount of salt and no oil, sugar or preservatives.
- Use a smear only of cold-pressed olive or coconut oil instead of fats to wipe the pan or wok. Eat no fried or microwaved food.
- There is no cane sugar in this daily regime. The sugars come from fruit, fruit juice, vegetables and a very small amount of honey (only one teaspoon daily).
- Thicken stews, sauces and gravies with wheatgerm, arrowroot or polenta, or use rolled oats that have been put in the blender to crumb (keep in a sealed jar). These can also be used instead of breadcrumbs as a coating for dry frying, or as a topping. Mix with apple sauce or other fruit to sweeten pastry and biscuits.

Say: *I hear what you are saying.*

- 50-75 per cent of the diet is *raw, fresh food* and all the food is unadulterated and unrefined.
- Drink six to eight glasses of fluid daily (five are juices).
- Let tap water stand before drinking it, or boil it to drive off the chlorine. When making herb teas, skim milk or soup, it is preferable to use rain water off a clean iron or colorbond roof (*not* an asbestos cement roof) or distilled water. A water purifier such as a charcoal filter, frequently changed, can also be used, but a reverse osmosis type is better.
- You can sterilise water in thin glass bottles by standing it in the sun for 6-12 hours. It will then be de-ionised and will not carry an electric charge, but only for about 24 hours.

As well as the food plan

- Read *Getting Well Again* by Dr Simonton. Make your own tape.
- Read and use my cookbook.
- Use a relaxation technique, meditation or prayer for 20 minutes, at least twice a day. Play your own or my tapes for affirmations daily.
- Exercise gently every day, to the limit of capacity without distress. Include deep breathing: five breaths five times daily (see page 383). Breathe from the diaphragm before filling the top part of the chest with air. Yoga and Tai Chi breathing exercises are suitable. Do *not* undertake jarring exercise such as jogging when you are feeling better. Walking is best— ask your doctor.
- If you are in pain do *not* undertake massage or chiropractic treatment without consulting your doctor. A bone scan may be necessary. Your pain *may* possibly be due to secondary cancer which can be made worse.

Note: Before reading about supplements (below), would those who are caring for a very sick person in the last stages of cancer please read the section starting on page 292. That person does *not* need supplements.

Why use supplements in such high doses?
See also appendix page 378

There are literally thousands of research papers about the role of vitamins and minerals in the working of the body and mind. I would have to write several more books to explain the dosage I use of the supplements. The facts are that they work—the patients who take them have a better chance of recovering. They feel better, they work better and their blood tests are better. Body and mind work better than when they were *not* taking the supplements.

With this improvement, the spirit becomes strong and the cancer very often loses its grip. If you want a little more information, one of the easiest books to read is *Cancer and its Nutritional Therapies* by Dr Richard Passwater. There are hundreds of others, but a word of warning: many popular writers about cancer diets do not have the knowledge to research their subject. Many make generalisations out of specific reactions so that some of what they write is untrue and misleading. If three quarters of a book is true and one quarter is trash, how will you know which is the trash? What I am telling you is all based on authentic research and has been proved beyond all doubt.

The person who has developed cancer has many unmeasurable deficiencies. There may be an inherited inability to absorb certain vitamins and other substances from food. There may be a need for more than the average amount—chemical needs vary enormously from person to person. We don't know and cannot find out what is wrong, so we take extra of every substance which we know the body uses to defend itself.

Vitamins are natural substances needed by everybody. Vitamin toxicity is rare, though vested interests constantly dwell on the 'terrible dangers' of taking too much. Vitamin A is usually the target now, though C was the popular scapegoat earlier, then B6 and B3. The effectiveness of supplements cannot be disproved, because they work. They cannot be patented because they are natural compounds. All that people wishing to make money out of expensive, patentable substitutes can do is to denigrate the natural product. Some drug

Say: *The best exercise is kindness and tolerance.*

manufacturers have a constant advertising campaign educating doctors about their products and sneering at the 'old-fashioned' natural healing compounds. Some are making both types of medication.

Supplements

If taken in the amounts prescribed, supplements can never be toxic. However, some people may have allergies to some manufacturers' additives. *Use the supplements strictly only as ordered*. The first six are detoxifying anti-oxidants that protect your body cells from invasion and damage by free radicals (see page 157).

Take vitamin supplements as follows:

- Vitamin A 10 000 i.u. capsules: one three times a day.
- Vitamin E, 250 i.u. or with Pectin: one three times a day
- Pro-Vitamin A, 10 000 units (Beta Carotene, 2 capsules twice a day = 40 000 units) or six carrots daily. This is *never* toxic but should cause yellowing of the skin. If this is excessive, cut down on red, orange, yellow and green foods and it will soon lessen.
- Vitamin C, from 12 000 mg up to 20 000 mg of non-acidic calcium or sodium ascorbate, gradually increasing to one rounded teaspoon three to five times a day (work up slowly to avoid diarrhoea). Start with ½ teaspoon in water and increase every two days to bowel tolerance. This will stop cancer cells growing and help to detoxify as well as prevent viral infections. Preferably find a powder of mixed ascorbates with bioflavinoids, usually called 'C-Complex' or 'BioC'. Read the list of ingredients before buying.
- Coenzyme Q10: one tablet three times a day.
- Selenium 50 mcgm: one three times a day or garlic capsules—three daily.
- Mineral and Vitamin tablet—1 daily—containing: Vitamin A, B1, B2, B3, B5, B6, B12, Vit C (Ascorbic Acid), Bioflavinoid, Rutin, Hesperidin, Biotin, Vitamin E, Folic Acid, Amino Benzoic Acid, Potassium Amino Acid Chelate, Calcium Amino Acid Chelate, Copper Amino Acid Chelate, Ferrous Fumerate, Magnesium Amino Acid Chelate, Manganese Amino Acid Chelate, Zinc Amino Acid Chelate, Kelp, L-Methionine, Glutamic Acid, and Betaine Hydrochloride.

- Zinc compound also containing magnesium, B6, manganese and others: one to three a day.
- Vitamin B5, pantothenic acid, 250 mg a day, or more for preventing 'nerves' and pain.
- Digestive enzymes: one to three tablets with each meal to use the good in your food.
- Hydrochloric acid and pepsin: one with each meal for those who have nausea, burping and bloating after eating.
- Thymus extract: one three times a day to make your white-cell defenders.
- Freeze-dried liver tablets, 4000 mg: one daily (or raw or cooked liver).
- B12 cytamen, 1000 mcgm preferably by intramuscular injection each week.
- Cold-pressed linseed or cold-pressed safflower oil or cold-pressed olive oil: 1–2 tablespoons daily overall (in soup, juice, salad, porridge or off the spoon before food), not cooked.
- Magnesium orotate: one tablet twice daily if not taking Epsom salts: ¼ teaspoon before breakfast.
- Lysine, 500 mg: one to three daily, if necessary for cold sores and herpes, but also to stimulate appetite.
- Acidophilus powder: ⅛ teaspoon three times daily with juice, *or* one tablespoon natural low-fat yoghurt with each meal.
- Lecithin granules (soya) in breakfast: one tablespoon; or one choline and inositol tablet three times daily.
- Dolomite tablets: two to six daily, unless serum calcium is raised.
- Dried vegetable powder as seasoning.
- Dried herbs for tea (loose rather than in bags).

There are some cookbooks, such as vegetarian and Pritikin ones, which include suitable food but it is necessary to eliminate from the recipes the substances I have not recommended; for example, pepper, condiments, canned food, soup cubes, margarine, colouring, flavouring, sugar, salt, preservatives, and so on. It is best to use our *Anti-Cancer Cookbook*.

Note: This program is *not just a food plan*. It teaches a physiologically effective lifestyle which is completely in accordance with any treatment your doctor may be giving you, and does not fight with surgery, radiation or chemotherapy. In fact, the program makes these treatments more effective.

How come I did all that and I still got cancer?

Recently I read an article by Claire R. Farrer, PhD, who is Associate Professor and co-ordinator for the Applied Anthropology Programs of California State University. It was entitled 'Stop Blaming the Victim—My Honest Opinion'. The gist of her indignation was that she developed cancer of the breast in spite of 'doing all the right things', or at least by doing none of the wrong things, which she calls 'popular notions of cancer-causing behaviour'.

Confusion arises because there is *no one cause*. There are only factors that exacerbate the formation of cancer cells and factors that inhibit them. Media articles naturally home in on the factors that affect the majority of people and so will cause the most sensational headlines. They leave out the great diversity of factors at work in people's individual chemistry and also the great variety of minds and spiritual values. Dr Farrer writes as follows.

> Look at my own history in regard to popular notions of cancer-causing behaviour, particularly regarding breast cancer:
>
> 1 **Cancer incidence is positively correlated with fat intake.** I am allergic to all milk and milk products and have been since birth. I was one of the first babies raised on soybean milk. I have never had a high fat diet, since I also am allergic to other usual fat/oil sources such as nuts and seeds. I have always eaten a lot of fruits and vegetables, often raw, and I have always limited my intake of meats.
>
> 2 **Cancer incidence is positively correlated with alcohol.** I have never abused alcohol and, while I do enjoy a glass of wine with dinner, it is not an everyday occurrence. I rarely consume hard liquor.
>
> 3 **Cancer incidence is positively correlated with stress.** (What disease isn't?) My stress level, if one can judge from blood pressure, is low. I am a productive scholar and an excellent teacher (hubris again, I suspect) who thoroughly enjoys her work.
>
> 4 **Cancer incidence is positively correlated with genetics.** I do have blood relatives who have died from cancer, both on my father's side of the family. No one in my mother's family has or has had cancer, save me. My sister and I share the same

parents. Why did I get cancer and she has not? This is an especially appropriate question, since my sister is not allergic to milk or milk products and has throughout her life consumed vastly more meat and fats than have I. I also have always been more athletic, which leads me to . . .

5 **Cancer incidence is negatively correlated with physical activity.**
As a young woman I taught dance and was an active performer. I also was a competitive roller skater. I skied, walked and swam, as I still do. I've never been a couch potato rolling around in my own lard.

In sum, I've done all the right things and none of the wrong ones and still had cancer. And I do not appreciate anyone, whether a lay person or one with initials after the name, telling me if only I'd done X or Y, or eaten this instead of that, I'd not have had cancer.

Let us realise that when research is reported in the popular press, it is usually simplified in the mistaken assumption that the general public cannot absorb complicated material. That fallacy, which teachers such as myself daily demonstrate is untrue, leads to the pop theories and fads we have all seen. Unicausal theories of any disease set as varied as is cancer are unsatisfactory.

Cancers are complicated, and while each of us should do what we can to eat properly, exercise and reduce stress, those actions alone will not guarantee that one will not be struck by cancer.

Whatever our own philosophy or belief, let us stop blaming the victims of any disease.

This excerpt was quoted in a newsletter which Dr Yolande Friare, writes every quarter for her patients. Dr Friare's note at the end of this article reads:

Feeling victimised by something or someone makes me think of: 'I feel sorry for myself' and if someone discovers the '*Why* I feel sorry for myself', we tend to hate that person, article, scientist,

Say: | *I smile a lot; laugh with me.* |

etc. In my experience, cancer may develop regardless if you smoke or not, eat well or not, drink alcohol or not. (Saint Therese of Spain, 1515-1582, died from what is believed was cancer of the uterus), and we are no more a 'victim' of cancer than we are of diabetes or muscular dystrophy.

There are several points to discuss here that will help people with cancer not to waste energy on taking sides. There is no *right* and *wrong* in how you feel, there is no *blame* and *criticism*. Let us just forget being victims, which makes for a negative picture of anger and fear in the brain, and give the positive, *victor* attitude a chance!

8 CLEARING THE MIND

If we have not quiet in our minds, comfort will do no more for us than a golden slipper on a gouty foot.

Anonymous

Understanding the brain—a new science

It was during the Korean War that great changes accelerated in the Western world's understanding of brain physiology. You see, for a hundred years or more, the world of psychiatrists and psychologists had been immersed in the aftermath of Freudian theories and the hypotheses burgeoning from them.

Psychoanalysis was very big business in America and still is, but the study of how the mind actually works had been mostly overlooked. On the other hand, the countries behind the Iron Curtain had been following the Eastern European line started by Virchow and Pavlov, according to which conditioned reflexes, even starting in the womb, dictated the behaviour of animals throughout their lives.

Giant steps had been made in understanding the external influences which governed the development of behaviour and the way changes could be brought about in it. These involved study of the brain physiology and chemistry, subjects which received very scanty attention indeed in the textbooks when I first started studying child psychiatry with the Department of Health in 1963.

The penny dropped during the Korean War when young American recruits were taken prisoner in the fighting and returned in a prisoner exchange, after a very few months, as profoundly indoctrinated and unchangeable communists.

The furore that followed involved questions in the US Congress and panicky accusations of ill treatment which were not substantiated by the erstwhile prisoners. They were beleaguered with questions, tests and experiments for years and finally were discharged back into civilian life, an embarrassment to the American forces, because they could not be deprogrammed.

From this episode the emphasis changed in the USA, not only to the study of the brain's chemistry and physiology, but also to psychic phenomena being studied in Russia. This had already been well established and understood throughout Asia and the middle East for several thousand years.

A promising young American doctor, Joseph Kamiya, had noticed that each part of the body has its own electrical output. If you hold a voltmeter in the hand for instance, you will see that it registers a tiny charge. In 1953 Dr Kamiya had made a machine, the 'electrocardiogram', which measured the electrical output of the heart. So, in 1958, he built the 'electro-encephalogram', which tested the output from the brain. Both of these machines were immediately useful in diagnosis and they are still important aids today.

Many dedicated researchers have been involved in bringing up to date the knowledge we need to understand the part played by the mind in every physiological function—including healing. Prominent in studying and reporting this work, both in scientific journals and to the public through paperback books, have been such astute researchers as Barbara Brown with Biofeedback, Joseph Kamiya, Elmer Green, Herbert Benson, José Silva and many, many others.

Dr Ainslie Meares, an Australian psychiatrist, was one of the pioneers in teaching people how to heal themselves. His most famous pupil was a veterinarian, Dr Ian Gawler, who recovered from the terminal stage of osteogenic sarcoma with the aid of prolonged meditation, the Gerson diet and psychic healing. Even so, Ainslie Meares was persecuted in Australia. When I attended his sessions in Melbourne in 1985, he had resigned from the AMA in disgust after his colleagues had boycotted him, persistently ridiculed his ideas on psychiatric practice and rejected the incontrovertible results of a lifetime's work as false. Though he died in 1987, attacks on his work are still published in the *Australian Medical Journal*. Such is the threat to established cancer therapies of self-induced healing.

Another great leap forward was made by Dr Carl Simonton and Stephanie Matthews Simonton, whose classical work at Fort Worth,

Texas, and in Arkansas still continues. Carl Simonton MD was a US Air Force radiotherapist who found that some of the terminally ill patients he treated were suffering more, emotionally, from the fear of dying than from the disease itself. He worked with his wife Stephanie Matthews, a psychotherapist, to give them a happier self-image and instil vivid pictures in their minds of the immune system destroying the cancer. It worked. The method they devised and applied resulted in remissions of cancer for up to 10 per cent of the terminally ill people who could work up the motivation to undertake the program. Not only did cancers go into remission, they said, but for those not able to recover, pain was relieved and the dying process became a peaceful, dignified experience.

Reading their book *Getting Well Again* was an inspiration to me in 1982 when I was feeling very guilty because I could not help my cousin through her fatal illness. Once I resolved to use visualisation in my own program, I learned to make up my own words and pictures in the guided meditations I use for my patients. They have found this most useful and satisfying because it brings *peace of mind*—one of the main ingredients in healing. *Getting Well Again* is part of the reading I recommend.

We are born with life energy and survival emotions

We are born with fear and anger. These are the survival emotions. If we were not fearful and angry at the forces acting on us in our passage down the birth canal, we would not take our first great cry to expand the lungs on entering the world. In fact, babies born by caesarean section have to be stimulated to breathe. That stimulus used to be slapping and pinching before newer techniques were used. Fear and anger are the 'flight or fight' emotions that give the message to the adrenal glands to make their hormones to change the tempo of the body.

We are also born with certain *needs* which help us to regulate these two possibly negative emotions. The need to love, the need to be loved and the need to please are very strong, too, in little children. Guiding and shaping those needs are the most basic parental

Say: | *I see the good in you.*

responsibilities, just as important as providing food and shelter for the young. It doesn't always happen unfortunately.

Families that fight, families that fear

'The child maketh the man', we are told in the Bible. Patterns of personal behaviour learnt in very early years determine to a great extent the way we manage our lives and our health. But it is often the behaviour of dominant members of our family circle who have the greatest influence on us. In one way or another the rest of the family must either accept, fight, manipulate, escape from or ignore the behaviour of the dominant person among them.

Some families are dominated by a father or mother who grew up in the milieu of financial insecurity during the Great Depression. Often unfounded fears of poverty and deprivation haunt their children, who have taken on parental attitudes at an age when they were too young to reason.

Another family attitude of fear that is seemingly impossible to shake off is the fear of cancer, and the belief that goes with it that death is cancer's inevitable outcome. Even the word will not be said aloud in some Mediterranean households, for fear of attracting the dread disease. The belief is that *'No one recovers from the Big C'*!

There are also families in which the dominating influence, from one or both parents, grandparents or others, is one of stoical determination. To discount all obstacles, to show no emotion, to deny any failure—these were ruling virtues in Victorian English society. This belief is: *'I'm going to beat this thing if it kills me'*!

You will recognise many different coping patterns if you look around you. There are households where everything is external and superficial, for example. Problems are a joke to be treated with laughter and ribaldry such as, *'Come on, Tragedy Queen, give us a smile!'*

In some angry and aggressive families, where squabbling is the rule, everyone marches around demanding action and someone to blame: *'You brought it all on yourself, you're to blame!'*

All are ways of trying to manage a difficult situation of change. In each of these examples the cancer patient may suffer. The assessment and treatment of the patient may be refused, or at least delayed, hindered by attitudes learnt so long ago that they are unrecognised.

The patient should be helped to understand these patterns—if he or she hasn't worked out solutions and told you about them. Otherwise patients may become depressed and anxious about the effects their illness is having on the family.

An astute and trusted counsellor may do much towards clearing the way so that the patient will be able to cope with family attitudes and make better autonomous decisions. We need more counsellors.

There are many lecturers now travelling round the world running seminars on self-awareness, self-parenting, overcoming early childhood trauma, raising self-confidence and self-esteem. These workshops can open the door of understanding to give us the first glimpses of the best path to follow. There are also many books on family dynamics and relationships. One seminar is not enough, an ongoing group or therapist is better. In Brisbane Kharmine Feez has developed a series of seminars and workshops, starting with 'Who Am I', of three days duration, going on to 'Being', for one week, and 'Soul' for two weeks. The aim of her program is to draw a person with low self-esteem into her circle of security, closeness, compassion and understanding by a series of spiritually based exercises and disciplines. It is a creative experience. I have seen some heart-warming changes in people who needed help resulting from this course.

Case comment: Jack and Jill

Occasionally, when one member of a close couple is desperately ill, the other is completely unable to accept the situation. Denial that there is anything serious wrong can make nursing and tending the sick person very difficult indeed. I think of the very sad situation of a couple I shall call Jack and Jill, who came from very different family backgrounds. They were not youngsters and Jack was an architect and Jill a part-time bookkeeper employed by the same firm for years. They were both inveterate seminar attenders and

Say: *I look beyond outward appearance.*

met at their church seminar on improving relationships. Both had been through divorces that left mountains of resentment and lack of trust in their wake. They decided to live together because there were deep psychological problems they thought they could help each other to solve. Physically their relationship was wildly successful but subconsciously it was based on the fascination of endless and fruitless analysis of feelings, with a strong element of sparring for control and emotional advantage.

They both saw their friendship as a challenge and a chance of happiness. At last they had found each other, they were soul mates! In spite of frequent wrangles, it seemed a satisfactory, if not ideal, situation to outsiders.

Jack, who had been marking time for some years in his business, was now moving ahead, advertising and drawing new plans for houses he wanted to build. He was poised ready to succeed. Jill was doing her part-time work in her usual efficient manner. Though they were not young, Jill was keen to start a family. They discussed the reversal of Jack's sterilising operation. Jack had an adult family, Jill had no children.

It was about this time that he started to lose weight and feel weak and ill. He developed a troublesome cough and a hoarse voice. At first he thought he was just smoking too much but when he coughed blood, his GP and then his specialist sent him to have a series of whirlwind tests. Within a week he was diagnosed as having a large cancerous area in one lung, with massive lymph node involvement very near the heart.

It was completely inoperable, the surgeons said, and moreover, radium would not help either. He was doomed. Jack refused the palliative chemotherapy offered, telling me that he and Jill had decided to fight the cancer and that he was about to heal himself with his mind. Positive thinking will do it, Jill said.

There is a great difference between positive thinking and denial. Jill could not accept that her newfound love and protector was desperately ill. She came to me to deliver long tirades against his thoughtlessness in shirking his household chores and not getting out of bed at his usual early hour. He was being lazy and not trying, she said. He shouted in anger when she cried and pleaded with him to pull his socks up and make an effort. She took it as a personal affront when he was too tired to take her out and when he complained that the food tasted bad. I explained what was happening to Jack:

that he just couldn't eat when he had no appetite, that the mass in his chest was pressing his food pipe, that the cancer toxins were flooding his body, that his cells were not getting enough oxygen so they were reacting differently, that the large, fast-growing mass in his lung was eating into the tissue and arteries could easily bleed if he exerted himself. She said she could hear what I said but she just didn't want to know all that.

Jill had been brought up in a family of fault-finding brothers in which sickness was considered to be a weakness. Jack's inability to perform with his usual energy raised her anger and resentment, not her tenderness and compassion. She felt unable to fetch and carry for him unless he could do the same for her. It had always been like that in her blaming, competitive, masculine family. She took up her job full time and paid a woman to come in to make his juices because she couldn't bear to be near him. She accused him of not loving her and not wanting to get well. He accused her of causing his cancer by her critical, perfectionist attitudes and aggressive, demanding tone of voice.

After his first haemorrhage he had several blood transfusions, but he would not stay in hospital, even though he knew that the constant squabbling at home exhausted him. He was back in the love nest, where both partners went on demanding the nurture and acceptance of each other that neither could really give. After the second, near-fatal haemorrhage, though they both remonstrated, I insisted that he stayed in hospital. The helper had left. He needed nursing care desperately. Jill did not want him to stay in hospital, even though she could not look after him. I explained to her that his breathing was better when he could get oxygen and that she might come home from work one day and find him comatose or dead in bed. She burst into tears, and accused me of being negative. 'You just can't let him die, I need him,' she said.

I was not being negative, just realistic. Because I could not offer her a cure and he could not follow the survival plan she was convinced I had given him up to die by suggesting to her that he should stay in hospital. She was telling me it was my fault; she had to have someone to blame.

In fact it was only in hospital that he gained respite from gnawing

Say: *I see the beauty within you and me.*

anxiety and finally found a tranquility without pain for the last journey.

What is your attitude of mind about healing?

What is your attitude of mind about healing? 'Self-induced healing', Solzhenitzen calls it. The attitude of mind is all important. To desire and to believe that '*I am making the choice to change my life*'— this succeeds, not 'Pity me, a poor victim.

So many people find that it is easier to rely only on an operation. The mind is there saying, 'I am helpless. *You* fix me. *You* have the skill. It is *your* responsibility. You change my body for me. I'm putting all my hope and trust in *you*'.

We are not taught to take responsibility because that means we 'take the blame'. Blame and criticism may block potential in life. Attitudes are changing, however. We are moving towards love and affection instead, which allows us to express the best in us. Learning and teaching should be based on love and a positive attitude, not on fear and punishment of failure. This is hardly a 'New Age' concept—it is all in the teaching of the Bible, the Vedas and Upanishads.

We are not just physical bodies. The body is our shell, but we are *much more*. We are not our behaviour either, since behaviour can change if we want it to. It is my job to help people realise this and to encourage them to do it. To encourage motivation in others reinforces my own strengths. However, it takes time, love, encouragement and dedication on my part and on theirs. It is my reward to see it happen and to see a person grow in self and vitality. I play just a small part in the transformation. The person may not survive, the body may die. But this is not the important part. We will all die.

Life force

The Life Force (Chi, Ka, Prahna) is recognised and heeded in most enlightened cultures of the world. It is not just energy; it is the part of us that *enjoys*. It is the love, the affection, the perseverance, the hope and the kindness which is inherent in us all. To lose it is to lose the will to live.

It is not only a measure of success for a person to survive physically, it is also a matter of growing in spirit, love and understanding, becoming close to God, the Source, or whatever you call that universal energy which is part of each one of us and of which we are all a part. It is the force that made the stars and the ants, the ripples on the water and the light in the sky, every leaf factory, every part of animal life, the sunset and the first smile on a baby's lips. Because we can see and recognise the light and beauty of dawn we can also know the darkness of night. Two sides—always the dichotomy.

For so long, many dwell in the darkness, the negative, the strife and the fighting. If the world as we know it is to survive, we must turn to the light, the positive, to love and happiness. Here is the opportunity to see that light.

Relax for better health

Relaxation, which is normally a natural part of each day, is very difficult for some people to attain in our fast-moving world. The left side of their brain overworks, which stimulates the adrenal glands to make too much of the 'go-go' hormones too constantly. This overproduction can lead to high blood pressure, gastric ulcers, migraine and other stress-related illnesses. The right side of the brain is the monitor for relaxation, and the two sides should work in conjunction. Often the left overrules the right. We must learn how to turn on the right, relaxation side.

From the electro-encephalogram, which measures the electrical output of the brain, we know that when we relax the brain has slower waves of electricity, called alpha rhythms. Here is what you do to get the pleasant and normal state of alpha, to calm your mind, settle your adrenal glands and enjoy better health. (Remember, there are no hard and fast rules. Relaxation is a natural state and everyone can do it. There are no failures; you just have to find out what method suits you best.

1 Find a comfortable position in a place where you will not be disturbed. Unplug the telephone and put the pets and children outside. If you wear spectacles, take them off, uncross arms and legs, keep your back straight. Lie on the floor, if you wish, or sit in a chair.

Say: *I choose to bring out my best.*

2. Close your eyes to keep out unwanted stimulation.

3. Take a deep breath, counting to three in your mind as you breathe in. You can say 'I am' to yourself as you inhale if you like. Let our your breath slowly, counting to nine, and think to yourself 'relaxing', as you exhale.

   Do this three times or more, thinking only of your breathing; cut out all other thoughts. If thoughts intrude, just let them float on through. Do not hang on to them and let them distract you.

4. Now let your muscles relax. Some folk can do this very easily and quickly, while others are so tense that they need to 'teach' the muscles what relaxation feels like. So, clench your fists very, very hard as you count to three. Then let them go and say to yourself, 'completely relax'. Close your eyes very, very tightly as you count to three, then let those little muscles round the eyes relax as you say to yourself 'easily relax'.

   Now consciously let all the tension go out of your body and say to yourself, 'naturally relax'.

5. Now put yourself, in your mind's eye, into your favourite place, special to yourself, and make it a place where you can feel peaceful, serene, safe and happy. Maybe it is some place you know, a bit of bush, a creek, a beach, your garden, or somewhere you make up in your imagination.

6. Let your senses expand there, notice every detail, notice the scents and the sounds and the crisp, clean air. Take a few moments to enjoy it.

   By the time you have concentrated on this pleasant scene for one or two minutes, you will be in your alpha level and you can use this level for any good purpose you want. Just going to this level for 10 to 20 minutes every day does give you physical and mental benefits—you will become kinder, more tolerant, more confident and more understanding of yourself and others.

7. If you have any positive messages to say to yourself, now is the time when your body and mind is in the most receptive and accepting state to incorporate them. Your body later acts successfully on the messages you give now. These affirmations or suggestions for health and encouragement can be very powerful in helping you undo any old negative habits you want to change.

8 Make a goal for yourself or a step to follow. Picture yourself in your imagination as having *reached* your goal and see yourself enjoying the successful outcome. Take time to enjoy this.

9 Now recognise this peaceful, comfortable feeling. Resolve to keep it with you. Count to five slowly, knowing that when you reach five you will open your eyes feeling relaxed, refreshed, alert and happy.

To reach your goal, you need about 3 to 6 weeks of regular, daily reinforcement with this relaxation and visualisation.

Thinking in pictures: teach your body to do your mind's bidding

Fairy-tale themes are revealing. They contain clues for future generations on deep and basic matters of the human soul, as well as details for overcoming practical problems.

One of the recurrent themes in ill health is the often subconscious belief that it is linked with evil doing; that it is somehow a punishment meted out by unseen forces, that it is the result of impure thoughts or excesses.

This is mirrored today in the subtle conversion to blaming impure food, air and water, so shifting the emphasis to forces outside the body over which, because we were ignorant of them, we had no control. We were therefore innocent victims (see 'Stop blaming the victim' on page 78).

Going deeper, these attitudes are usually based on feelings and emotions that pattern our reactions to life from a very early age, when we were too young to think out cause and effect, probably before the age of five. At this age, we make these patterns not by intellect but by observing what behaviour gives us approval or disapproval—from our loved ones, our parents, our brothers and sisters and the significant people around us.

We need the emotions of *anger* and *fear* for the physical body to survive in the world. But though we are expected to express these emotions freely when we are very young, we are also expected

Say: | *I feel comfortable with people.* |

to learn to control them as we grow older, so that they will not embarrass those around us.

We learn to desensitise ourselves to sudden changes of emotion by using our intelligence to understand cause and effect so that we become more tolerant.

I remember that my older son was particularly curious and inquisitive as a baby, but unexplained noises terrified him. As an infant he cried every time I turned the vacuum cleaner on or flushed the toilet. But by two years old, when we had helped him to understand the source of these noises, he had to be firmly dissuaded from repeatedly pressing the pedals to keep on making the noise. Having learnt to control his fear, he wanted to go on repeating the feeling of satisfaction and power that it gave him.

When we can't gauge cause and effect, fear may remain as an undercurrent in the way we behave. Patterns persist. The person who is afraid of doctors, because of an unpleasant childhood experience, may put off seeking advice about a condition until it is far too advanced to treat successfully. Unexpressed fears and angers are so often converted to physical ill health.

Anger at having physical discomfort and unmet needs usually causes crying in a baby and tantrums in a three year old. As long as there is no secondary gain to encourage the continuation of this behaviour, it eventually finds its expression in more useful strategies. We grow out of bad habits if they don't work. But anger that is suppressed can lead to many physical problems, even to cancer.

The situations that drain the body, mind and spirit most potently are those that have no solution: the frustration of feeling helpless, unloved, unfairly treated, hopeless and powerless, is the worst.

We cannot live without stress, it is part of our make up; but stresses in life can be cumulative. There is usually a compromise between the mechanisms we have learned to cope with different stressful situations—which can then become exciting challenges—and those we learn to bury and not express. The latter may often do no harm at all, but sometimes they may contribute to such ill health as stomach ulcers, arthritis, high blood pressure, cancer and many more.

Usually, because its expression has caused us pain in the past, we learn hidden ways of dealing with unpleasant emotions. For example, we are taught not to show anger openly so we do it in many subtle expressions that point to the part of the body where conversion may take place. 'He makes me sick', 'She's a pain in the neck', 'What are you griping about?', 'You give me a pain', 'He makes me blow my top', 'A spineless creature', 'Stiff upper lip', 'A sight for sore eyes'—there are so many common sayings that suggest the self-image. The mind works continuously in the waking hours. It gives us thousands of messages every minute. Most of them are not recorded consciously; the body receives them through the autonomic nervous system and reacts automatically. These are the ongoing systemic actions such as the heart beating, the lungs breathing, the stomach digesting and so on. The somatic nervous system records environmental influences and allows us to change the pace of these so that other hormones can take over to stimulate voluntary action. The different parts of the nervous system are integrally related, working together in harmony with the brain.

But it is the mind that gives the voluntary messages and it is the mind that is controlled by thoughts. The thoughts give the messages in words and pictures. We 'think' of them in words and pictures that effect our emotions and our subsequent actions and reactions. There are many sayings that have recorded this through history. The most famous is from the Bible: 'As a man thinketh in his heart, so is he'.

Sad thoughts make a sad person, fearful thoughts a fearful person, angry thoughts an angry person. These are truisms but it has only recently been proved that *what we think has a direct effect on the immune system. Thinking happy thoughts boosts it up, fearful and angry thoughts paralyse it.*

The pictures you give yourself help you to heal. Visualising a successful outcome helps you to succeed. Words and pictures are tools we are given in our physiology—let us learn to use them to the full!

Chris: Case comment

In your visualisation of the immune system eliminating cancer, it is essential to finish the confrontation by seeing yourself return to

Say: | *Anger is a waste of energy.*

your healthy state. You must *dispose* of the cancer cells so that they are not left in the body. They can be carried out and away by any means you can imagine. Make sure you make up the scene of your being *healed* to your satisfaction.

Chris, who had cancerous fluid in her pelvis after uterine cancer was removed, came to see me after some months absence. She said she was a little fearful of visualising because she felt it had been responsible for a new metastasis. She told me that she had previously visualised the cancerous fluid coming up out of the pelvis like a gush of oil from a well. In her visualisation she had removed it completely from the original site but she hadn't disposed of it. A large tumor developed under the skin in the midline at the base of the chest. It was irradiated by her radio therapist but it did not reduce in size until she resumed visualisation and tamed the oil gush by rolling the product out of the body in barrels from the depot under the skin. What you see symbolises what you get!

Affirmations

The words we say and the positive word messages we give ourselves are responsible for our successes also. One of the first pioneers in the field of slogans to help keep the mind and body healthy was a Frenchman name Emile Coué. In the time of the great depression of the late 1920s, these two famous slogans of his kept many desperate people from committing suicide. 'Every day and every way things get better and better' and, 'I am the captain of my soul, I am the master of my fate'.

Lawrence Le Shan was another pioneer in this field who observed the differences that personality and attitude can make to healing (see bibliography). What you *say* can change your life!

We now call these positive messages 'affirmations'. I recommend that they are said, sung, hummed, shouted or just thought in the head as many times as possible during the day and night—with feeling and thought. You could concentrate on one for a day. Here are a few I use and there are more on every second page of this book. Say them!

> I make a choice to live.
> I make enjoyment a priority in my life.
> I release all fear by gaining knowledge.

I focus my mind on my healthy self with confidence.
I accept that there is much I can do to help myself to feel better and I do it.
I feel proud about my own self and the way I manage things.
I forgive myself and others for any nastiness of the past.
I reject negative thoughts.
I know that my spirit is free; it never dies.
I am an excellent survivor.

To gain the most useful and strongest effect on the body, mind and spirit, it is best when saying these to use the alpha or theta levels of awareness. These are the natural levels of electrical output the brain uses in childhood. As adults we use them for relaxation. We go in and out of alpha and beta all day long. In alpha level the mind, particularly the right brain, is more receptive to words and pictures. Follow the method discussed on page 90 any time at all when you have fifteen minutes to yourself but, for healing, use the pictures listed below.

- Close you eyes and sit quietly, breathing and relaxing, for two minutes. Then imagine or visualise your problem area in any way you like, symbolically.
- See the treatment you are having, or have had, first breaking up any pain, then strengthening the defences, destroying or chasing out the cancer.
- Now see your immune system cells as big, active, powerful and strong; scouting round the body and finding the trouble spots and healing them. Mopping up any debris, leaving the place clear and clean.
- Now see yourself really healthy and well, congratulating yourself for succeeding against all odds. See yourself getting the prize or the medal for good healing; feel exhilarated; know you are winning.
- Now set a little goal for the rest of this day—something you know you can do and want to do.
- Give yourself a pat on the back for the good things you have already done or thought today.

Say: *Fear paralyses; love releases.*

- Determine to keep that peaceful feeling with you.
- Slowly come back to beta, counting to five. Open your eyes.

A few points about visualising. Some people can only see clearly what they are interested in. We all visualise without realising it all the time. You may only see colours or a fleeting image—it doesn't matter. The *thought* will have the same effect as the picture.

Don't expect to have the same symbols each time, although you may have favourites, of course. Some times are better than others, too. It's hard to manage if you are very tired—you go straight to 'theta', which is sleep. Try to make your symbols *active*, a broom sweeping, water washing, etc. *Expect* to succeed; don't think negative thoughts; think some affirmations, if you like, as the symbols do their work. All the people in our group like to draw what they see. Do it—it is fascinating. You don't have to be an artist. Imagine the cancer as weak and easily removed or overcome. Use colour in your thoughts—bold, strong colours for the immune system and paler, weak colours for the cancer.

Open eye meditation on colour

Shirley McLaine has made a very beautiful video called 'Inner Work Out' for meditating with the eyes open. The colour changes are magnificent. See it if you can.

You can find a picture or a design that appeals to you through its colours, and concentrate in a relaxed state just on one part of that visual image. Some use a candle flame or a 'mandala', a picture of Christ, the cross or some other symbol. Ten to twenty minutes of stillness with the colour in mind can give you a deep sense of safety and peace. Some mandalas are shown on the colour pages.

Interpretation of drawings

Though the spirit rules, the mind communicates our thoughts and feelings to us in many ways. The mind 'speaks' to us in words, and when the chatter of every day is lulled away by relaxation or light meditation, communication over a given topic comes easily. The body and mind are in contact all the time, but unless we are in tune we don't heed the messages.

New patients with cancer go through a guided meditation with me so that I can introduce them to communication with their cancer and their immune system.

Then they draw in colour the messages they have received about the control that the immune system has over the cancer. All I ask them to do is to choose two or three colours, make the cancer weak and the immune system strong, and show in their own terms the cancer being overcome.

Eight pictures taken at random from some of the hundreds of files which contain a drawing are shown on the colour pages.

Say: *I speak and act with love.*

9 REVIVING THE SPIRIT

I do not merely want to possess a faith; I want a faith that possesses me.

Confidence and self-esteem

I have found books published by Unity Church of Denver, Colorado, most helpful in times of trouble. *Positive Thoughts for Successful Living* by Jim Lewis for example, is full of wisdom in a simply written, flowing style that calms anxiety and restores confidence. I particularly like this part from a little chapter entitled 'Developing Spiritual Confidence':

> You are more than just a human being limited by your genetic make-up and your environmental and educational influence. In Truth, in Reality, you are a spiritual being endowed with unlimited potential and possibilities. This is true regardless of what your present situation may seem to be. Establishing this truth in your consciousness will make you feel confident, for you will feel that you are worth something after all.
>
> You have far greater capacities than you have ever realised. You will have to believe this regardless of what appearances seem to indicate. If you accept your limitations, you will have to live with them and be miserable and unhappy. If you accept the truth about yourself, then you can rise above your limitations and have the happy, successful, healthy life you should have.

You may think what he says is self-evident; I didn't really believe it for many years. When I was a child it was considered conceited and wicked to love yourself. 'Self-praise is no recommendation'; 'know your place'; 'don't be a big head', 'show off' or a 'smart alec'. These were all put downs that kept children from being assertive. I was a timid and self-effacing child.

I had always been interested in God and me. My elder sister was my closest and most constant companion when we were children. We discussed who God was, obviously different from little baby Jesus, who was very believable and real to children in a large family. Sitting on the back steps of our home one early morning I was sure I could see God in a pink cloud hiding behind some dark ones in the sky. That was as abstract as I could be at four years old.

We didn't go to Sunday School but we enjoyed the Band of Hope concerts at the beach on Christmas holidays, where we were given holy pictures and other little signs of being good children loved by God.

Although I was educated at church schools I could not believe that we were born sinners so I would never sing that part of the hymns that said we were helpless and foul creatures.

When I was fifteen I became very interested in the questions that philosophers raised about religion. I read a large part of the Bible and also about the Buddha. Much later I read the teachings of Gurdjieff, Teillard de Chardin and Satya Sai Baba. I didn't study these as a zealot, but concentrated only on where I disagreed or what enthralled me as a fascinating new thought. So it was also with the dozens of other works of the mind that have occupied me long before de Bono's textbooks on how to think became popular as tools for self-education.

I am very grateful to those many authors for the tolerance and understanding I developed with book learning. With the life lessons gained in our competitive family they helped me to overcome the many setbacks I have had in my life. But there was always that 'I'm not OK' feeling which Tom Harris talks about* and Jim Lewis calls lack of spiritual confidence.*

I had used hypnosis successfully in my work. I had been to a term of Transcendental Meditation and I had recovered from a period

---

* Thomas Harris, *I'm OK, You're OK*, Pan Books, London, 1979.
Jim Lewis, *Positive Thoughts for Successful Living*, Unity Church, Denver, 1979.

Say: *Patience reflects my comfort within.*

of a reactive depression after my marriage broke up, but I had always resisted the urge to go to self-awareness classes because of shyness and inability to discuss personal matters with anyone.

Then, because of my success in building the sun-powered Eukey complex, I was often asked to speak at functions where alternative power and building methods were being discussed. In August 1981 I spoke at the 'One Earth Gathering', put on at Queensland University by Lionel Fifield and the Relaxation Centre of Queensland team. Lionel gave me a complimentary ticket to Bert Weir's 'Centre Within' course, as he did to all speakers.

The synchronicity of the events that lead up to that were very obvious to me, so I went. That weekend was the beginning of a transformation for me. The scales fell from my eyes and I realised that I *was* an 'OK' person after all. There was a lot of work to be done to keep believing that. Negativity kept creeping back in whenever I stopped the meditation (personal prayer) techniques that I was learning to make an intrinsic part of my life.

The affirmations at the foot of these pages are some of the messages I have found helpful over the years. You may too. Amuse yourself by making up your own.

A wide range of authors, tapes, workshops and lectures are available for you too. I have been back to the Centre Within and to the personal growth courses many times, not only at the Relaxation Centre of Queensland but with José Silva, William Glasser and others.

For all those years I was searching for faith outside myself, when what I was trying to prove was that I had faith in myself. 'Don't sell yourself short, conquer the crime of self-depreciation, concentrate on your assets', says David Schwartz in *The Magic of Thinking Big*. Listening to and concentrating on what God tells you inside is the invigorating factor, not listening to that negative voice that magnifies the fears of rejection by others.

It was after one such deeply meditative program that I had a revelation, a profound experience during and after a retreat. I made my commitment then to do this work. The decision did not seem to be mine alone; I knew I was led and that realisation made me very very happy.

Try it for yourself. *Know* that your spirit is perfect and that it will never die. *You* are not your behaviour. *You* can change your behaviour and your habits if you don't like them. *You* can shape your own reality, make a life that suits you, even if you are not physically well at the moment. It may be difficult but, with the bright goal of what you want life to be ahead of you, you can make it. What you think is what you get.

The spirit rules

The mind does the spirit's bidding, through words and pictures, only in the way you have taught it how. If the mind needs new tools, find them through meditation and prayer. Learn to use them by practice. *You can change your life.*

Your body does the bidding of the mind. It has been taking the brunt of everything that is heaped on it, not only from within but also from the environment. It may be a big task, but God is with you. Homeostasis—or the urge to return to the normal and the perfect—is part of God's law. All you need to start is faith and belief in yourself. God made you perfect. Emerge from your chrysalis! Let the good part of your body win! Make the shining new body you are growing overcome any problems, see the colours of your beautiful wings that allow the dreams of your spirit to soar!

Quality of Life Support Group

Pam, from our Quality of Life Support Group, wrote the following for you to describe how her faith and belief have helped her to manage what was a very large cancer of the lung.

> Recently I had occasion to visit my oncologist who told me he got a shock to see my name in the appointment book. My reply was, 'Please explain'. He proceeded to tell me he thought I would have been long gone. (In August 1990 he had wanted to fit me with an implant and feed the chemotherapy into my body over a two-year period. I declined and, very shortly afterwards, was seen by Dr R.)
>
> The oncologist asked me what I was doing and I replied, 'I have managed thus far by embracing these three factors in my life: God, Dr R. and myself.'
>
> There is a tremendous amount of work to be done by the

Say: | *My inner self rejoices.* |

patient and for me it works. Stress only hastens the disease so avoid it at all costs. Care for yourself. Maybe this will be a new skill you will have to acquire. Diet and meditation are vital to my recovery. God is a loving father and wouldn't yours want you to be well again? Of course he would! Trust in Him!

Bill Jackson describes in his own words how he has conquered two potentially lethal forms of cancer of the lung and the brain.

I have approached my cancers as a challenge. Although initially I was afraid, these feelings have gradually lessened as I have got to know more about my cancers.

I don't see myself as anything extraordinary, having the same foibles as most people. Aspects of my personality are stubbornness at my worst, but fierce determination at my best.

I believe in the regime that my doctor has put me on, it makes common sense. It has been working for me since January 1988. In addition I get along very well with my doctor and I like to think that my ongoing treatment is a team effort.

I have an offbeat sense of humour: I enjoy telling jokes, especially one liners, and quips and making people laugh. This comes from my childhood and used to take the pressure off myself. These days I still use it to lighten my load.

I was single-minded, I even had tunnel vision initially about my problem, eliminating as much stress as possible and meditating. It does not work for me all the time but I keep going.

If any one asked me for advice about cancer I would say: Find out all you can about treatment and medication. Read books about the subject. Ask questions and when more come to mind, keep asking. It gives me a sense of satisfaction to know that I am in charge of my life.

Nobody has all the answers and we have all got to go sometime, but I don't want to leave without feeling I have given it my informed best shot. Lastly I find it very difficult to give up life, and it is probable that this, amongst lots of other things that I do, is why I am well after initial problems in July 1987.

Rosa Di Francesco has written to encourage others who have cancer. Without any treatment except the original operation, she overcame cancer of the ovary that had spread to her lungs. Here she describes how she did it.

I felt so privileged when asked to share my experiences about healing my body. The most important factor that helped me through my illness was my faith in the Lord, knowing that what He had to offer was all loving, caring and positive, not negative as I had previously thought.

Through prayers I was guided to ring Dr R., who encouraged me to meditate—eliminate stress, eat sensibly and most of all to continue on with a positive, loving, caring and forgiving attitude.

I had to change my lifestyle in accepting things which I could not accept before. I also found acceptance a key factor.

Having a suporting husband and very caring family and friends has also helped me.

I don't allow any of my thoughts to dwell on the past. I was grateful that what happened was a learning experience for me and felt that we are all human and nobody is perfect. Having to forgive myself and release myself from guilt, fear and anxiety was also important as it removed any blockages I may have had.

I continue on praising and thanking the Lord for all the things he has given me, especially at the weakest moment in my life.

Say: *Pain is going, going and will soon be gone.*

Part Three

ON THE TRAIL OF DISCOVERY

10 TAKING THE ROAD TO AMERICA

Making a film of the blood

In 1986 I was asked to write a chapter concerning my work with cancer groups for a book called *Victory Over Cancer*, by Leonie McNabb and Alan Ryan. Another participant in this publication was Dr John C.A. Dique MB, BS, FRCPA.

I knew Dr Dique when I was a student in 1945 and in February 1987 I met him again because of this book. Dr Dique, who was a leading pathologist in Brisbane for many years, is now retired. He was one of the first pathologists to recognise the lethal Rh antibody reaction which killed so many babies in utero or neonatally before it was understood.

Dr Dique came to Australia in the early 1940s from Goa, on the west coast of India, as a young research pathologist. His research was at the Brisbane Women's Hospital, where his particular expertise was with mothers and babies with Rh incompatibility. He trained himself in the extremely delicate task of venepuncture (intravenous therapy) of the new-born. He was the first expert in the world to save children who would otherwise have died, by complete exchange transfusion of their blood with compatible blood, often from the father. He received world acclaim for his work in this field. He also ran the Pathology Department of the Mater Hospital for many years with great energy and success.

Dr Dique was very interested in the research of Dr Virginia Livingston in the USA and had heard that I had visited her clinic, so he asked if I would like to present a paper at the Mater Clinical Week in September 1987, to introduce Brisbane pathologists to an organism, now called 'Progenitor cryptocides', that was her particular interest and which I had been studying in the blood of cancer patients.

We discussed the format of such a paper and, since I had an

excellent microscope with good resolution in the dark field, I suggested that I should make a film of the Progenitor cryptocides organism in human blood.

With the disappointing experience of the previous poorly attended lectures I had given to my colleagues on the subject, I thought that a visual presentation of the organism's life history might stimulate their interest more than a wordy lecture. So I proceeded to contact people at the Clinical Sciences and Pathology sections of the Royal Brisbane Hospital who could help me with their knowledge of video microphotography.

Since I did not have a Government grant or any higher degrees in bacteriology, my requests for aid in that section were refused. However, with the help of other friendly experts, I finally received a reply to my letters asking for assistance from the Queensland University Audiovisual Department. The directors of this section agreed to help me technically to make a film of the blood, which was finally finished in May 1987.

Since I had no credentials in bacteriology, it was useless for me to describe in my own words the intricacies of the lifestyle of the progenitor cryptocides. I went back to the symposia and many research papers on this organism in the compendium collected by Dr Virginia Livingston and her late husband, Dr Afton Livingston. The first part of the film was a precis of excerpts from their work and the research of Doctor Irene Corey Diller.

I used fresh blood from a patient with metastatic cancer of the prostate as a basis for the demonstration of the cancer organism, and fresh blood from the staff of the Audio-Visual Department to show the common harmless forms that occur in healthy people.

Knowing that I would need to quote Dr Virginia's writing in this film, I telephoned her and confirmed that she would have to see the finished product before giving me permission to use her words.

My mother was most interested in the work I was doing, and even though she was in poor health and in the process of publishing her last book, *My Life*, she insisted on going through the transcript with me to make sure *she* approved also. Even though, at 93 years of age, she had recently undergone a cataract operation, she was able to see the film and encouraged me to continue with my plans to visit Dr Virginia again.

I was in some conflict about going away because she was not

in good health, but after seeing the film she gave me her blessing and insisted that I went. Taking my farewells on 3 July 1987, I was fated not to see her alive again. She died of a heart attack while I was in the air flying home on 26 July.

Since 1984, I had been a life member of the Cancer Control Society (CCS). It is a non-profit organisation based in Los Angeles, dedicated to the investigation of cancer, its causes and treatments. I had corresponded with the indefatigable secretary of the society, Lorraine Rosenthal, who runs the office from her own home and has a remarkable store of knowledge about old and new work in the field of cancer.

I had bought much of my reading matter on unorthodox and new methods of treatment through the catalogues and magazines she sent. It was through these magazines that I read of the work of Contreras, Gerson, Manner, Livingston and many other medical doctors. Every year a seminar is held at which the people who are doing new work may be asked to lecture on their methods and their outcomes. It is an open forum. A researcher is allowed to speak his or her mind and present results without fear or favour and without the prohibitions of Food and Drug Administration interference.

I had been yearning to go to one of these seminars to meet and hear the people whose work I had read. Now was my chance, since I had to go to the USA to show the film to Dr Livingston anyway.

The moving force behind the band of Cancer Control Society workers was the energetic naturopath and nutritionist Betty Lee Morales, who had a most successful health farm at Eden Ranch, outside Los Angeles. There she not only helped people to recover their health in the country atmosphere, but also made and distributed a huge range of natural supplements. She lectured widely and had been on the same platform as my mother, lecturing on nutrition at a seminar in Perth some years earlier. Mother knew her well and urged me to visit the ranch and pay my respects when I was over there. So I rang Lorraine and booked a room at the Hyatt Wilshire Royale, only a few blocks from the seminar venue at the famous Ambassador Hotel, Wilshire Boulevard.

Say: *It costs nothing to smile.*

The tedious flight through New Zealand and Honolulu, the long haul through customs and shuttle service in Los Angeles, all were swept into insignificance by the excitement of going to this seminar at last—so much to see, do and learn.

The Cancer Control Society annual convention

At the Royale I looked out of my window onto a blank wall—I could not even see the Los Angeles smog but I could hear the shots in the car park below and the sirens wailing in the night. Next morning, I started off up to the Ambassador, wondering how many of the people walking in the same direction were going to the same destination. Many were. We turned into the neat shrub-lined paths of the formal garden and marched into the grand entrance hall, famous in early films as the place where stars meet and romance begins. It was rather tired and dowdy now, like an old playboy resting on his laurels.

Past the shops and restaurants the tables for registration were crowded with hundreds of people. I bought tickets for everything! The lectures, the tapes, the banquet, the meeting of doctors after the main seminar and the bus tour of the Mexican clinics the day after—six days of excitement!

An extremely noisy sort of regulated mayhem took over until the big doors into the huge auditorium closed and the lectures started. All around the area, flanking the sea of chairs, were booths for the therapists and their staffs. The booths flowed out into courtyards and alcoves, and round into the main foyer. Workers on health food stalls were preparing their wares for the breaks: books, pamphlets, brochures, billboards and placards were everywhere.

The President, Norman Fritz, opened the Convention and I learned immediately that mother's friend, Betty Lee Morales, had died a week previously, in the midst of the preparations. It was to have been the grand celebration of her seventeenth year as President. Everyone was sad about her death, which had occurred, as far as I could gather, after a stroke. She had been a woman of great courage, foremost in the dispute of the right of ordinary citizens to *choose* the treatment they wished to receive. The main war she had waged was on the prohibition of laetrile—an extract of apricot kernels that had been used and investigated for years in Mexico but which was banned, on flimsy supporting evidence, by the Food and Drug Administration, in accordance with their policy of decrying anything except surgery, radiation and chemotherapy in the treatment of cancer.

Laetrile

This product, also known as B_{17}, amygdalin, benzaldehyde and by other names, was first studied by Dr Ernst Krebs and Dr John Beard in 1936. The 'trophoblast theory' hypothesises that immature foetal cells called trophoblasts are in our organs but stay more or less dormant unless stimulated to grow. The stimulus could be any type of stressor—carcinogenic substance or hormone imbalance. Thus formed, the cancer cells continue to grow, unattacked by the body's defence immune system because the cancer cell membrane has the ability to secrete a blocking agent, fibrin, which prevents the white cells from recognising it as an abnormal substance. The theory is, briefly, that trypsin, a digestive enzyme, dissolves this fibrin coat and allows amygdalin or other anti-cancer therapies to destroy the tumour cells.

There are plenty of inconsistencies in the hypothesis but the telling factor is whether the therapy worked or not.

It was usually, but not always, administered with lifestyle changes in diet and stress control so evaluation of the results of laetrile alone was impossible. Certainly some did recover and people continue to do so. Maybe those who recovered from their cancer did so because of factors other than the amygdalin. Who knows?

Betty Lee Morales amassed a mountain of information on laetrile and presented it to the congressional enquiry with great vigour. The cause she championed was of *the little persons's right to enquire*. By asking for information on the results of laetrile usage, the open forum brought into public view those brave therapists who had the real good of their patients at heart. Castigation, not approval and praise, was their reward.

In any case the battle that was waged was a political hot potato that led nowhere for laetrile—it is banned in the USA and in Australia. What the controversy engendered was a consolidation of the drug

Say: *I don't need pain; I let it go.*

firms' hold over permitted cancer therapy by a rash of new, harsher legislation. The doctors who did not toe the line were charged as criminals and many lost their licences to practice medicine in the 'land of the free'.

On her Eden Ranch Betty continued to teach people to use nutritional methods for obtaining the medication they needed. Her motto was 'the consumer has a right to know'.

The Gerson story

I knew that Dr Virginia Livingston would not be speaking and presenting her recovered patients until Saturday and would not be arriving until Friday, but Charlotte Gerson had already set up her display. I made my way to her booth in the first break to renew our friendship.

I had read the book *A Cancer Therapy: Results of Fifty Cases* by her father, Dr Max Gerson MD, in 1984. His philosophy and the results of his treatment impressed me so much that I visited the Mexican Clinic at La Gloria in 1984 so that I could see at first hand if the results were worthwhile and, if so, how to administer the treatment to the carefully selected patients of mine who might benefit from it.

On that first trip to the USA I had enormous trouble understanding and using the telephone systems which were all so different from Telecom Australia. After many fruitless attempts phoning the numbers of the Cancer Control Society's list, not understanding the sound signals, I finally telephoned an after-hours number late at night and Charlotte Gerson answered. It was like a door opening at last. She is such a kind and helpful lady, so dedicated to helping anyone who in genuinely interested in her father's therapy. While staying in San Diego at that time I went to La Gloria with Charlotte five times over two weeks and stayed there at the hospital for four days.

The building was a reconstructed former motel in attractively green grounds, so different from the surrounding country, which was dry with red-grey dust. It contained more than twenty-five rooms for patients, plus a guest wing with nine units. The doctors who ran the establishment were the brothers Ortuno, Dr Yolande Merenda and an American, Dr Rogers. Charlotte Gerson visited three times weekly to talk to patients and discuss their progress with the doctors.

I was allowed to sit in on these lectures and discussions if the patients gave their permission and by doing so I learned much.

The preparation of the Gerson food was particularly important and I welcomed the diet there at La Gloria. It was nutritious and tastefully prepared.

I found Charlotte Gerson to be an excellent teacher who expounded her father's principles with great enthusiasm and conviction. There were many successful results, which was surprising when you realise that every person with cancer went there diagnosed as 'terminally ill'.

One of the questions often asked at the Convention, and which I am asked repeatedly, is 'What is the success rate with your treatment?'

What an unanswerable question! There are more than 120 different types of cancer. Which one, of what type, at what stage of invasion, how treated, what prior treatment had been given, what motivation does the patient have to get well, what drugs are being taken from elsewhere, what age is the patient, and 'success' in what period of time are you envisaging? When all these questions are answered, then *maybe* a guarded guess at the possible recovery figure might be given. No two patients are the same, and cancer is unlike any other disease (see page 31, 'The Trouble with Statistics').

Nevertheless, every therapist in every cancer clinic I have visited seems to answer this question with, 'Oh, about 70 to 80 per cent success rate'. This means *nothing*. Success of what?

With the care, kindness, positive thinking, detoxification and diet that most people receive in most therapies in most of the clinics, I am sure 70 per cent or more will feel better very quickly and may think they are cured—even for the first six months. By that time they have gone home from the clinic, so that if regression takes place the clinic never hears about it. The majority of newspaper success stories have been given to the paper by the patient or family in that first flush of feeling so much better. *Sustained improvement* is the only real test.

What is so satisfying about the work of the Gerson Institute is

Say: | *Cheerfulness lightens every load.*

that recovered cases are followed faithfully year after year and *recorded* honestly, so that we have some real stories of success or failure.

The Gerson Institute is situated at Bonita, California, and is not a hospital. Its journal, *Healing,* is published annually by Gar Hildebrand, to keep subscribers up to date with the work of the institute and of cancer treatment generally.

Charlotte Gerson spoke on the Gerson Therapy developed by her father, Max Gerson, MD. She was born and had her early schooling in Germany. She left in 1933 and continued school in Austria, France and England, then attended Smith College after coming to New York. She helped translate her father's books and writings into English. She sometimes helped at Dr Gerson's clinics, attended his lectures, supervised nursing and joined him in making rounds and in discussing cases. As President of the Gerson Institute, she lectures widely and currently teaches physicians who operate the Gerson Therapy Hospital.

Dr Max Gerson is famous for his revolutionary healing therapy for cancer and other diseases presented in his book *A Cancer Therapy—Results of Fifty Cases.* Dr Albert Schweitzer called Dr Gerson 'one of medicine's most eminent geniuses'.

Charlotte made her usual impassioned and articulate presentation at the convention. She followed it by introducing fifteen people who had recovered for five years or much longer from 'incurable cancer' by using the Gerson Therapy. This was a most moving and dramatic presentation in which each person gave the story of recovery in simple and heart-warming terms. There was no subterfuge—it had been a hard-won struggle.

For my own part I have always chosen the people who could fulfil the strict criteria necessary for administration of this therapy most carefully. It is by no means easy.

So many come to me when they have been told 'there is nothing more that medical science can do'. That means that they are very sick indeed and have been given the 'go home and make your will' treatment. They are desperate and will try anything. I take it as a sacred duty to evaluate carefully every case and prescribe this difficult therapy *only* to those who may benefit from it.

You will notice that no less than four of the case histories of recovered terminally ill patients in this book had been using Gerson

Therapy for part of their treatment before they went onto the much simpler Cilento Survival Plan.

The Livingston Medical Clinic

In May 1987, when I phoned from Australia to tell Dr Virginia Livingston about the film, she had invited me to stay with her for a week in San Diego after the Cancer Control Society Convention. She had at that time a magnificent home overlooking Whalewatch bay at La Jolla. This was the culmination of the fortune she had made in her real estate interests, *not* in her medical work. The top floor, with its 180 degree expanse of picture windows and tasteful polished wood furniture, has been the venue for many famous dinner parties bringing together, as Dr Livingston likes to do, interesting people from all over the world who have contributed in any way to the increase of human knowledge, especially about cancer.

The second floor contained sitting rooms, a TV room, a huge library, an office, a private study and two generous guest suites. Every detail of convenience and elegance had been thoughtfully designed by Dr Livingston herself. Books are my passion, so to be housed so graciously on that floor and given permission to use the library was a great delight.

Dr Livingston's husband, Dr Owen Wheeler, was not at all well at this time, so she spent many hours each day tending him. They were very close in his illness—just as in the days when they first met and her vaccine helped him overcome the lymphoma that had nearly killed him then.

Every day I would go to the Immunology Clinic with Dr Livingston's secretary to learn as much as possible about the successful administration of her program. The helpful, warm and friendly people at the Clinic gave an atmosphere of confidence and healing, even though almost every patient I saw there was considered to be terminally ill. I renewed contact with the office, kitchen and nursing staff and with the laboratory team who make the precious autogenous vaccines from the patient's own organisms. These were the patient people who, in 1985, first identified the Progenitor

Say: | *A glad heart makes a cheerful countenance.* (Proverbs 15)

cryptocides organism for me, giving me several photographs of it in my own blood, taken under one of the big dark field microscopes. Now, two years later, I had gone on to study the organism myself.

One day I sat in with the new Medical Director, Dr Ken Forror, while he interviewed patients returning for check-ups and explained to those on their first visit the intricacies and expectations of the medical immunology program. He takes infinite care in his assessments, using compassion but firmness in pressing home the need to comply wholeheartedly with the diet, supplements and injections.

I was privileged to see one young lady who had been away from her vaccines for three years while travelling around doing seasonal work fruit picking. She returned because she wished to get married and wanted to know whether it was wise to have a baby. She had been told when she left the Clinic three years before that her cancer of the cervix was in remission. However, though the x-rays and scans were still clear, an examination of her blood showed some bad forms of the Progenitor cryptocides. So the doctor advised her to go back to her program strictly for three months before she repeated the test to make sure she was fit and healthy, and then to stay on it in a modified form *always*, to prevent recurrences. With a little planning and forethought, this is not a hard task and makes for a long and healthy life. The food at the Clinic is so healthy, tastefully prepared and reasonable that I would like to eat there all the time.

I also spent a day with a computer expert, Mr Mole, who introduced me to the Pennsylvania Quality of Life Scale and the database he was working out for Dr Livingston's research.

As for the Pennsylvania Inventory, which purports to investigate quality of life, I have never seen a more negative document. Maybe it was devised by people fearful of cancer; it seems geared to put patients in a depressed mood. Here are some of the questions:

'Tick on a scale of 1 to 10 how unhappy you have felt today?'
'How much pain today?'

and so on in the same negative vein. Why not put 'How many times have you counted your blessings, or felt you were improving, or taken a new step in helping yourself get well today?'

I decided not to use the inventory even if it put me out of line and out of the data-collection pool for this particular research. The results, if they ever come out, will be a very poor indication of 'quality of life', you may be sure. The people who wrote it do not realise that, without the verve and stirring of the spirit necessary to fight for survival, there would be *no* recoveries from cancer and *no* quality of life to research. What a waste of time, money and effort to distribute these down-putting, depressive forms. No one who has survived cancer would be keen to fill them in and those who are struggling with the disease would be made worse by even reading such rubbish.*

Dr Virginia had arranged a luncheon party at the exclusive La Jolla Yacht Club to introduce me to Dr Joseph Issels as a prelude to his viewing the film I had made. With me was Dr Suzanne Henig, a Professor of English at San Diego University and researcher for some of Dr Virginia's books. We were seated at a long table beside picture windows, overlooking a beautiful garden and the well-patronised beach to the calm blue water beyond. Everything was formal and perfect. What I recall most were the floors of polished hardwood, the snowy white table linen, the finger bowls with floating petals and the ice bucket incorporating its frozen peach blossoms.

But I was frustrated. I was placed so far away from Dr Issels and Dr Livingston that I could not hear or participate in any of the discussions of their work. Frau Issels was speaking mostly with those who could understand German, but she told me that Joseph had retired from his famous clinic in Germany and they were now in the USA staying with their son in Florida and looking for an American home.

Dr Issels, the vaccine and dead teeth

The only chance I had to talk to Dr Issels was during our walk through the gardens back to the car park. I asked him if he was

---

* I am not denigrating the Pennsylvania State University. Its students are renowned for carrying out excellent research programs which have added to our understanding of many human problems, not only in medicine but also in social welfare, psychology and anthropology.

Say: *I am at home in this world of kindness.*

still making his vaccines in Germany. He said the scientists he had trained were still making it and that he was using it not only as injection and by mouth, but through the skin as well.

'First you must rub the skin briskly with a towel until it is very red. When the antigen is applied to the area of erythema, it is taken into the skin by the increased circulation and can make an antibody.'

We were at the car park being directed to different cars for transportation back to Dr Virginia's home.

'I wanted so much to discuss this further', I said as we were leaving. 'But, of course. When we return to the house,' he called as the door of his limousine was closed.

We never did have that chance, however.

Dr Livingston had been asking him about his rationale for tooth extraction, since it was well known that no patients with untreated carious teeth or root fillings were admitted to his cancer treatment programs. Every mouth is alive with countless organisms of many different sorts, 'good' and 'bad'. Each time we exert the pressure of chewing, organisms are pushed into the tissues around the tooth. When there are dead teeth or inflamed gums, as in pyorrhoea and gingivitis, pathogens can be forced directly into the blood stream through the capillaries. Bad forms of the progenitor cryptocide organism are increased in the blood of people with these conditions, so making them more prone to cancerous changes.

A doctor and his wife had been watching the film, sitting close to Dr Livingston. He had recently had a heart attack and an operation for cancer of the prostate, and was in the process of going through Dr Livingston's program at her clinic. Since they knew no one in San Diego and were staying in the clinic car park in their mobile home, she was extending her hospitality to them in her usual generous way.

Another visitor watching the film was Dr Livington's dentist from La Jolla, who had his consulting rooms close by. Dr Livingston wanted to know if the doctor with the cancerous prostate had dead teeth in his head. As soon as the film was finished, she was busy arranging with the dentist to x-ray him and remove dead teeth if any were found. In spite of the doctor's weak protests, the dentist and I were asked to marshal him and his wife to the dental clinic forthwith for the examination and x-rays. So again I had no chance to resume my conversation with Dr Issels.

The worldwide call of a simple lifestyle

Over the next two hours, while the men were fulfilling these demands, I had a chance to talk to the doctor's wife. She was his second wife, a trained nurse, and a good deal younger. They had been drawn together through their mutual interest in a New Age philosophy of Elizabeth Prophet, I think, although they never actually discussed the name of their leader. There seem to be several large groups of people who believe there will be a holocaust, possibly nuclear, at the end of this century. This, they think, will make the waters rise all over the world and cause famine, pestilence and the end of civilisation as we know it.

With this firm belief they had sold up his well-established general practice and moved with others of the group to the backwoods of the mountains of Montana. There they were building a home designed for self-sufficiency, with the help of neighbours, in a communal arrangement. All their hard-earned savings had gone into the communal melting pot. His grown-up family were against the marriage and the move, though they were still on speaking terms—just.

To make the decision to uproot everything at the age of fifty-eight and leave his life's work, through fear of the future, must have been a tremendous period of personal conflict, stress, uncertainty and desperation for the doctor. The chemical changes engendered by that stress no doubt caused his cholesterol levels to change, his coronary arteries to block, and his immune system to break down. Coronary artery occlusion, myocardial infarction and cancer of the prostate were the outcome. His personal holocaust had already arrived.

They were most intersted in the houses I had built at the Sun-Powered Eukey Complex SPEC), particularly one of stone, one of wood slab and stringy bark, and one of pressed earth and mud bricks. Also they thought the wind generators, methane digester and solar equipment I had set up there would be most useful in their new lifestyle. My motivation in building the Eukey complex, raising an angora goat herd and forsaking the city pollution, was

Say: | *Most of me is perfect—I'm working on the rest!*

to live closer to the earth, in tune with nature. I find this is a strong basic urge in many people today. It is not 'dropping out', it is dropping *in*—to hard work and independence that satisfies the soul. These people I could understand.

Luckily for the doctor, when the dentist developed the x-rays they were all clear, so no teeth needed to be pulled. The dentist drove home, but Dr Issels and his wife had already left.

Most of the people who had been there to see the film had departed by the time we returned. However, it was acclaimed as a success by Dr Owen and even met with Dr Livingston's approval. Better equipment for microphotography of living unstained organisms is no doubt available today, but this film is a remarkably effective teaching aid for those who doubt Dr Livingston's words. This was the first of four occasions I showed the film in America.

One night Dr Livingston arranged a dinner party for several distinguished people from the San Diego University, the Loma Linda University and her own church. Our mutual friend, Dr Henig, was also there to fill me in with the background information on these people. Evidently Dr Livingston and her husband were considering selling the magnificent mansion in which they lived. It was far too big for the two of them. The housekeeper was the only other person living there. Dr Livingston has an extremely acute mind and a tendency to insomnia. The secretary arrived by 8 a.m. most mornings, by which time Dr Livingston had made many phone calls to act upon those plans she had thought out during the early hours.

They had decided to give a quarter of the money they would receive for the sale of the huge house to a university to endow a laboratory and to tutor a research fellow for studying and using her inventions.

Knowing from a personal disappointment in 1956 how grants can be diverted and mismanaged by unscrupulous people for their own ends, Dr Livingston was making a careful appraisal of those principals among the contenders for the grant, who would administer it. She wanted to make sure the money would be used to further her own important work for the good of humanity and not be frittered away on just another new building.

So the contenders for the donation and their wives, present at the dinner, were watched carefully for their reaction to the film. The dinner was, as usual, sumptuous. Because Dr Livingston is

Adventist by faith, there was no alcoholic liquor served, which helped to prevent the postprandial somnolence that could occur when the lights were turned low to watch the film. Even so, those who had only feigned interest in the subject did go to sleep, and were duly noted, no doubt!

After this viewing, Dr Livingston gave her formal permission for me to use the film in Brisbane at the Mater Clinical Conference in September.

Is light important to health? Dr John Ott

Another film shown that evening was 'Health and Light' by Dr John Ott. It opened up for me a whole new scientific study that I had never investigated. He had been a speaker at the Cancer Control Convention I had just attended, but I had missed his presentation. His booth afterwards was so crowded for the rest of the seminar that I had bypassed it. I was keen to study his work so that I could better understand his discoveries about the effect of different light frequencies on us, as well as on the rest of the animal and vegetable kingdom (see pages 245 and 246).

We know that every substance in the universe has a vibration. We have been endowed with receptors, our eyes, our skin, and our pineal glands, among others, which can sense the vibrations that we call light. There are profound effects on our psyches as well as on our physical selves, from these vibrations, even though these effects are rarely monitored or recorded by us. The unpleasant effects of glare and strobe lighting and the healing uses of infra-red and ultraviolet are the extent of most people's interest in the subject.

John Nash Ott is Director of the Environmental Health and Light Research Institute in Sarasota, Florida, and President of John Ott Pictures Incorporated. After twenty successful years as a banker in Chicago, he turned a life-time hobby of time-lapse photography into a full-time career in photobiology.

Dr Ott's pictures show that variations in the periodicity, intensity and wavelength distribution of light energy control certain plant growth processes such as setting of buds, opening of flowers,

Say: *I claim a healthy heart and strong bones.*

determination of sex and maturing of fruits. He points out similar responses in light entering people's eyes and stimulating the retinal-hypothalamic-endocrine system.

Citations and awards have come to him from horticultural, scientific and medical societies, including an honorary Doctorate of Science from Loyola University, and the grand Honours Award of the National Eye Research Foundation. His work in the horticultural field has been recognised by a host of societies. He is the author of a number of technical papers published in the proceedings of the New York Academy of Sciences, the National Technical Conference of the Illuminating Engineering Society, the Fourth International Photobiology Congress at Oxford, and others.

Since studying the literature on the healing effects of different light frequencies, I have started to incorporate light into my treatments. It is early days yet, but with careful observation and recording, and using the experience of others in this field, perhaps there will be some useful and authentic results to report in time.

Showing the film in Brisbane

The sequel to this trip to the USA was my presentation of the film at the Mater Hospital in Clinical Week, September, 1987. It was obviously an embarrassment to the hospital's pathology department but, because Dr Dique had been an honoured head of the department for so long, no one could deny him the time to present his protégé.

I was given the very last session of the week, when almost everyone had left. It followed a lecture on the costs of the premature nursery. Of the few nurses and doctors still in the lecture theatre, many walked out when they heard the words 'cancer-causing organism'. This was heresy they didn't want to hear.

The chairman was a keen young pathologist, but after he had thanked me publicly and was helping me pack up my film he said, 'You know, Ruth, they weren't organisms you photographed. We pathologists all know they are only granular debris from old leukocytes.'

It is such a pity more specialists are not interested in the history and research of their subject. In another section we will find some of the discoveries of the many people who spent their lives researching the cancer organism.

Part Four

PHYSIOLOGICAL SIGNPOSTS

11 WHY DON'T WE ALL GET CANCER?

We all make cancer cells, whether we are healthy or sick. We don't all get cancer because most of us make antibodies against it.

The immune system recognises what is 'of the body' (self) or 'not of the body' (non-self) by the 'markers', the amino acid, molecules, polypeptides and polysaccharides on the cell membrane of each cell. Immune-system cells attack only the substances that are 'enemy' or non-self.

Consider an enemy plane flying overhead. You know it is an enemy by its shape and by the flag on the wing—the marker. In a fog you couldn't see them and the plane would be impossible to identify, so it would not be attacked. This bears some similarity to what goes on in the cancer cell. According to Dr Lawrence Burton, a researcher into cell metabolism, the immune system makes a substance known by Dr Burton and his team as a 'blocking agent' on the surface membrane, which camouflages it from the natural defenders. Much work is being done now to identify these substances, which may be the same as those called 'cancer antigens' or markers. We can test how much and how many cancer antigens are in the blood stream. The cells protected by these blocking agents will not be recognised and so can go on growing in a little nest, undisturbed by the immune system defenders.

Most of us make substances in the liver which destroy the blocking agents. Since their discovery around 1970 by Dr Burton and his co-workers, the anti-blocking agents are still extracted and purified and given by daily injections at the Immuno Augmentive Therapy (IAT) Clinic in Grand Bahama. There have been some excellent results from this clinic, but diet and lifestyle changes are necessary too. Of the terminally ill patients I have treated who have gone on to IAT, only the one who continued on my program in conjunction survived longer than the text-book prognosis (see page 389).

It used to be thought that there was just one anti-blocking agent—called 'macro 2 globulin'—made in the liver. We now know there are many more substances that work in the fantastically complex field of immunotherapy.

In 1985 I participated in a cancer seminar in San Diego where I was privileged to hear Dr Saul Green talk about his part in the discovery of the *tumour necrosis factor* (TNF), with his team at Sloan Kettering Memorial Hospital in 1975. Bio-engineering techniques make it possible to use the substances of the immune system now being discovered in greater numbers every year. So far only animals have had the benefit of the 'synthetic' TNF. Since our body will make it naturally in the liver when stimulated to do so by antigens or vaccines, I prefer to use them. I know that they work. We must carefully gauge the use of the expensive genetically engineered substances, which are being produced in many countries, in relation to our bodies' multifaceted needs.

In January 1992, on the television science program *Quantum*, there was an interesting segment describing the painstaking research over twenty years by teams of scientists from Melbourne University and the Walter and Eliza Hall Institute.* Headed by Professors Bradley and Metcalfe and others, the researchers have isolated Colony Stimulating Factors (CSF) which stimulate stem cell production. CSF can now be mass produced to stimulate the replication of stem cells from blood in huge numbers. These are the very same types of cell which are harvested with difficulty from the patient or donor for bone marrow transplants. We can now use stem cell transplants from blood, as well as marrow.

In sixteen progressive countries, following this work, the system is being used successfully for treating patients with lymphoma, Hodgkins disease and other lymphatic disorders. The Australian Government has not passed it for use in Australia, although the discoveries were made here.

---

* Work is continuing still. Dr Lloyd J. Old, of Memorial Sloan Kettering, in collaboration with Elizabeth Carswell's team, Dr Seth Rudmik of Biogen, Dr Stephen Sherwin of Genetech, Dr Anthony Cerami of the Rockefeller University and others continue to unravel the inter-relationships of TNF and the interferons in destroying cancer cells. (See *Medical Journal of Australia*, Vol. 143, 11 November 1985, p.451.

Putting natural processes of defence in jeopardy, upsetting the balance of hormones or biochemical transactions, may be counterproductive in the long run, by causing gross anaemia or kidney or liver damage or, at least, severe side effects that are destructive to the already beleaguered immune system. The years of painstaking work that went into the discovery and production of a useful biological tool may be cancelled out by the insensitive clinical use of the product. So it may be with the interferons, the interleukins, TNF, the peptides and other wonderful discoveries of this century.

In none of the many articles I have read on the clinical trials of these substances has the nutritional status of the patient been taken into account; yet it is all-important. Without the right nutrients in abundance, our main defender, the immune system, cannot function. This brings us on to new questions.

Say: *I claim good health, I am healing now.*

12 WHAT IS THE IMMUNE SYSTEM?

When I was a medical student in 1943 we were taught in very simplistic terms about our defenders and their methods of attack on the substances coming into the body that are 'not self'. The whole subject has become incredibly complex. Researchers, vying with each other to discover more, wrote over 7000 papers on the topic in 800 journals in 1980 alone. The field is expanding just as rapidly today. What is written then is now either common knowledge or obsolete. Ideas and understanding are changing so swiftly that what was contained in my student textbooks is kindergarten stuff. For established biologists and medical practitioners, self-education is becoming more and more difficult, with a flood of new terms and jargon that attempt to describe new-found mechanisms of action in the minutiae of obscure changes in cell and molecular chemistry. A new speciality, immunotherapy, has been born.

Nutrients needed in the production of cellular and humoral immunity

In the table opposite are some of the vitamins and minerals necessary for the proper development and maturing of the cells of the immune system. *The foods that contain them* are on pages 133 and 134. Make sure you add some of each group to your diet daily.

My explanation of the immune system will be necessarily brief and basic. Look at the table again; it may help.

There are two types of defence, *cellular* and *humoral*. In *cellular immunity* members of the T cell group of lymphocytes attack cells, germs and biological irritants.

In *humoral immunity* the *antigens* (or foreign not-self substances) are destroyed by *antibodies* made by the B cells of the lymphocyte

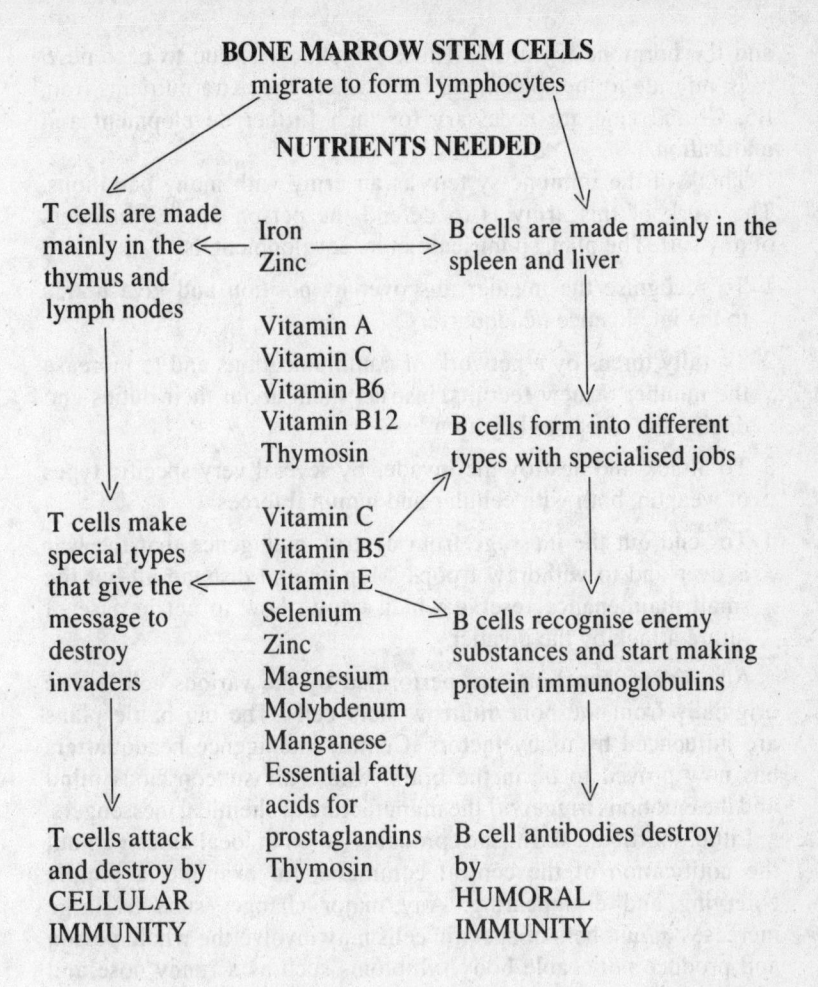

BONE MARROW STEM CELLS
migrate to form lymphocytes

NUTRIENTS NEEDED

T cells are made mainly in the thymus and lymph nodes	Iron Zinc	B cells are made mainly in the spleen and liver
	Vitamin A Vitamin C Vitamin B6 Vitamin B12 Thymosin	B cells form into different types with specialised jobs
T cells make special types that give the message to destroy invaders	Vitamin C Vitamin B5 Vitamin E Selenium Zinc Magnesium Molybdenum Manganese Essential fatty acids for prostaglandins Thymosin	B cells recognise enemy substances and start making protein immunoglobulins
T cells attack and destroy by **CELLULAR IMMUNITY**		B cell antibodies destroy by **HUMORAL IMMUNITY**

group. The antibodies latch onto the surface markers of the offender like magnetic mines and blow it up. All the lymphocytes start life in the bone marrow where the mother cells, called *'stem cells'*, start to develop different characteristics with the stimulus of the following nutrients: Vitamins A, C, B6 and B12; trace minerals, iron, zinc

Say: *Judge not and you will not be judged.* (Luke 6)

and the hormone thymosin. Those lymphocytes, due to become *B cells*, migrate to the spleen and liver, where the extra nutrients iron, B6, C, and zinc are necessary for their further development and maturation.

Think of the immune system as an army with many battalions. The work of this army is to defend the person against invaders of any sort. The plan, so intricate in its development, is:

1 To recognise the invader, discover its position and give notice to the intelligence headquarters.

2 To rally forces by a network of communications and to increase the number of new recruits, instruct them about their duties and deploy the troops to key areas.

3 To attack and destroy the invader by several very specific types of weapon, both with cellular and humoral forces.

4 To send out the message from central intelligence that the war is over and to withdraw troops. Mop up and disband all but the small maintenance reserve which knows how to act in case of future attack by the invader.

All of these functions are performed by the various cells made originally from the bone marrow stem cells. The big battle plans are influenced by many factors. Central intelligence headquarters has now proved to be in the brain, where the subconscious mind and the emotions trigger off the manufacture of chemical messengers.

Little, shortlived skirmishes probably go on in local areas without the notification of the central command; for example, a pimple emerging and disappearing. Any major changes such as large increases in numbers of specific cells may involve the whole person and produce noticeable body symptoms such as a runny nose and sore throat when someone is getting a cold.

If any part of the system fails, the battle plan may go awry and the invaders may gain the upper hand for a time, such as happens when we are suffering from an infectious illness. With many viral infections the maintenance reserve forces remain strong and are always on the alert, so that future attacks are repulsed at the point of entry. We seldom have mumps or measles again; 'one attack confers lifelong immunity'.

More and more actions of B cells are now known. B cells receive chemical messages from all over the body, but in particular they work in conjunction with the generals, the *macrophages* made in the liver. Macrophages ('big eaters' or 'mouths') are chief cells that have many actions. They recognise tissue signals to organise the different army patrols to do special tasks. B cells attack foreign agents (*antigen* or Ag), first recognising them by the surface markings that show they are 'not self'. They make an *antibody* (Ab) to these that can combine with the foreigner's surface membrane markers, inactivate it and destroy it.

In the womb, each one of us is given the antibodies our mother has manufactured but, by about fourteen weeks of age, a baby is breaking down its mothers' antibodies and starting to make its own with B cells in the liver and spleen. The B lymphocyte that has learnt an antibody program can become a carrier for that reaction and is then called a *memory cell*, that will be in reserve.

This has nothing to do with memory in the brain. It means these cells have a memory bank to use as a blueprint for manufacture of more of these particular defenders, should the same antigen enter the body again. *Plasma cells* are other B cells which assist in this manufacture of an even more specialised defence corps.

There are T Lymphocytes of many types

Going back to the stem cells: another battalion of immature T cells migrate from the bone marrow to the thymus, spleen and lymph nodes where they are made and trained in large numbers under the influence of *thymosen* from the thymus gland in the base of the neck, behind the breast bone. As mature or '*activated cells*', they have many and various tasks.

The following are some of the many types of T cells.

- **Effector T cells.** Some form natural killer cells (cytotoxic lymphocytes) that can destroy any cell with a foreign marker on its surface; for example, virus-infected cells. Others form delayed sensitivity T cells that react against Ags slowly. Helper T cells promote the maturing of B and T cells when the message

Say: | *We are all learning and growing.*

goes out for more troops to make more antibodies. T helper cells enhance the responses of B cells.

- **Suppressor T Cells** block this message and stop further manufacture once the crisis is past—otherwise the body would be flooded with one type of cell. Some antigens can stimulate too many suppressor T cells so that B cells are inhibited or confused and antibodies won't be made in the right way. This can cause the rest of the system to react against it in an *auto-immune reaction*. The antibody (Ab) is a substance that causes a lymphocyte to recognise a foreign molecule on a cell surface membrane. It is a polypeptide made from a glycoprotein.

Each species of animal and each human has antibodies that are specific to that individual. This is why we cannot transfuse a person with another's blood unless it matches and why we cannot use the blood of animals. It is also why one person rejects another's tissue in organ transplants. *Haptens* are molecules, usually small, that do not make an immunity reaction themselves but which help an antibody to form. An immune response, described by Professor Hans Selye as the *'general adaptive response'*, can be induced against many, many substances, not just microbes; for example, red blood cells, pollens, drugs, grafts and foods.

Professor Herman Eisen, writing in his textbook on Immunology, explains that *the immune system's response to distinctive antigens of tumour cells may ultimately contribute to the control of cancer.*

In fact we know that it is this response that gives us all our antibodies right now against cancer. We all have cancer cells in us. It is those of us who make antibodies against them who do not develop the disease.

Some good food sources of vitamins and minerals

Vitamin A: Beta carotene	Liver, egg yolk, fish oil: dark green leafy vegetables, all yellow, orange and red fruits and vegetables
Vitamin B$_1$:	Liver, brewer's yeast, all unrefined cereals, nuts and seeds, wheatgerm, legumes
Vitamin B$_2$:	Liver, milk, brewer's yeast, eggs, kidney, cereals, nuts, mushrooms
Vitamin B$_3$:	Liver, kidney, fish, brewer's yeast, eggs, wholegrains, legumes, nuts, mushrooms
Vitamin B$_5$: (pantothenate)	Liver, egg yolk, soybeans, some fish, brewer's yeast, cabbage family such as broccoli, mushrooms, royal jelly, whole grains, nuts
Vitamin B$_6$:	Liver, kidney, wheatgerm, seeds, fish, brewer's yeast, legumes, oatmeal wholegrain, nuts
Vitamin B$_{12}$:	Liver, kidney, oysters, fish roe, eggs
Vitamin C:	All fresh raw fruit and vegetables, especially citrus, strawberries, watermelon, cantaloupe, cabbage and fresh green leafy vegetables
Vitamin D:	Sunlight, fish liver oils, egg yolk, sprouts, milk
Vitamin E:	Wheatgerm, oils of nuts, cereals and seeds, fish roe, egg yolk
Magnesium:	Wheatgerm, nuts, legumes, whole grains, all dark green vegetables, dolomite, milk
Potassium:	All fresh fruits and vegetables, all legumes, oatmeal, potato, nuts, sweet potato, avocado, banana, apricot, mushrooms, molasses, fish, milk
Calcium:	Milk, yoghurt, cheese, dolomite, legumes, seeds, bonemeal, green leafy vegetables
Sodium:	Celery, kelp, salt, cheese, seafoods
Sulphur	Garlic, onion, mushroom, cabbage family, celery

Say: *I study all sides of the questions to find real truth.*

Selenium:	Liver, brewer's yeast, wheatgerm, egg, onion, garlic, kelp, goat's milk
Zinc:	Liver, oatmeal, legumes, fish, seeds and grains, leafy vegetables
Iron:	Liver, brewer's yeast, legumes, egg yolk, green leafy vegetables, wholegrains
Copper:	Liver, brewer's yeast, eggs, heart, prunes, almonds, legumes
Essential fatty acids:	Oils of seeds, grains and beans, especially cold-pressed linseed (flax) oil, safflower, olive, corn
Folic acid:	Green leafy vegetables, liver, kidney, eggs, legumes, brewer's yeast
Biotin:	Brewer's yeast, sprouts, liver, kidney, milk, whole grain, rice, eggs
Paba:	Brewer's yeast, whole grains, yoghurt, liver, kidney
Bioflavinoids:	Pigment and pith of fruits and vegetables, buckwheat, citrus
Chlorine:	Lecithin, brewer's yeast, liver, legumes, whole grain, milk, eggs, brains
Inositol:	Lecithin, brewer's yeast, citrus, nuts, whole grain
B_{15}-pangamic acid:	Brewer's yeast, seeds, whole grain, liver, kidney

(See also nutrients needed for production of immunity, page 129.)

13   WHAT IS A VACCINE?

The immune system has a reserve corps of B memory cells that carry hundreds of thousands of antibody programs. Ever since infancy, our defences have been repelling threatening substances that come to us from our food, air and water, by ingestion, by inhalation or by direct contact with skin or mucous membranes. Some antigens are congenital, which means that they are already in the tissues when we are born, given to us through our mother's blood in the womb.

So it may be with the many viruses and other organisms such as rubella, AIDS, herpes, toxoplasmosis, rheumatoid arthritis and the cancer organism. Many of the organisms do *not* manifest themselves in the infant. Rubella (German measles), for instance, does not affect the baby adversely unless it is contracted between the eighth and twelfth week of foetal life.

Many organisms are *pleomorphic*, which means that they have numerous forms, many of them harmless. A non-active form of the germs' life cycle may be passed through the placenta and may never change into a form that causes ill health in the host.

When we consider the cancer organism, however, we see that it has many different forms. The cell wall deficient 'L' forms are the common, harmless forms which most of us have in our blood. When the blood or body tissues are altered in various ways—probably to an alkaline Ph among other changes—then the organism can change to other forms. One most often seen which heralds a stressed and vulnerable state of the body is the *motile rod*. Some researchers, such as Glover and Von Brehmer, considered that if motile rods persisted in the blood, as seen under the dark field microscope, the person would manifest cancer within two years.

When I was studying the cancer organism intensely, between 1984 and 1987, I looked at blood from each patient and from myself as often as possible. If there were many motile rods I advised the person to have a vaccine made to educate the immune system to recognise and destroy that form of the organism. In 1986 I was working too hard, so I had many bad forms in my blood. When I was in America I had a vaccine made for myself and used it for a year. Within three weeks of starting that vaccine all the bad forms disappeared.

You see, the body may originally have only the 'L' forms, which are not recognised by the immune system as 'nonself' because they have no cell walls to carry identifying markers. When a new form is made (see diagram), such as a thallus, a spheroblast or, particularly, a motile rod, then the body should recognise it as 'nonself' and make an antibody against it.

No doubt we usually do this early in life. Sometimes a child develops cancer, a child who has not been severely ill before in any way. The supposition is that the cancer cells had been growing very slowly in an unrecognised immune-deficient child, or that some external stresses had made a constant alkaline environment and so a gross change to bad forms. Repeated courses of some antibiotics and some other drugs, *plus* inappropriate nutrition, have been known to do this.

Case Comment: Bobbie

I remember Bobbie, who died of leukaemia at the age of two and a half years. He had been in and out of hospital being treated with course after course of chemotherapy cocktails—that is, combinations of chemicals—from the age of eleven months.

He was the youngest of four children in a loving and stable family. His mother had toxaemia of pregnancy and recurrent thrush (see case histories page 339) while carrying him. As an infant he had thrush in his mouth and as a skin rash and had cortisone ointment for it. Toxaemia, thrush and cortisone are all insults to the immune system's antibody-making capacity. His mother did not have enough milk so he was bottle fed, thus gaining none of her antibodies. No baby supplements were given. At two months old he had his first ear infection, for which the doctor gave antibiotics. This was followed by a cold that went to his chest and was treated with more antibiotics.

One infection followed another and in the first ten months of his life he had six courses of antibiotics, not one of them given with any protective acidophilus yoghurt or vitamin B and K supplements, or any blood tests to see what the immune system was doing.

At eleven months he lost his appetite altogether and became extremely listless and very pale, with gross bruising of the skin. Blood tests showed acute myelocytic leukaemia.

Bobbie had no chance. His lymphocytes, right back to the stem-cell stage in the bone marrow, had suffered one insult after another. They tested the family for bone marrow transplant compatibility but it was too late. The chemotherapy and the disease had knocked out his platelets so that he was bleeding almost every day. Repeated transfusions trying to keep him alive only made his little liver and spleen swell to enormous size, reacting to the donors' blood cells. The doctors who saw him every day were very kind and knowledgeable people. The family had done everything possible for this much-loved child. They had followed the treatment their doctors had prescribed from the very moment of his birth.

Who can use a vaccine?

Would Bobbie have been saved by a vaccine? Probably not. Why? Because his immune system could not have been stimulated to make antibodies against cancer fast enough between courses of antibiotics, which depress it. The *autogenous vaccine* is a culture grown from the person's own cancer organism in its bad form. This is done by isolating the organism from the blood, urine, faeces or cancer tissue and growing it in a special medium with very exact environmental factors which eliminate every other type of organism. At a certain stage the culture is killed and sterilised by mixing with an antiseptic, standardised for strength and put into ampules for injection. The whole process is done under strictly sterile conditions to avoid any contamination.

If the immune system is not making any antibodies against the bad forms and the killed and purified autogenous antigen is given, it may start to make some. Making antibodies against the cancer

Say: | *I treat myself and others fairly.*

organism may stimulate the body to react against the cancer itself, too, and bring the natural killer cells into action against it. In the first and second stages of cancer the vaccines are very useful. Read *Where There's Hope*, by Patricia Gilshenen, a patient of mine who recovered from anaplastic lung metastases, after six years of battling, with the help of her autogenous vaccine and our nutritional plan.

Before each visit I ask each patient to have a blood test to gauge what the white cells are doing. Of course the cells can only be looked at under the pathologist's microscope when they are dead and stained by dyes that show up various features of the cells. They are also counted in a standard fashion, so that the results in percentages are comparable with those of any other laboratory. Many important points for management can be gained by studying these simple quantitative results.

More Cells

The white cell count is not only measured as T and B cells but also by the appearance of the cells, which can be recognised by their proper names and what work they do.

- **Neutrophils** are large cells with a nucleus containing several lobes. If these contain granules they are called granulocytes. They are part of the T-cell cellular defence system and may ingest germs and other debris.
- **Lymphocytes** are smaller and may belong to either system. There are many different types and stages of development.
- **Monocytes** defend us against viruses and may be precursors of lymphocytes. In patients who have infections, the viral element of herpes, cytomegalovirus and others of the Epstein-Barr family may be recognised inside the living monocytes when examined under the dark-field microscope in freshly shed blood.
- **Eosinophils** are usually present in increased numbers when a patient has an allergy. The granules in them are large and very bright when viewed under the dark-field, but large and pink when dead and stained with eosin which is pink. An increase in these often suggests that the patient is having allergic reactions to something, since these cells destroy histamine, the cause of allergic symptoms. They are also increased as a response to some types of chemotherapy and to some parasites.

14 BIOLOGICAL PRODUCTS IN TREATMENT

Biological products are being used more and more frequently to stop the changes the cancer makes in its march forward.

Antiblocking Agents

Macro 2 globulin and other fractions from immune serum are used with some success against certain cancers by Lawrence Burton in his clinic in Grand Bahama I.A.T. (see page 00).

Biological products developed synthetically from in-the-test-tube observations of cancer cell behaviour—growth and inhibition—have had a great vogue since patents have been awarded for their manufacture.

Alpha Interferon

This is a small, soluble, protein complex produced and released by a cell that has been attacked by a virus. It starts other non-infected cells producing anti-viral proteins that stop viruses replicating.

Type I interferon is made by leucocytes in the human liver but commercially it is made by bacteria such as *Escheria coli*.

Type II immune interferon is made by specially sensitised Ag-stimulated lymphocytes with specific antigens, so causing antibodies to form. It can activate lymphoid tissue to make these antibodies against cancer cells in certain circumstances. Carcinogens and steroids (cortisone, oestrogen, etc) can depress the making of interferon. Produced from the *Escheria coli* bacillus it, and its commercial artificial product immune interferon, is being used in Australia and other countries. It was discovered by English scientist

Clerk Isaacs. Like so many substitutes for the real thing, the artificial form can cause severe side effects not engendered by the natural product in its normal tiny amounts. If only it could be given in conjunction with a sound nutritional and stress control program, it may yet be helpful as a palliative agent.

It is probable that the anti-tumour effect of immune interferon is caused by its capacity to stimulate natural killer cells into action. Interferons work synergistically with TNF which activates the macrophages in the liver to stimulate the natural killer cells, found in great numbers in the spleen. They can be also activated by Interleukin 2.

Interleukin 2

This is a leukotriene, made in the human liver but commercially produced from the action of bacteria such as *E. coli*. It is the substance that activates natural killer cells. It calls them to battle and directs them to recognise 'non-self' cancer cells. In a sterile environment white cells are removed from the blood, incubated for three weeks with this artificial reagent and returned to the body as killers. This process may work better if other factors, such as blocking agents made by the cancer to inhibit it, are controlled. It is made in the USA, Japan and Europe, experimentally so far.

Organ extracts

The endocrine system is produced by organs of the body known as ductless glands, which have been studied intensively since the last century. The complicated system of hormones and enzymes these glands produce is responsible for the efficient chemical reactions that govern work in every organ of the body.

Many of the hormones are peptides—the tiniest soluble molecules of protein breakdown. The best known endocrine glands are the pituitary, pineal, thyroid, parathyroids, thymus, adrenals, pancreas and gonads (sex glands). The manufacture of raw products needed for these regulatory hormones and enzymes depends on many organ factories such as the liver and spleen.

Extracts of thymus, pancreas, liver, spleen and thyroid, for certain patients in varying amounts, are part of the Cilento Survival Plan.

The person with cancer who is not making any or enough can be helped by these substances, made naturally by the body organs, and taken by mouth.

Modern doctors may scoff at such 'unscientific' technology—giving the whole gland when they believe that 'the active principle' has been isolated. Unfortunately, we know only a fraction of what substances are actively present and what relationships they have to one another. When we isolate and refine what some scientific school has discovered as the useful substance, we often throw the baby out with the bath water.

There are many more active ingredients that we have *not* yet discovered that are adjuvants. Other cultures have known and used parts of animals in the treatment of illness for countless years, back to antiquity. Carnivores (don't forget that humans *are* carnivores) will eat certain organs preferentially and by tradition, depending on need.

The Australian Aborigines had a strict division of parts when a kangaroo or other large animal was being eaten. The elders received the brain, the men the muscle meats, the pregnant women the liver, and so on. Many people look on 'offal' as 'awful'—this abhorrence is learned behaviour from early childhood. Its source goes back many generations and can be traced to beliefs deeply embedded in warlike traditions—the food of warriors was red meat. Other organs were for lowlier mortals, were 'dirty' or for the sick.

Yet for invalids, the menu has always included broths made of other organs, bones that make a jelly; milk puddings, junkets and custards; coddled egg, steamed fish and brains. A surprising number of doctors mistakenly believe that patients on my program must be starved of protein, whereas there is ample protein *of the right type.* Many urge our mutual patients to 'build yourself up with some good fillet steak'!

The cancer organism is grown in the test tube on beef broth, mutton broth or ox blood, so I don't encourage red muscle meat

Say: | *You lighten up my day.*

in the food plan. It is a wonderful culture medium for the growth of the cancer organism.

Most of the organ extracts are now available commercially. Because we don't know all the active substances we should use the whole organ if possible. For instance, thryoxine is not the only useful ingredient in the thryoid gland, though it is one of the only ones we can standardise for dosage and is therefore the most useful today.

The many critics who claim that glandular substances are changed and made useless by digestion should note that, in spite of their theories, many glands taken by mouth when accompanied by digestive enzymes actually work. Each acts in accordance with its use in the body, to a greater or lesser extent.

Though you can see the connection here with the rules of homeopathy, in which 'like treats like', it does *not* follow that treatment is simplistic. It is important to use the right dosage of these extracts in an acceptable pill or injectable form. I notice the clinical improvement particularly in patients who become debilitated by radiation or chemotherapy. They pick up remarkably quickly and also withstand their treatments very much better when they take some of these natural biological products. It may be the turning point into remission of their disease.

Wobe Mugos

Wobe mugos is a compound of proteolytic enzymes from animal and vegetable sources. One pill of the substance contains calf pancreas, thymus, pisum sativum, lens esculenta and papaya. I give some of these substance as part of my supplement program, but *separately* so that dosage can be controlled to suit the individual patient.

Liver Juice

Liver juice is unequalled as a boost to the immune system. The liver is the kitchen of the body, home of many different sorts of cells, all with varied tasks to perform. Among the many hundreds of transactions it monitors is the making and breaking down of our sex hormones out of the raw product, cholesterol. It also detoxifies substances harmful to the body and excretes the products of detoxification into the bile to be passed out into the intestine for elimination. An even more important job that the liver performs is the manufacture of macrophages, tumour-necrosing factor and other substances that allow the immune system to function in its task of destroying damaging substances, such as cancer cells, in the body.

The macrophages and other white cells that are contained in the liver are still *alive* in fresh raw liver and the anti-blocking agent and tumour-necrosing factor are still present if the liver has not been frozen. These are all destroyed in the process of cooking, drying or freezing liver.

The aim in taking raw liver juice for those with cancer who are not making sufficient for the body's needs is to gain these substances.

Calf's liver is used because it is not as strong tasting as lamb's fry and it makes a thinner and more palatable juice. Also, calves do not get liver fluke, a parasite that is not uncommon in sheep in some parts of Australia and may be contracted by humans. Fresh young unfrozen liver, when juiced with carrot, tastes of carrot. It may also be juiced with apple for those who find carrot unpalatable. Also, young animals have not been subjected to so many toxic substances.

Liver extract by injection, liver tablets and cooked liver as food are still very useful substances, if available, but do not contain the *live* cells.

In the first half of this century Dr Max Gerson, who found liver juice so important for his patients believed that the only way of making liver juice was to use the grind-and-press type of machine, such as the Norwalk juicer, which did not heat the substances going through it or alter their electrical potential. In his day, the slow and clumsy centrifugal juicers tended to do this.

However, the grind-and-press juicers are now far too expensive for most people to buy and the centrifugal ones are not only cheap but also have a less destructive effect on the substances being juiced than they used to have. People are getting better using either nowadays. The liver juice must be strained and then drunk almost

Say: | *I am tolerant and understanding.*

immediately it is made, however, or it will oxidise and some of the important items in it will be destroyed.

Those who do not like the taste may take liver juice without tasting it by using the following methods.

- Make and stand aside a small amount of carrot, apple or grape juice *before* starting with the liver. Hold the nose and drink the liver and carrot juice down promptly. Then, before releasing the nose, clear the palate by drinking the apple chaser. Then take another breath. Alternatively, just drink the juice down and then take the chaser without taking a breath, if lung capacity is large enough to do that.

It helps to know that the substances extracted from fresh liver cost $680.00 a day to have by injection, *if you could get them*. That makes it taste much better!

Protamide

Protamide was a proteolyte enzyme processed from the glandular layer of a hog's stomach. It was a very useful form of treatment in the past, especially for scleroderma, herpes zoster and auto-immune conditions. As with staphage lysate and wobe mugos, it was banned by the Food and Drugs Administration in the onslaught against immunological forms of treatment in the 1970s. The effectiveness and safety of these products have never been questioned. They stimulate the manufacture of interferons, interleukins and leukotrienes in the liver and spleen. These are all substances made by the body to increase our resistance to disease.

Thymosin

One of the key glands for the immune system is the thymus which sits at the top of the chest and is particularly large in childhood.

Thymosin, a peptide enzyme/hormone made by this gland, stimulates the migration and maturing of lymphocytes. It is essential for a strong immune system. Even dried extract of the thymus gland has been found effective in stimulating the activity of lymphocytes, so restoring a flagging immune system.

In the politics of medicine it is widely suspected that the rapid advent of commercially produced antibiotics spelt the demise of these harmless and efficacious healing substances.

Herbs for healing

Herbs have been used for healing since prehistoric times. Some animals use them too. I noticed a dog eating grass to help itself vomit round worms. It wasn't my dog.

Goats are the most amazing in that they are very good at recognising useful and poisonous substances by scent. They have thousands of bytes in their smell computer and in their own natural state refuse to eat or go near things that would harm them. When raised in artificial circumstances and taught to eat foods that are convenient and cheap for us to feed them but which often contain carcinogens and chemicals, they lose some of this sense. They are then susceptible to more diseases. The same happens to animals crowded into 'feed lots' of any type. Disease is the natural outcome. Unless vaccinated against it soon after hatching, 25 per cent of battery chickens die of cancer. How analogous this is to our crowded take-away food outlets in city life!

Herbs have been used to beat cancer since before written history. I have grown them since childhood, when my fascination with botany first started. When I was very small I used to sit beside our chook pen and feed the hens green leaves and pieces of grass through the bird-wire. They were very, very discriminating in what they took from me. I used to find caterpillars for a rather picky magpie who hobnobbed with them too. He wouldn't eat the leaves I found. When my older brother grazed his knee falling off his bike, I hurried round the garden, picked some green grasses, bruised them in my hands and rubbed them on the hurt area. The friend who was with him asked what I was doing and he said, 'Oh she's just treating it with herbs to stop the bleeding. She's going to be a doctor when she grows up.' I was three years old at the time. What my admired and beloved brother said must have programmed my goal pattern

Say: *Your happiness is infectious.*

from that early age. What better confirmation! I was helping, I had gained his approval and that of his friend too. I didn't recall that incident until I started studying herbal medicine with Denis Stewart many years later. I had to ask my mother where we had lived and how old I was when we had that chook pen.

I now use herbal medicines for selected patients, not only for cancer but also for high blood pressure, heart troubles, acne, allergies, migraine, candida, auto-immune diseases and nervous disorders.

The many experienced teachers I have to thank in studying herbal medicine include Denis Stewart, Kerry Bone, Michael Tierra and David McLeod. There are dozens of books on the subject, some exclusively about cancer treatments such as John Heinerman's *The Treatment of Cancer with Herbs*.

The Hoxsey Biomedical Clinic

In 1986 and 1988, I visited the Biomedical Clinic in a grand old building on top of a hill in Tijuana, where herbal medicine is used to treat cancer and other diseases. It is best to arrive there early because, as in most of the Tijuana clinics, it is 'first come first seen' for the many patients who crowd in each morning when the buses arrive from across the USA border.

Sister Mildred Nelson, who has run the clinic for many years, originally worked with cancer researcher Harry Hoxsey in the USA. I found the herbal formula* originally used by his father in my father's British Pharmocopaea of 1911 as 'trifoliatum compound'. The book *You Don't Have To Die*, written by Harry Hoxsey, gives the story of how his father used the herbs and also gives a resume of the troubles the family went through in establishing the clinics, finally culminating in the move to Mexico.

Mildred Nelson came to work with Harry Hoxsey first after he treated her mother, who had cancer. It was too late to cure the disease but Mildred was impressed by his results. After Harry died,

---

* The Hoxsey herbal formula contains potassium iodide combined with some or all of the following herbal substances: licorice, red clover, burdock root, stillingia root, barberis root, poke root, cascara, prickly ash bark and buckthorn bark. The amounts of the substances in the formula are varied to suit the type of cancer and the state of the patient.

Mildred continued to see patients. By that time she had gained vast experience of cancer to add to her nursing knowledge. I found her a very knowledgeable, honest and down-to-earth person. She was most hospitable and helpful to me in answering many questions and she allowed me to 'sit in' while she treated the lumps of several patients with either the yellow or the red paste*, depending on the type of cancer they had.

She explained to them in detail how to take the herbal mixtures and the program of return visits, if necessary. There is not much prohibition in the diet she advocates. She makes sure that the restaurant attached to the clinic has simple but nourishing food at a low price.

There were four Mexican doctors employed at the clinic when I was there. The examination and treatment of patients is thorough and the therapeutic equipment is sound. I 'sat in' with Dr Arriola, who spoke English, after gaining permission from the patient, from Mildred and from Dr Arriola himself. I also had a long discussion with Dr Guierrera and went to a clinical panel conference on the treatments necessary for the patients who attended that morning. This is a very similar procedure to clinical conferences in Australian hospitals. I couldn't understand Spanish but the doctor explained.

When clinic facilities are insufficient, patients are referred to a Mexican hospital where these doctors can attend them or refer them to other specialists. So much is obtainable in Mexico, there are so many open-minded physicians who are now in the forefront of examining promising treatments, not only for cancer, MS, SLE, rheumatoid arthritis and heart disease, but also for AIDS.

This has brought hundreds of thousands of desperate people to Mexico, seeking the medications reported as useful by anecdotal experiences but which have been put aside in the USA without any trials. Of course, unscrupulous people are selling supposed 'medicines' that are really useless on the streets at black-market

---

* Yellow paste: arsenic sulphide, yellow precipitate, sulphur and talc.
  Red paste: antimony trisulphide, zinc chloride and blood root. Escharotin: trichloro acetic acid.

Say: *I enjoy your company.*

prices. But most substances that are available on prescription from doctors have a favourable research background, although they have not been produced commercially elsewhere.

The prescribed Mexican pharmaceuticals are standardised and carefully produced under government supervision. Some of the herbals Dr Guierrera used were unknown to me. They came from native plants of the area and are not available in Australia.

Interest in the medicinal qualities of Australian plants is increasing. No doubt there will be useful additions to our herbal medication from the recently completed textbooks, *Australian Traditional Medicine* from the team led by Dr Ella Stack, and *Traditional Bush Medicine* by Tim Low.

Twice when I went to the Biomedical Clinic I had lectures from the medical director there, an energetic doctor who called herself 'Dr Friday'. She described the tests she was giving for candida yeast in the bowel to four or five of us at a time. Then she went over the life history of the organism and what to do with the medications we were given to control it. About half the cancer patients she tested were sensitive to the fungal form of the candida organism and so needed treatment.

Dr Yolande Fraire is no longer at the clinic. She has started her own consulting in Tijuana, mostly general medicine with a special bias towards treating cancer patients. She has very good results. Every time I have visited there I have been invited to sit in with her and I have learned much. Many of the substances she uses are not available in Australia. Some which we could make, such as Staphage Lysate, are no longer being advocated by the Food and Drugs Administration in America and, following our copy-cat mode, are not advocated here either, even under licence.

Dr Fraire has good results with Wobe Mugos and other natural treatments. She gives practical advice on everyday lifestyle in the wholistic, old-fashioned way, as we have been trained to do as family doctors. She still sends me the delightful newsletter she writes for patients full of research news, jokes, practical hints, witticisms and her own astute philosophy. I treasure that.

Is chemotherapy harmful to the immune system?

Many people ask this question and the answer must be *yes*, and some types more than others. What has become unequivocally apparent over the years is that my patients, who are on a basically simple and physiologically sound food plan with vitamin and mineral supplements essential to the immune system, *withstand and recover from the side effects of chemotherapy much better than those without the program.*

Patients who have had chemotherapy before and then after the food plan and supplements tell me how much difference it makes. Their oncologists also tell them how remarkably well they manage their treatment. There are many who fear to tell the oncologist that they are taking my program in conjunction with his or hers, for fear of getting a dose of negativity or denigration. Some, however, have found an oncologist who is open-minded and willing to go along with nutrition and stress control.

It is very heartening for me to find that the climate among chemotherapists is changing. In 1983 there was not one who was willing to listen to the facts, for fear of being thought 'alternative', 'on the fringe' or a 'medical heretic'. Now there are four oncologists in Brisbane alone who have quietly promoted dietetic advice, support groups and psychological counselling in meditation or relaxation techniques. Even if they have not read the research literature or been to seminars on these subjects, they cannot fail to see the difference it has made in our mutual patients. Their longest survivors are on my program too.

B_{12} *Cytamen*

B_{12} cytamen, as weekly injections, given as a medication, *not* as a treatment for anaemia, has proved to be one of the best supports for a white-cell count knocked down by chemotherapy. In fact B12 1000 helps the whole haemopoietic (blood-making) system to remain stable since it probably acts as a catalyst in many body transactions. It picks up the appetite, promotes more energy, dispels depression

Say: | *I look forward to meeting people.*

by enhancing brain enzyme manufacture and is completely non-toxic.

With people who have cancer, the stomach is often not making enough 'intrinsic factor' to digest the B12 out of food or even out of a tablet. I find it really only works efficiently if given by injection.

What about radium?

Radium also upsets the haemopoietic system as a whole, particularly when parts of the bone marrow and internal organs are irradiated. Destruction of cancer cells and normal cells occurs due to vast showers of free radicals (see page 157) released by radiation and these are disposed of much better and more quickly if the patient is taking Vitamin E, Selenium, Co-enzyme Q10, and Germanium in appropriate dosages. These should be continued, to sustain the supportive effect on normal tissues, for some weeks after the radium treatment is finished.

I have not found the same degree of open-mindedness among radiotherapists as among chemotherapists so far. Perhaps it is because the past president of their society here was so much against any infringement of his discipline (which he thought was the only one) by any other modality. I had a long talk to him about nutrition, meditation and herbal medicine in 1983, when he visited Stanthorpe on a lecture tour. He told me that in the seventeen years he had led the radiotherapists association he had eighty-seven doctors under his control. He said he was happy that he had taught them all to 'close ranks' against any of the 'modern quackery' creeping in to undermine what he thought was the only cancer treatment worth using.

Though now retired from active dedication in his field of expertise he still has an important voice in the 'watchdog' committee, as it is called. He started this group of doctors, nurses and paramedics some years ago for the very purpose of putting down those he calls 'medical heretics'. The committee has a close association with a sister group in California which has been responsible for the persecution and deregistration of innovative doctors by the Food and Drugs Administration.

There is usually one watchdog at any lecture I give, so I am careful to welcome him and give him the notes on the talk, if I have any. Maybe if the notes are read, another mind might be opened.

Chemotherapy and radiation are both useful, often life-saving therapies that have stood the test of time in aiding the body's fight against *some* cancers. I have great rapport with and admiration for the caring and careful specialists who use these modalities. I spend much time explaining the pros and cons to patients who are fearful of undergoing such treatment.

But, through it all, it is the patient who is the healer. The bulk of the cancer may be removed, burnt out, poisoned or slowed down, but the body must still develop the strength to recover itself and to offset the damage that these treatments have done.

What we should realise is that these modalities of disease treatment are no more 'alternative' to orthodox treatments than baking is to roasting—one is just as wholesome as the other. Everything can work together for a good result. It is the patient who must choose the therapist who can help most.

Nutrition, supplements and stress control are *essential* for this, and never forget that, for the body to survive, we also need *mind* and *spirit*.

Who are the healers?

Doctors are the traditional healers. We hold a time-honoured place in society for good reason. Training for the basic degrees of Bachelor of Medicine, Bachelor of Surgery (MB,BS) requires in Australia eighteen years of study and practical work just to be judged fit to tend to a sick person. The preparatory primary and secondary school teaching, before the arduous seven years of medical training, is just as crucial in shaping the attitudes of the doctor-to-be as the professors teaching later on.

Choosing the profession denotes a desire to help others, for it is choosing too a lifetime of hard work and heavy responsibility. In the last thirty years, with group practice becoming the norm, we are losing the feeling of belonging in the community that used to give support, trust and stability to the family doctor's role.

The fine ideals of service and solace to the suffering, that have always been part of healing through the ages, are in danger of being swamped in the maze of regulations and reports imposed by the

Say: *Nothing nasty gets under my skin.*

changing methods of government.

I am proud to acknowledge that doctors still uphold the best of the healing methods and compassionate attitudes they know in spite of officialdom. Our Society, the Australian Medical Association, is like an industrial union that gives us a voice in the political arena. There are other Societies that have been springing up in the last thirty years but though they may represent some extra points of view it is the A.M.A. that still has the traditional power to direct us however we might grumble at times.

It is the medical profession that also takes the brunt of the fear and anger that many people are experiencing due to the escalation of cancer and other diseases. There is still a persistent simplistic and ignorant idea that doctors should be able to cure everything and that doctors should be responsible if the disease is *not cured*. I hope this book will help people to take back some responsibility in understanding their condition and doing their part in helping themselves to heal.

Part Five

THROUGH THE MAZE OF CANCEROUS CHANGES

15 WHAT ARE STRESSED CELLS?

I have discussed some of the causes of stressed cells—the precursors of cancerous changes—but what are they, and how do they change into cancer cells?

Much research is going on in many parts of the world on these subjects. What I am recording is the outcome of facts gleaned from the scientific papers and books of dozens of knowledgeable scientists in different disciplines, from cell biologists to agricultural biochemists. If we gather such information and study it with an open mind, symptoms and patterns of action sometimes emerge.

So let us go back to the physiology of the cell, particularly the cell with a nucleus. There are over 150 different sorts of tissue in the body, all made from the one cell that we consist of when we are conceived. That is a miraculous beginning.

Of these, about 120 types of tissue have cells containing a nucleus. This is a complicated structure, like a computer, which holds some intricate working parts that program it and tell the cell as a whole what to do. It is a change in the electrical magnetic mechanism of the cell membrane, plus a fault or breakdown in the programming department of the nucleus that allows the cell to grow out of control.

How can this happen? We must go back to the energy source to make more discoveries.

Energy source

We know that all matter is vibration, even seemingly solid substances are made up of atoms with specific vibratory fields. These are made up of infinitely small, negatively charged particles called electrons which move round the positively charged nucleus of the atom. Each substance or element has its own specific number of electrified particles. The number and structure of these is the basis of the Periodic

Table or list of elements of the earth's structure, which the Russian Mendileev spent his life composing. Each atom, with its electricity-charged electrons, creates a tiny magnetic field which can now be measured.

But where does the energy of these particles originate? The search for the origin of life has been the ongoing fascination of countless diligent investigators from before written history. Universally it is believed to start from the energy of the sun.

The sun's energy is poured onto the earth in units called photons. We see it simply as sunlight but it is much more. These tiny particles of pure energy live forever and are constantly in motion, separately or coalescing into partnerships that resonate, changing frequency and colour, making bridges between their pure energy and the elements of earth.

The way the sun's energy as photons is trapped by an atom depends on the frequency of the vibratory electrons of the atom. A photon vibrating at the same frequency can be taken into an atom's tiny electrical circuit, so changing its magnetic field. At an appropriate time that proton can be released, so giving energy up again.

The collection and distribution of electrons is the basis of energy production in all living substances, using the elements carbon, hydrogen, oxygen, nitrogen, phosphorus, sulphur and many trace elements in the myriad combinations that make up matter. The human being is the highest form of this resonance between electrons and the photons of the sun. It is the fatty acids which facilitate this link.

Fatty Acids

Fatty acids consist of groups of atoms that have trapped photons to form together in chains by electrical connections called single and double bonds. The double bonds are very active because they have extra energy to impart.

- **Saturated** fats, such as animal fats, have no double bonds. They are stable and very inactive.
- **Monounsaturated** fats have one double bond and do have some activity.
- **Polyunsaturated** fats have two or more double bonds and are very active; they are concerned in the basic chemistry of every cell.

The energy these fats contain in their double bonds comes from the ability of plants to capture, harness and store the sun's photons by their chlorophyll. Oil from seeds, grains and beans is the main food which contains these most valuable substances. But not all polyunsaturated oils are the same, as we shall find later. Two of them, linoleic and linolenic fatty acids, are *essential* for humans since we can't make them by our own metabolism and must take them in our food.

Other factors influencing the pre-cancerous change

We know that the membrane that surrounds the nucleus of a cell has protective potassium ions in it, while outside, in the fluids of the body, there are sodium ions. If the ratio of potassium inside the cell to sodium outside the cell is upset, the electron flow and magnetic fields may change. What the loss of this charge means basically is that the antioxidant properties of the free radical scavengers in the cell membrane may no longer protect the cell from damage. A leaky membrane can let in foreign particles, such as toxins and viruses that travel in via protein molecules and damage the inner working of the cell.

Free radicals

Free radicals are unpaired oxygen electrons occurring from substances with a molecular structure that has been damaged. These free electrons attempt to stabilise themselves very reactively by linking with another free oxygen electron from another molecule, so damaging it and generating another free radical, and so on in a chain reaction that is extremely destructive to cell metabolism. Free radical cascades are the basis of many, if not all, degenerative diseases.

Essential Fatty Acids

Essential Fatty Acids (EFAs) are the initial substances necessary to start the conversion of oxygen in the atmosphere to the energy factor of every living cell.

Say: *I give myself a pat on the back.*

When we breathe in air it is the EFA in the cell membranes of each tiny lung alveovus that attracts, captures and transports oxygen *in* and carbon dioxide *out* of the body. It is the EFA that carries the oxygen through the red blood-cell wall and helps it combine with the iron-containing 'heme' to form the oxygen carrier, 'haemoglobin' in our red blood.

Other essential substances in these transactions are vitamins A, C and E and the trace elements selenium and, probably, germanium. In fact it is the *oxygen-holding capacity* of the cell membrane with these substances in it that protects the working mechanism of the cell from invasion by disease-causing bacteria, viruses and fungi. They cannot live in the presence of oxygen.

The cell membrane

One to 2 per cent of each cell in the body consists of cell membrane, through which all transactions take place. It is composed of two EFA layers combined with amino-acids—phosphatide, loosely connected to allow essential vitamins to intersperse through these two (see diagram in the colour section). The electromagnetic field engendered here creates a negative charge on the outer surface of the cell which repels invaders. Changing the electric charge may change the permeability of the membrane.

Unfortunately, in countries where fast food is common, EFAs are very often denatured by heat and chemicals during the extraction process. They do not carry a repelling charge. Why and how does this happen?

EFAs are able to form a loose bond with the sulphur-containing amino acids. These combine because they can resonate at the same vibration as double bonds of cold-pressed oils containing the right EFAs, thus releasing energy to form an electron cloud which can flow along the fatty acid chain. Oils extracted by modern methods, with superheated steam and chemicals, do not have the right vibrations.

It is this electrical flow that we can sense or feel in heart beat, nerve signals, muscle contractions and all electro-chemical transactions in the living body. It is also this flow that keeps the cell cycle of replication and growth in order by taking part in the *contact inhibition* properties of a cell.

Contact inhibition

We have now learned to measure the electrical output of the heart (ECG), the brain (EEG), the muscles, nerves and so on. One of the newest and most exciting techniques is at the very cell face, monitoring the cell membrane potential and the magnetic field electrons with Nuclear Magnetic Resonance now performed by computer and called Magnetic Resonance Imaging. Electrons are discharged haphazardly unless there is a magnetic field to direct them.

Contact inhibition means that cells don't clump together. When cells have contact inhibition there is some separateness of their membranes, with channels that allow ions and small molecules to pass between them.

When cells lose this capacity to separate they can then clump together so the electrical flow is lost, oxygen cannot enter the cell and cell respiration is upset. The *contact inhibition of normal cells controls overgrowth*, but it can be overcome by many external factors.

Harry Rubin, a cytologist at the University of California, Berkeley, has shown that *cells infected with a* **cancer virus** *will lose their contact inhibition, change appearance, lose conformation and grow on top of each other instead of in a single layer. He used viruses known to cause cancer in animals for his research.*

Cell cycles, the replication cycles of each cell, occur at different rates in each kind of tissue and take place in definite phases. These phases are governed by external as well as internal factors. Whatever factors cause clumping of cells can also promote cancerous overgrowth. First the controlling contact inhibition of the cell has ceased. This decreases its oxygen source and starts the cell on its abnormal reproduction cycle which leads to cancer. There is much evidence that variations in the ion exchange, that is the electrical flow, of the cell's external environment can dictate cell cycles. The cell membrane is not just a wall or a skin. It is an active, responsive, communication system whose changes can be passed on into the interior of the cell. The membrane potential is vital to cell health.

Say: *I am an interesting and helpful person.*

The ongoing work of Dr Caroline Mountford

In September 1991 there was a documentary on *Quantum* the ABCTV program, discussing the work of a young medico at Sydney University, Dr Caroline Mountford. She has been studying the profiles of cell membrane components and their electrical activity for nine years now. Having been refused grants by the government-run National Health and Medical Research Council, she has now received funding from the USA and Germany.

She is particularly interested in the way the fats in the cell membrane behave and especially in the activity of the triglycerides, which are the oily substances formed in the transition of sugars into fatty acids.

She has found that cancer cells develop a sugar, *fucose*, on the cell membrane. It can be identified by magnetic resonance imaging and so can be used in diagnosing even the most minute cancerous change in a tissue. Her work has been verified by other doctors at the Royal Prince Alfred Hospital in Sydney and also by Dr Ian Smith of the National Research Council, University of Canada, Vancouver.

'You can't do experiments on dead cells', Dr Mountford says. She describes swirling spheres of triglycerides in the live cell membrane of cancerous cells apparent on magnetic resonance imaging. Though this may be heresy to the conventional pathologists, who diagnose cancer by dead cell histology at the moment, in years to come it will be the usual and best non-invasive method of discovering cancer in the body.

Research into Essential Fatty Acids (EFAs)

Many researchers, biochemists, physicists and others have studied the cell, each adding a part to the jigsaw.

Much work was done by German scientists, Liebig, in 1842, Pflueger, in 1872 and Hoppe-Seyler in 1876, who showed that oxygen usage in the body was dependent on oils and proteins in the food. In 1858 Lebedow found that starved dogs fed a high *protein* diet *or* a high *fat* diet alone very quickly died. Yet when 'good' fat and 'good' protein were fed together the dogs quickly recovered. The 'good' fat was flax seed oil; the 'bad' ones were animal fats. Rosenfeld, in 1899, showed that eating animal fats caused obesity and fatty degeneration of the liver, and his further work in 1902 found that high carbohydrate diets, with either low or high protein, did the same. To his surprise he found that not all fats caused obesity. At that time, however, there were no techniques to discover and separate the chemical structure of fats and oils.

This also hampered the work of Thumberg in 1911, Meyerhof in 1920 and Szent-Gyorgy in 1924. These great chemical researchers all worked on the properties of linoleic EFA and the oxygen-carrying capacity of sulphur-containing amino acids. Another Nobel prize winner in the field was Otto Warburg who, in 1926, found that *oxygen inhibited cancer growth*. Although he studied many oils, he looked in vain for the right ones he knew must be involved.

Interest in the question waned and it was not until Dr Johanna Budwig took up the challenge that great progress and practical application was made.

The discoveries of Udo Erasmus and Johanna Budwig

In 1987, after an exciting week at the Cancer Control Society Seminar in the Los Angelos Ambassador Hotel, Lorraine Rosenthal had arranged a special meeting for doctors, researchers and other cancer therapists.

We each gave a round-the-table introduction of our interests. It was such a gathering of eager, enquiring and well-informed minds that Norman Fritz and Gar Hildebrand (the chairpeople who ran it) had trouble keeping order among the many speakers in lively discussions.

A tall, fair young man took our attention. He passed around samples of a special oil he was sponsoring and held up a book he had recently written which he proceeded to explain.

This was Udo Erasmus BSc, MA, MS, PhD, educator, counsellor, consultant and author of what I consider to be the definitive work in English in its field, *Fats and Oils**. His teacher and mentor for

---

* Alive Books, P.O. Box 67333, Vancouver, Canada, 1986.

Say: *I am kind and loving.*

this subject was German researcher Dr Johanna Budwig, whose many published papers are in German.

My mother, who kept up with the latest work in many fields, told me in 1974 about Cis and Trans—fatty acids in commercially made products that were damaging our food supply. She was at that time fighting the National Heart Foundation's edicts about the efficacy of margarine through her writing in the press. Much to her disgust, I continued to use margarine for some years but, as a concession to her ideas, I took wheatgerm and vitamin E to counteract the ill effects of the trans fatty acids in margarine. Later I learned by my reading that she was right.

Dr Erasmus has this to say about his teacher:

> Although her doctorate is in physics, Dr Johanna Budwig of West Germany also has a vast knowledge and understanding of chemistry, biochemistry, pharmacology and medicine. This broad base of knowledge, coupled with her ability to conduct meticulous, painstaking work in the pursuit of answers, has enabled her to break new ground in the understanding of the link between oils and proteins. Among the breakthroughs made by Dr Budwig are analysis techniques that are so sensitive that the fatty substances in a single drop of blood can be identified. Using these techniques, Dr Budwig systematically analysed thousands of blood samples from sick and healthy people. She found that the blood samples from many people with a variety of problems were characteristically deficient in linoleic acid. Substances made up partically of linoleic acid—phosphatides and certain lipoproteins were also absent.
>
> Dr Budwig also found the presence of a yellow-green protein substance in the blood of the diseased individuals, and the lipoprotein used to make haemoglobin was missing, resulting in anaemia. To Dr Budwig this provided two explanations of the lack of vitality associated with so many disease states. Oxidation, a part of the respiration process which produces the energy used by our bodies, depends on both oxygen and linoleic acid. If haemoglobin levels are low, there will not be sufficient oxygen. Because linoleic acid plays a vital part in many energy functions and is also used in the creation of haemoglobin, if there isn't enough of it, energy production will decrease.
>
> In every instance, it appeared to Dr Budwig that a number of conditions involved a deficiency of EFAs. She reasoned that if a

problem is even partially caused by an E.F.A. deficiency, perhaps a diet rich in linoleic and linolenic acid could relieve some of the symptoms.

Using her knowledge of the inter-relationship of oil and protein, Dr Budwig fed patients a mixture of skim-milk protein and fresh flaxseed oil. The skim-milk protein is a rich source of sulphur-containing proteins, and flaxseed oil is the richest source of essential fatty acids. She then monitored the resulting changes in the patient's blood.

Her findings were dramatic. The yellow-green pigment slowly disappeared, to be replaced by increased haemaglobin; phosphatide and lipoprotein, anaemia was alleviated and vitality increased.

After making this breakthrough, Dr Budwig continued to explore other aspects of the oil-protein relationship. She discovered that the lipoproteins of the active body tissues (the liver, brain, glands, etc) always contain highly unsaturated fatty acids and sulphur-rich proteins. She also demonstrated that many drugs, such as barbiturates, sleeping pills and painkillers, break the natural association between oil and protein.

The toxic fatty substances she discovered are formed during the hydrogenation process, which is used in the manufacture of margarine and shortening. This seemed to implicate the commercial fats and oils industry, and these companies viewed her work as a threat to their livelihood. When she refused to suppress information showing the dangers of commercial oil processing, she lost the laboratory facilities she was working with and the fat research journals refused to publish her findings.

Because Dr Budwig found her attempts to further her research being thwarted, she decided to open her own health practice. She later stated, 'This is the best thing that could have happened. It forced me to apply my theoretically sound knowledge practically, on humans, on the cases doctors had given up as hopeless.' Dr Budwig has written several books detailing the cases she has treated successfully.

The basis of her treatment is the oil-protein combination she developed, made up of skim-milk cottage cheese and fresh-pressed

Say: | *I have good advice to give others—through my experience.*

flaxseed oil. She also includes carrots (for their carotene content), whole grains, nuts, and some herbs, along with fish high in the Omega-3 fatty acids.

So now you see why cold-pressed linseed and safflower oils are part of my food plan and why hard animal fats and cooked oils of any sort are not.

Lecithin

Lecithin, a very useful substance which is part of every cell contains choline, inositol, EFAs and phosphatides. It is an essential ingredient of the human body, with many uses. Of the brain, 37 per cent of the white matter and 47 per cent of the grey matter is made of this substance. It keeps cholesterol soluble so that it cannot collect in the arteries as plaque, to cause arteriosclerosis. It has strong emulsifying properties so it can dissolve gall stones and kidney stones if taken over a long period. It helps the liver to detoxify toxic products of metabolism, and the choline it contains is essential for the proper functioning of the liver. Dogs fed a diet deficient in choline develop cancer.

Soya bean lecithin contains both essential fatty acids Omega 3 and Omega 6, but lately commercial interests are breeding hybrids that contain fewer EFAs and more saturated fat so they will have a longer shelf life without going rancid.

Lecithin is the fat emulsifyer in bile. It breaks the food fats down into more easily digested particles. Most importantly, it keeps the cell membrane pliable, allowing the electrons to flow.

I use it successfully as a supplement in my treatment of psoriasis and arthritis and in the 'High B' breakfast in general. It is especially important for cancer patients and is part of the breakfast mash in the Survival Plan.

The dangerous lipid peroxyl radical is quenched by vitamin E, probably in conjunction with A, while the water-soluble free radicals are inactivated by vitamin C. All work together for protection of the cell. Various studies have shown that cancer is more prevalent in people deficient in these antioxidant vitamins. This is why they and the essential fatty acids are part of my program of supplements which improve the nutritional status.

Studies in other disciplines have shown that almost all modern fast-food and long-shelf-life, pre-packaged food diets are deficient in many nutrients. It is difficult to choose food that has been grown on soil free of artificial fertilisers, pre-emergent sprays, insecticides and pesticides, but we must search diligently for food that is not laced with chemicals of one sort or another.

More people are becoming aware of food values now and are asking questions, demanding full disclosure of the contents of processed foods and choosing more carefully.

Adrenal overaction and stress

Adrenal overaction can deplete nutrients and therefore add to the burden of stressed cells. The adrenals are our stress glands, our survival glands, which monitor the 'flight or fight' reaction. If we could not have altered our metabolism to flee from a dinosaur or fight a foe, we would not have survived. To do this, the adrenal hormones are made within a few seconds of a crisis occurring. They are poured into the bloodstream so that the heart beats faster, the breathing increases, the muscles tremble ready for action, the pupils dilate and the emotions quicken. All other unnecessary action and use of nutrients stops to give survival hormones first priority.

This reaction can take place even if the crisis is not life threatening. Fear and anger will call forth these changes, but so will anxiety, depression, resentment, irritability and many other lesser emotions. If the process goes on in a chronic fashion, then the adrenals will continue to have first priority for the nutrients coming into the body and other essential mechanisms, such as immune system defences and proper digestion, will be left short of nutrients and 'run down'. We all know how being depressed and 'overdoing it' can lead to the common descriptions of feeling 'washed out', being 'run down' or 'burnt out' and catching everything. 'The surly bird catches the germ', as someone said! If it goes on long enough, it can also lead to cancer.

The adrenals use up many of the nutrients that other cells need— cells of the immune system for instance, which should be making antibodies against cancer for cells of the target areas. All these

Say: *I forgive others and they forgive me.*

need vitamins A, C, E, selenium, magnesium and potassium. These are some of the substances also needed for making adrenal hormones.

Case Comment: 'Little Dorothy'

I think of our classic survivor, 'little Dorothy', now aged 85 years. She had cancer (lymphoma) first in 1952, when she and her husband Joe suffered a financial setback after years of hard work. They overcame this and Dorothy recovered. One by one all of their seven children left home. Then, in 1981, Joe died suddenly. They had been an inseparable couple, working side by side through many hardships. Though cherished by her absent family, Dorothy lived alone to mourn her mate, feeling depressed and sleeping and eating poorly.

Within eighteen months Dorothy's lymphoma returned. Her daughter came down from the country to bring her to our support group—she was too depressed to come on her own at first. Learning to eat better, overcoming shyness, making new friends, taking the supplements, participating in prayers and meditation and having some radiation—all worked together to raise her spirits and her healing energy again. She is over her cancer again and comes to the group each week to help others by her experience. She is not a shy little wallflower now, either, telling us about the new clothes she loves to sew and the exploits of her twenty-seven great grandchildren.

So no matter what your age, old cells can regenerate to make good new ones; that is another lesson from little Dorothy. During our life span, all the cells in our body die and grow again a set number of times and at different rates, depending on their tissue type. For instance, a cut on the face heals twice as fast as a cut on the foot; the broken bone of a child heals twice as fast as a fracture of the same bone in an adult; red blood cells will be replaced every 120 days; regeneration of nerve cells may take from three to six months.

Free radical damage makes cells grow at the wrong rate, causing aging or death of cells which can then be replaced by scar cells, improperly formed cells or cancerous cells.

Radiation and chemotherapy cause vast showers of free radicals, which may kill the cancer cells but can also cause damage to good cells if they are not protected by ample supplies of antioxidant protective supplements such as vitamins A, C and E, beta carotene, selenium or coenzyme Q10. My patients take these supplements regularly, but particularly before, during and after radiation or chemotherapy, both to protect themselves and to enhance the effect of these treatments.

Say: *I handle all problems successfully.*

16 HOW DO STRESSED CELLS BECOME CANCEROUS?

Free radical damage may go on for years in the *initiating* stage of cancer development before another change, the *precipitating* or trigger factor comes into play to start the nuclear growth factor running out of control. Some researchers into the physiology of the genes that make up nuclear D.N.A. have found the very ones whose damage has initiated this cancerous change. The extremely complicated study of *oncogenes* is still going on amidst controversy about the meaning of the thousands of facts that have been discovered.

Varmus, Bishop and retroviruses

The Nobel Prize in Physiology and Medicine for 1989 was shared by scientists J. Michael Bishop and Harold E. Varmus of the University of California. They were awarded the prize for the discovery that *retroviral oncogenes* are derived from similar genes in normal cells. These 'cellular oncogenes' are the ones concerned in the cell growth pattern of the cell. The change from a normal program of growth to an out-of-control pattern starts by damage to one or more of these genes. It is probably damage to the growth-patterning genes that makes them into 'oncogenes'. Damage can be caused by the factors described in the section on 'what causes stressed cells?' on page 155.

More than sixty oncogenes which can result from damage to human DNA in the initiating stage, have been described so far. These do not *cause* cancer, but they can be precursors if a precipitating factor or trigger activates the oncogene to an abnormal growth pattern subsequently.

Bishop and Varmus discovered that *viruses* (retroviruses) *inside*

the nucleus of a cell can activate the oncogene. This could be the
final step in the explanation of the cancerous change.

It was the study of the genes of the cancer-causing virus that
Peyton Rous found in chickens in 1911 (see page 206) that led
Bishop and Varmus to further research. It was known that this virus
contained a gene which was necessary for tumour development but
not for viral replication. This means that the virus could not reproduce
itself without using the growth program of the cell nucleus that
harboured it. To make the cell growth faster, the virus needed to
stimulate the host cell's own growth gene. In 1976, Bishop and
Varmus, with D. Stehelin and P. Vogt, found that one gene of the
cell nucleus was practically identical to the viral gene. They found
that the retrovirus had picked up and modified a normal cellular
gene and turned it into a potent viral oncogene, a growth stimulator.
Since then it has been shown that viral oncogenes of other retroviruses
also have cellular counterparts.

It was the study of tumour viruses that led to the discovery of
cellular oncogenes. But what went before this? It has been *known*
that viruses cause cancer since the late nineteenth century.

Other researchers
Professor Antoine Bechamp

Professor Bechamp (1816-1908) called the cancer-causing
organisms 'microzyma' in his monumental papers of the 1860s. He
believed these particles were the essence of all life.

Hundreds of other scientists have studied cancer-causing viruses.
As mentioned before, the work most often studied was that of Peyton
Rous of the Rockefeller Institute who, in 1911, demonstrated that
Mareks disease, a widespread sarcoma of chickens, was caused by
a virus. He was ignored because the warring factions of medical
opinion were (and still are) so divided about the cause of human
cancer that no one was concerned about chickens. Because of these
differences, Rous did not receive recognition for his discovery until
1966, when he was awarded the Nobel Prize, two years before his
death.

Say: | *I help others and they help me.* |

Surely no one can now gainsay the painstaking scientific research of so many other notable virologists and bacteriologists. Here are just a few whose work has shown to me beyond any reasonable doubt that *the final precipitating over-growth factor in the oncogene is caused by a virus or by a pleomorphic organism in its 'viral' form;* that is, in a form so small that it will pass through a Seitz filter and also a cell membrane when it is damaged.

Louis Pasteur

In the 1870s Louis Pasteur won a battle in the infant science of microbiology. He considered that microbes were the cause of all diseases; that each disease was caused by an unchanging organism. He and Bechamp fought bitterly over their beliefs, both of which had value but neither, we now know, could be generalisations.

When lethal vitamin deficiencies were studied in the 1920s, the focus of science changed and another facet of disease took the heat out of both arguments. Many hundreds of scientists and others have added facts since then that will help us to see the whole picture more clearly.

Professor Hans Selye

In what he called 'General Adaptation Syndrome', Selye described the interactions of the pituitary, adrenal, thymus, lymphatic and gastrointestinal functions with the immune system. In his classic books *Stress of Life* and *Stress without Distress*, he wrote that many diseases result from *conditioning factors* that may go on for years, culminating in a final *precipitating factor* or *stress* that results in the clinical manifestation. He discusses the stresses as physical, nutritional and emotional.

So much research shows this: *in a healthy body, in a healthy environment, cancer cannot grow*.

Hippocrates

As far back as Hippocrates, the famous physician of 500 BC, clinicians had noted that only those who were susceptible contracted certain diseases. Selye dissected the holistic factors that pull down our defences to make us susceptible to infections and other ills, particularly implicating disturbed adrenal reactions and exhaustion of endocrine systems. *Alarm, adaptation* and *exhaustion* are the three stages he recognised and described in conjunction with physical findings. He described how cellular response to multiple stresses mirrored our ability to withstand pathological changes in common organisms, and how keeping the body in the best possible condition will put us in harmony with the multiple environmental factors that could otherwise cause disease.

René Dubos

Dubos, a leading microbiologist of the Rockefeller Institute, summarises: 'In the body of normal individuals, under usual conditions, ubiquitous microbes do not cause any trouble but *persist in a latent form*. But they can be bought into a state of activity and thus become a cause of disease when some disturbance occurs to upset the equilibrium.'

Dubos, who was born in France in 1901, had suffered in his youth from two environmentaly moulding forces which directed the course of his life—typhoid and rheumatic fever. Being unable to follow a physically active career, he first distinguished himself in studies of soil microorganisms in agriculture. In 1927 he joined the Rockefeller Institute in America where, over the next forty years, he made many important discoveries in microbiology, including the first clinically useful antibiotic. His ecological philosophy developed from his childhood walks in the French countryside into his study of organisms in relation to their environment. He proved many times that the important element in disease is not the infection but the external or internal stresses that alter resistance.

Dubos found that organisms could change their shape and their performance of such functions as enzyme production as an adaptive response to their nutritional needs. In his PhD work he demonstrated that environmental characteristics such as pH, moisture, oxygen availability and surrounding chemicals determine which microbes grow and what activities they perform. He believed that this principle applied to viruses, germs, people and nations. 'Each one of us is born with the potentiality to become several different persons', he said, 'but what we actually become depends upon the conditions

Say: | *I carry out the plans I make.* |

under which we develop. These conditions, furthermore, are often largely of our own choosing.'

Through the tragic death of his first wife in 1942 from tuberculosis, René Dubos questioned Pasteur's 'one germ, one disease theory. After a lifetime of research he concluded that 'microbial disease is the exception rather than the rule. Why do pathogens so often fail to cause disease after they have become established in the tissues?' He discovered that germs such as tuberculosis had forms and strains that caused disease and forms and strains that did not. He standardised the weak strain of non-infectious tuberculosis called 'Bacillus Calmitte-Guérin' (BCG) giving the whole world a way of *preventing* disease. He was a lively, persuasive and imaginative genius in the pioneering of immunology and cell chemistry.

It is not necessary here to précis the history of microbiology over the last 150 years. There have been so very many concepts and hypotheses and so much has been discovered by intuitive and dedicated workers, then lost and rediscovered in the context of new evidence. Each is a step towards understanding the miraculous intricacies of nature and the human species.

A revolutionary discovery that caused a furore of anger and rejection in the medical world may later be accepted. A hypothesis may become common knowledge, while the one who dies in proving it is very often forgotten. So it is with the germs, the viruses, filtrationists and antifiltrationists, pleomorphic (many forms) organisms and the 'one germ—one disease' theories of bacteriology.

17 THE ROLE OF PLEOMORPHIC ORGANISMS

Pleomorphic organisms need some explanation, since they have at last been recognised, though mostly ignored, by clinical bacteriologists. Pleomorphic organisms have two or more definite forms during a life cycle. Very often they have a form in which they lose everything but their genetic material. They are then called 'Pleuro-pneumonia-like organisms' (PPLOs), 'L' forms or 'cell-wall-deficient organisms' (CWDOs). Many have complicated life cycles with oxygen-dependent (aerobic) and anaerobic forms. Because of these variable qualities, culturing and staining is difficult and classification is a nightmare. This is probably why most laboratories will not take the time or the trouble to undertake the slow and meticulous job of growing them for study.

Lida Mattman

The recognition of CWDOs, even though grudging, by modern pathologists has been largely due to the dedicated investigations and teaching of Lida Mattman. Though retired, she still holds classes in microbiology at Wayne State University, where she held a professorial chair for many years. In her untiring work on the TB microbe, she uncovered its life cycle, showing that bacteria can develop forms as small as viruses (CWDOs) or as large as red blood cells (the largest cell structures). The acid-fast stain she devised is very valuable in identifying these forms. So it is also with the cancer microbe. Let us hope that some of her pupils will carry on her work without the fear of ridicule and ostracism that silences many (see page 231).

174 *Heal Cancer*

Forms of the cancer microbe as seen by some researchers

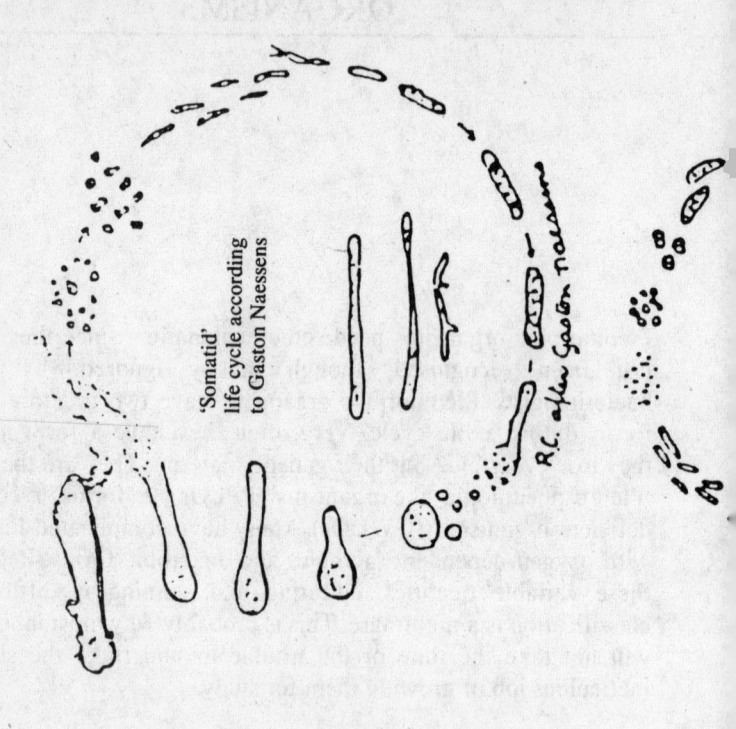

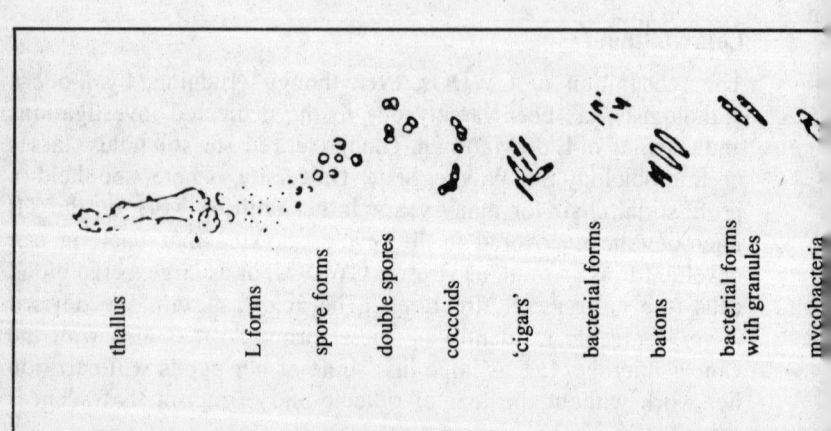

'Somatid' life cycle according to Gaston Naessens

R.C. after Gaston Naessens

thallus | L forms | spore forms | double spores | coccoids | 'cigars' | bacterial forms | batons | bacterial forms with granules | mycobacteria

The Role of Pleomorphic Organisms 175

The cancer microbe according to Tom Deakin and T. J. Glover

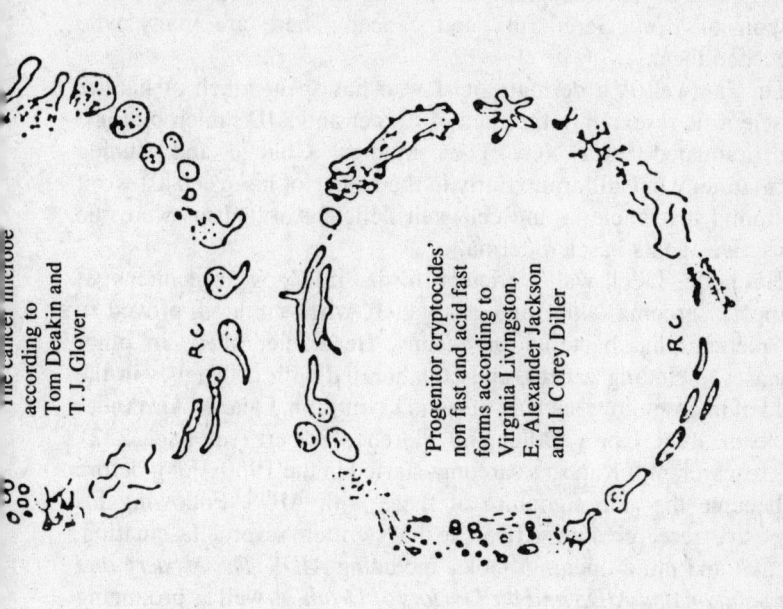

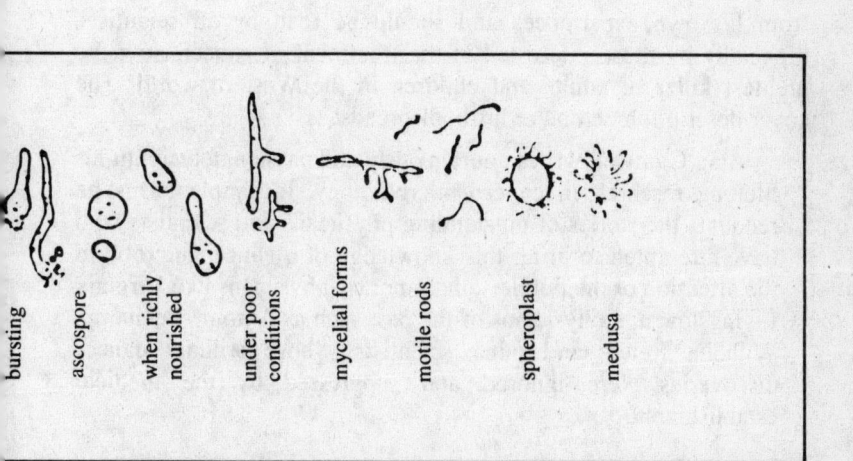

'Progenitor cryptocides' non fast and acid fast forms according to Virginia Livingston, E. Alexander Jackson and I. Corey Diller

bursting

ascospore

when richly nourished

under poor conditions

mycelial forms

motile rods

spheroplast

medusa

Alan Cantwell

Doctor Alan Cantwell MD (1934–) has been another researcher who gained from her teaching in studying the pleomorphic microbes responsible for scleroderma and cancer. There are many who preceded them.

Dr Cantwell is a dermatologist who has spent much of his life in scientific research in the field of cancer and AIDS microbiology. He graduated from New York Medical College and studied dermatology in California. Early in the course of his specialist work he found that bacteria and cell-wall deficient organisms were the causative agents in scleroderma.

He noticed cell-wall deficient forms in biopsy specimens of Kaposi's sarcoma (skin tumours) which, when cultured, proved to be pleomorphic bacterial organisms. He studied these in other diseases, including cancer, and collaborated with colleagues in the field of microbiology such as Virginia Livingston, Eleanor Alexander Jackson, Irene Corey Diller and Florence Seibert (see page 222). His research into Kaposi's sarcoma started in the 1960s, long before it became the skin signature of those with AIDS. Following his intensive research into AIDS, he has written several fascinating, factual and mind-opening books, including *AIDS, The Mystery and the Solution* and *AIDS and the Doctors of Death*, as well as producing over thirty published papers on cancer and other immune-deficiency diseases. His revolutionary book, *The Cancer Microbe*, is written from his own experiences and should be read by all scientists, especially by those interested in the treatment of cancer, now the greatest killer of adults and children in the Western world. The cover description on one of his books reads:

> 'Alan Cantwell writes courageously and passionately about his lifelong research in cancer microbiology. In simple terms he recounts the stories of outstanding physicians and scientists who have attempted to bring this knowledge of a cancer microbe to the attention of the public: contemporary physicians like Virginia Livingston; and physicians of the past such as Antoine Bechamp, Wilhelm Reich, and other scientists, whose brilliant cancer discoveries were ignored and suppressed by the medical establishment.'

Clara Fonti

Clara Fonti of Italy also found specific organisms in all cancer tissues. She developed a method of culturing organisms from the blood of cancer patients on broth and beef extracts. She grew organisms *only from the blood of cancer patients*, whereas the blood and tissue of healthy individuals and of those with other diseases was negative for that organism. Over a long lifetime, she developed two specific strains of the cancer organism and recognised differences in the organisms obtained from sarcomas and epithelial tissue. Fonti wrote a fascinating book, *Etiopatogenese del Cancro* (The Etiology of Cancer). A review of her book by Dr Virginia Livingston includes the following:

> The first chapters discuss the evidence for the parasitic theory of cancer. This is followed by a chapter on transmissibility of cancer, with citation of some thirty cases, observed during the author's clinical practice, of apparent direct transmission from one individual to another, either by contact or close association. Analysis of the data is presented in tables showing tumour types, duration of contact, previous illnesses and survival after exposure. To further explore transmissibility, this intrepid investigator inoculated herself in the chest wall with fluid from a metastasising mammary carcinoma. After a few days there developed an erythematous papillary eruption between her breasts. Gradually a nut-sized lesion formed in the left breast with numerous small ancillary papules. Three different histological examinations of tissue taken from these lesions in different laboratories proved them to be baso-cellular epithelioma (cancers). Photographs of the tissues are given in the book. Over a period of several months the neoplasms regressed. The author's blood, presumably containing antibodies, was transfused to a patient with multiple abdominal metastases, resulting in an amelioration of the patient's condition.
>
> The author discusses numerous clinical observations that led her to hypothesise that the blood is the carrier of a specific organism that is the causative agent of cancer. Her first attempts were to discover culture techniques which would grow the agent and demonstrate it by means of staining reagents. These formulae are given in detail in the text.

18 EARLY VACCINE MAKERS

William Mervyn Crofton

Crofton was born in Dublin in 1905 and was at one time a lecturer in special pathology at the National University of Dublin. Later, in private practice in London, he came to believe that cancer was caused by a pleomorphic organism. He saved the lives of many by using therapeutic *immunisation with the patient's own autogenous vaccines*, made from killed microbes of cancer tissue, to prevent and cure diseases including cancer. He also isolated a specific microbe from all cancer tissues. His colleagues ignored his work. When he was ninety years of age the British Government made him an honorary director of the Crofton Leukaemia Trust of Northern Ireland, faint recognition for his lifetime of work in the field.

E. Villequez

While I was staying with Dr Virginia Livingston she gave me permission to study one of her most treasured books. It is a most descriptive document of the cancer organism: *Le Parasitisme latent des cellules du sang chez l'homme, en particulier dans le sang des cancereux* by E. Villequez. (Libraire Maloine, Paris 1955). This French/Spanish researcher worked at the University of Dijon and in the 1950s studied the cancer organism in blood extensively by dark-field examination. He exchanged cultures of the organism with Dr Irene Corey Diller and other researchers in Germany and Italy. His information coincides with theirs, but with his time-lapse photographs he was able to trace the development of pleomorphic organisms: 'microbacillus,' the L forms, in the blood cells of cancer patients to the bacillary, coccoid, mycelial and spore forms. (See pages 174–5.)

Dr William Russell

Russell was a Scottish pathologist who in the 1890s demonstrated specific germs occurring in all cancer tissue. He defined certain particles he called 'Russell bodies' which have been noticed by many other workers and have never been explained. They are suspected of being one of the pleomorphic forms discussed by Villequez (see Dr Livingston's Compendium, page 396).

Dr James Scott

Scott was a Scottish obstetrician who came to New York in 1921 to seek treatment from Dr John Glover. He was an outstanding surgeon in St James hospital, Butte, Montana, at the time. He was enthralled by the cancer organism Glover was using for vaccines and serum. He worked with Dr Glover and finally left his surgical career to study and use anticancer serum.

Dr T. J. Glover

Glover spent many years isolating and growing organisms from thousands of cancer patients to make serum. To make this he injected the culture into horses, in the same way as antitetanus serum is made. He and his assistant, Tom Deaken, were able to induce verified cancer remissions in many of the people who used this serum subcutaneously for two years. The antiserum, when given to cancer patients, resulted in decreased toxicity of the cancer; the change of a thick, foul discharge to a thin, clear one; reduction of the tumour mass; and, in many of the less advanced cases, complete remission of the tumour. After publishing 'The Bacteriology of Cancer' in the *Canada Lancet and Practitioner* in 1930, Glover retired under a barrage of disfavour from the medical world. James Scott took up the fight to press for recognition of this cancer treatment and spent the rest of his life in unsuccessful attempts to teach his colleagues about Glover's serum.

Wilhelm von Brehmer

In the 1930s a German scientist, Wilhelm von Brehmer, repeatedly demonstrated a wide range of stages in the life cycle of a pleomorphic

Say: *Today is a day of great good fortune.*

organism he isolated from cancerous tissue. He called it 'syphonospora polymorpha'. In 1934 von Brehmer described this organism at a new species he had isolated from human blood. He detailed its possible relation to tumour genesis. After many years of study of the organism, he was led to believe that he had discovered the long-sought *Grundkrank* or basic illness. His work had been interrupted by World War 2, but after 1946 he worked in a new research institute that was established in Berlin. Further investigation of the organism at that institute involved examination of focal infections of teeth and the possible relationship of subinfections to tumour production. Von Brehmer postulated that syphonospora becomes involved in the development of malignancy only when the pH of the blood becomes alkaline. (Some others think it is when the body becomes acid.)

Following this research, **Dr Joseph Issels** and **Dr Hans Neiper**, both working in Germany, insist that their cancer patients have all dead teeth removed (see page 118).

For many years von Brehmer conducted a clinic at Bad Kreuznach in Germany, where he treated patients by means of therapy based on these observations. Primarily, therapy involved treatment with the product of pooled cultures of 'syphonospora' isolated from different types of cancers. This product was known as 'Tozinal'. A marked feature of treatment was a dietary regime which von Brehmer believed could make the patient's blood more acid. This is similar to the program used by Dr Livingston, who was his pupil. He and his co-workers claimed marked improvement and some permanent remissions in patients so treated. Von Brehmer also made routine dark-field examinations of patient's blood.

Von Brehmer spent much of his life studying the organism he called syphonospora, elsewhere described as Mycobacterium, M. tumor faciens, M. avium, Coryne-bacterium, Somatids, Agens, Krebs virus, Microbacilli, Microzyma and Progenitor cryptocides, among other names. Many eminent researchers presented their work in this field at the Sixth International Congress of Microbiology in Rome in 1953 (see page 224).

Livingston's Compendium

Among the many reports about the association of bacteria with cancer, some of the best-documented papers and accounts from the following investigators are published in *The Compendium*, compiled by Dr Virginia Livingston: Crofton, Fonti, Gerlach, Inoue and Singer, Livingston (Wuerthele Caspe) Alexander-Jackson, W. and I.C. Diller, Mori and White, Mazet, Stearn, Villequez and von Brehmer. *The Compendium* (available from the Livingston Medical Clinic, 3232 Duke Street, San Diego, USA) lists a wealth of references to the scientific papers of these and other researchers into the cancer-causing organism from its earliest recognition. The many names given to the organism may seem confusing, but this is probably explained by its tendency to change to forms that mimic other bacteria, depending on the medium employed, the temperature, pH and other variables in culture methods. Though the stages described by Glover, von Brehmer, Villequez and Gerlach are similar to those described by Virginia Livingston and her co-workers, it seems unlikely that there is a fixed progression of stages, because direct microscopic examination and time-lapse photographs show transformation from one form to another at times, without intermediate stages.

Say: *I make good goals and I achieve them.*

19 WHY IS THERE SO MUCH DISSENTION IN RESEARCH?

In the early 1960s the district around the village of Heguri in Japan had the highest incidence of cancer in the country with one person in three dying of the disease. Dr Ki-ichiro Hasumi (see page 211) undertook the gigantic task of inoculating the whole village population every year for three years with his anticancer vaccine. The outcome made medical history: not one of those he injected developed cancer while nineteen of the control group did.

In spite of the conclusive nature of this classic epidemiological, immunological study, the medical profession paid it little or no heed. It was 'as a voice crying in the wilderness'. This was a time when radiation was very much in vogue and hailed as the saviour of humanity. The disastrous side effects of its indiscriminate use were then unknown. Other therapies were dropped or ignored in the rush to the one in favour. As when chemotherapy became fashionable, there is often violent controversy, not just among commercial interests but among the scientists themselves.

It is only human to disagree, and thinking scientists all through the ages have fought vehemently for their own particular ideas. Rigid thinking has in history led not only to ostracism and persecution, but also, from time to time, to martyrdom and death in the cause of proclaiming what a researcher discovered.

Antoine Bechamp disagreed violently with Louis Pasteur, Virchov with Robert Koch, Lida Mattman with Virginia Livingston—the list is endless, and rightly so. Without that vehement faith in their own goals, researchers could never continue to work.

In their psychological make-up, researchers have several attributes in common and it is these very characteristics that make it possible for them to devote their time, money and energy to pursuing the elusive proof of their beliefs:

- They have that conviction and desire to find the answer.
- They have a creative ability for new thought and ideas.
- They can pull apart and examine what they have observed.
- They can relate facts to each other and see a pattern emerging.
- They have the determination to go on believing what their 'gut feelings' and intuition (that is, the right brain) is telling them, in spite of opposition.
- They will test and retest with great tenacity to substantiate their hypotheses, for a lifetime if necessary.

Many, like Semmelweiss, Goldberger and Gye, to name just a few, have martyred themselves in causes that were never accepted until after they had died. Others gained from their knowledge.

It is that tenacity and faith in their own beliefs and theories that drives the researchers on, but it also makes it difficult for them to accept the beliefs of other researchers if they differ.

Belief that is too vehement or hope that is too fervent may become a left-brain interference that hampers the proper evaluation of results. It may also cause bitter dissention, hostility, anger, tension and depression, those negative robbers, that stultify any free thought in those who are opposed to change.

Innumerable research hours have been spent in understanding how cancer forms, how it interacts with the body and how it is reversed. To declare that we have no knowledge of these things simply demonstrates either ignorance of the work of our dedicated forerunners or plain fear of ridicule by the current orthodoxy in 'scientific thought'.

The cell discoveries of Emanuel Revici

At the 15th Annual Cancer Convention, arranged by Lorraine Rosenthal and her helpers of the Cancer Control Society, the man who was proclaimed 'Hero of the Year', Dr Emmanuel Revici, was due to speak with Dr Lawrence Taylor at 11.15 on Sunday, 5 July 1987. I was disappointed that Dr Revici, then 91 years old, was not able to attend through illness. Dr Taylor delivered Dr Revici's address 'Cycles in Cancer Treatment' for him. I had heard about

Say: *I choose to enjoy life NOW.*

the work of this Rumanian-born medical genius and pioneer, but knew little of his teaching, except that it involved the chemistry of the sterols and the essential fatty acids in the body.

Emmanuel Revici MD came to New York from Rumania in 1946. Though his continuing work in cell pathology has been recognised and used in Europe for forty years, he has never had any work accepted by American journals. One of his discoveries is an anti-bleeding agent, Hemostipticum Revici, used widely in Europe. He researched selenium in the 1950s while investigating the elements contained in mud, where he considered life started. His philosophy of opposites, the positive and negative energies inherent in all things, ties in with Chinese and other Asian traditions of Yin and Yang. He was the first researcher to understand and lecture on the free radical scavenging potential of *selenium* and its role in the health of the cell membrane, in the 1960s.

Revici had a broad overall concept of physiology which enabled him to see the *immune system competency and the needs of every cell as the basic factors in freedom from disease.*

Revici's medical work at his Institute of Applied Biology in New York covered a huge field. He turned his attention particularly to the chemistry of the nucleus, the cytoplasm and the cell membrane. He delved into the changes that can take place in the ratio of fatty acids to sterols, in health and disease, in a body defending itself against the attack of bacteria, viruses and toxins, both internal and external. He found that when the cell membrane loses its omega-3 fatty acids, it loses its repellent electrical charge.

He put his discoveries to work successfully for years in the treatment of addictions to narcotics, alcohol, tobacco and other drugs, as well as to the treatment of infections, cancer and later AIDS. Here was the old story. His products were not secret and they were available, but they were not cheap. He was not a threat to the drug firms and the medical establishment until he was successful in treating cancer. Then the publicity nettled his colleagues and, in spite of the testimony of over 2000 successfully treated patients at the Congressional Hearing, political pressures made physicians withdraw support from his clinic and the Food and Drug Administration did not pass his medications for testing. Revici uses adrenal gland extracts, selenium, and essential fatty acids in a careful balance of anabolism (building up) and catabolism (breaking down) of substances. As early as May, 1955, he gave a paper to his colleagues at Beth David Hospital, New York, entitled 'The Control of Cancer with Lipids'. His work followed on that of his predecessors, William Koch, John Glover, Max Gerson and others. He was also a contemporary of Dr Johanna Budwig and recognised her work.

Revici traced the development of cancer in the cell from the change of electrical potential at the cell wall, brought about when the lipids of the membrane are affected by stressors or toxins. This change causes the nucleus to lose its potassium shield so that viruses can enter. He further delved into the changes of ion and the base electrolytes—the pH of the intra- and extra-cellular fluid—and how this can be influenced by products of the cancer cells to cause pain. He has proved overall what others had hypothesised in a piecemeal fashion by this explanation of the mechanism of pathological change and how it can be turned around if only the therapy is instituted when cancer is still in the secondary, not the tertiary, stage.

In 'Control of Cancer with Lipids' he says:

> 'Pain due to local and/or alkaline changes may be relieved; the systemic changes may return to normal; vascular changes, especially bleeding, may be controlled; and finally the atypical growth of cells may be controlled or arrested. When all these effects are achieved, the malignant tumour can be regarded as having been returned to a phase of non-invasiveness.
>
> 'All of these changes have been observed following adequate lipid treatment. Moreover, in many cases significant diminution in the size of tumour masses and even their complete disappearance have been observed. Theoretically, such objective changes in the size of malignant neoplasms can be in part accounted for on the basis of alterations in cellular lipids, the body apparently having relatively ample means of defending itself against non-invasive cancer cells. One indication of this is the observation that so-called 'cancers-in-situ' have disappeared without any treatment.'

Revici is also careful to point out that the Revici method is not always successful.

Say: *I love the world—and the world loves me.*

He discovered that there are distinct physical changes in the body lipids (fats) with alpha beta, gamma and x-rays, and with hormones and chemotherapies. After a critical point is reached in administration of these, the waste products created by them cause irreversible changes in the lipids which, if more is given, will lead to death, not from cancer but from its supposed remedies.

Many recovered patients claim that his therapy with lipid and lipid-like agents has alleviated cancer and brought some into remission. It can work successfully in combination with radiation and chemotherapy, as the Cilento Survival Plan does, helping to maintain the immune system rather than to destroy it.

Revici is an old, frail man now, too old to fight any more. Unfortunately his centre was recently closed by the Food and Drug Administration. I am so glad he won an award from the Cancer Control Society. He sent a touching speech which was read by Dr Taylor on his behalf.

It was from Revici's work that I learned to put selenium and spleen extract, as well as Dr Budwig's cold-pressed flax (linseed) oil, into my program—with great success. His theories explain and bring together *all* other concepts.

Since we are on the subject of cell metabolism it is appropriate to discuss briefly the work of two professors whose astute observations and scientific skill paved the way for further understanding of the degenerative changes that cause disease.

Otto Warburg and William Koch

Professor Otto Warburg was the pioneer who developed methods of studying oxidation of tissues. His classic biochemical experiments established anoxia of the cell—the inhibition of cell respiration or, in other words, fermentation—as the basic change. This he called the 'Pasteur Effect', after the work of that supreme observer whose work on the chemistry of fermentation in wine opened doors in so many minds. In fact the work of Antoine Bechamp in this field was the basis of Pasteur's experiments and led the way for Otto Warburg, who received the Nobel prize twice in the 1930s for his investigations into the physiology and metabolism of cancer.

Another giant step was taken along the way in the work of William Koch MD, Professor of Physiology at Detroit Medical College, Wayne State University. His many papers and published works record the advances of our understanding of cancer up to 1958. His investigations were the first that showed the effect of free radicals in the jigsaw of cell destruction. He had intimate knowledge of the work of Glover, who described the cancer bacteria in such detail in 1923.

William Koch was trained as a biochemist and undertook original research into the function of the parathyroid gland. He received his BA in 1909, his MA in 1910, and a PhD in 1916 from the University of Michigan. He gained his MD from Detroit College of Medicine in 1918.

Through his vast knowledge of cell chemistry, he understood that the way to prevent cancer and stop the progress of the disease was to:

1 remove the poisons that caused cell damage;
2 capture and defuse the free radicals, which he found were the catalysts in the destructive process;
3 oxygenate the body cells in every way possible.

In fact, that is the recipe for curative *success* in every cancer therapy, whatever methods are used to reach these goals.

William Koch developed a synthetically produced carbonyl compound with high oxidation-reduction potential which he used very successfully as a therapeutic agent, not only in cancer but in many other diseases caused by poor oxidation in the body. He called his product 'Synthetic Survival Reagent' or SSR. Its chemistry and actions are described in detail in his book *The Survival Factor in Neoplastic and Viral Diseases*.

Given by a small injection, the carbonyl compound caused a chain reaction, under ideal conditions, which could destroy free radicals and allow the cells to reconstitute. It put many cases of cancer into remission. Medical therapists all over America started using SSR with excellent results. By 1940 the drug companies, especially ones making antipsychotics, had started a vendetta against him because SSR could also reverse dementia.

I will not go into the sordid history of his destruction by the

Say: | *The best in life is mine from today.*

usual means of discrediting and denigration by money- and power-hungry assailants, but his product is no longer made. Koch spent the rest of his life in Brazil where, rumour has it, he was murdered.

This clever and courageous man was a contemporary of Dr Max Gerson. They worked along the same lines and came to the same conclusions. In treatment, their management of cases was very similar. It reads as though William Koch corroborated in chemistry what Max Gerson had discovered by nutritional means in a more organ-based clinical method.

The therapy of Gerson, Budwig and Revici is absolutely based on three principles but, instead of using SSR, the detoxification, oxygenation and reconstruction is physically done by dietary means.

So far we have seen how the body manages environmental stresses, how the mind manages emotional stresses and how the cell membrane and the cell nucleus react. What about the actual body of the cell? How does that become part of the cancerous change? Or does it?

20 INTERNAL CELL DEFENCE, PEPTIDES OR ANTINEOPLASTONS

Since the 1960s intensive work has been going on in various research centres on the proteins that the body needs. First their chemistry was broken down to the amino acids they contain. Then these were found to be made up of molecules called 'peptides', forming part of the cytoplasm (body protein) of every cell. There are probably hundreds of these and they all have different characteristics and uses in the body.

Stanislaw Burzynski

The Polish microbiologist Stanislaw Burzynski took on the formidable task of separating the different ones for study. He started his research at thirteen years of age in his mother's kitchen and obtained his MD and PhD degrees while researching peptides in Poland. Reaching the USA in 1970, he was funded in further studies by the National Cancer Institute and Baylol Medical Research Institute. He continued his work in isolating over 116 peptides from the body of cells with a nucleus in the urine, blood and tissues. *Many of these peptides were concerned with the initiation and inhibition of cell growth.*

What Dr Burzynski discovered in 1967 was that our bodies can and do direct potential cancer cells back onto their normal path through 'messenger' peptides that bond to cancer cells, feeding them the complex information they need to normalise and fulfil their original functions.

These peptides, or 'antineoplastons' as Dr Burzynski has named them, are components of a separate biochemical defence system that is completely different from our immune system. Without this corrective system, asserts Dr Burzynski, we would soon succumb to the cancer-causing forces that are continually triggering abnormal cell development. His research indicates that cancer sufferers typically have a lower level of these peptides in their blood than healthy individuals.

Following the 1986 Nobel Prize for Burzynski's work on peptide growth factors, peptides have been regarded as exciting chemicals in the development of new medicines.

Each of the ten formulations of antineoplastons has been submitted to Phase 1 clinical trials and some to Phase 2. Results revealed that a majority of patients went into complete remission, partial remission or stabilisation of their cancer.

Stanislaw Burzynski is the author of 143 scientific publications, a presenter of scientific papers at major international conventions, and has been awarded nineteen patents covering sixteen countries for his antineoplaston treatment. Other groups have replicated and expanded his preclinical work, including researchers in London, Japan, Italy and China. Also, independent clinical studies with antineoplastons are being conducted with patients in Japan and Poland. Although treatment is expensive and, at present, hospital orientated, we will see more use of these substances in conjunction with surgery, chemotherapy and radiation for people with cancer in future.

The peptide defence system being so intensively studied in these universities undoubtedly comes from the protein in our food. But which proteins?

Some proteins produce the 'good' and some the 'bad' peptides, we could suppose. But it is some of our multiple enzymes which determine how much we make of what peptides? And is it the *lack* of some of these enzymes that determines the deficiencies of the protective ones, so causing a person to be 'cancer-prone'?

And these enzymes known to us already? Are they the non-specified substances that Edward Howell, William Kelley and others keep referring to when they talk about the 'live enzymes' in raw fruit and vegetables? If so, are these some of the good things apparent but not yet studied in the raw, fresh and unoxidised fruit and vegetable juice that is the basis of my program, the Gerson program, the Moerham therapy and so many others?

It is possible that the tribes who don't get cancer who live almost exclusively on animal products—like the Masai, Wurtana, Boran and the Inuit (Eskimo)—have a food chain that supplies the defending peptides already made in a simply assimilated form from the animal foods? Feed these people our western style foods and by the next generation they are just as cancer-prone as we are. Could it be that some of these peptides are the ones that keep the cancer organism in its cell-walled state or quiescent mode and stop it making growth hormone?

It would all tie together wouldn't it? We need so many more enthusiastic researchers to find out. These are the cancer answers we should be seeking. One person in three is now getting the disease, and half who get it still die from it. Is this ordained genocide? Can we do something about it?

Yes, we can. Hundreds of recovered people have proved it and not just in the few ways I've discovered here. But only those willing to run the gauntlet survive. Will you be one of them? Will future millenia term this the 'Age of Homo barbaricus technicus' and space invaders ponder how this whole species disappeared, leaving as much trace as one little polluted leaf fallen from the great Tree of Life?

Stages in cancer formation

Please study this connecting link before embarking on the next part of this journey.

Normal cells defend themselves by using the right nutrients to make double phospholipid protein membranes which don't let injurious substances through into the cell, by keeping a constant electrical charge and by destroying invaders with special vitamins and minerals.

The initiation stage of cancer
Stressed cells are made if defences fail.

Stressed cells have lost the vitamins, minerals and nutrients which protect them and their electrical charge. They have been invaded by toxic substances which get through their damaged membranes to deplete the working mechanism and alter the cell program.

Say: *Every day and every way I get stronger and healthier.*

Causes of stressed cell development are deficiency of necessary nutrients, contamination of food, air and water by toxins, escalation of cell stressors by radiation, toxic chemicals, drugs, hormone imbalances, chronic irritation, repeated trauma, invasion of germs, viruses, fungi or depletion by stressful emotional factors.

Alteration to stressed cells occurs to membranes by wrong fats, proteins and sugars, to the nucleus by the formation of abnormal DNA and genes (presently called oncogenes), to the body of the cell by altered or deficient peptide formation.

The precipitation stage of cancers

Damaged cell environment then allows for the entrance and interactions of the *cancer organism* in its harmful form. The DNA oncogenes may be reprogrammed now to make the growth hormone that initiates uncontrolled growth of the cell, making *cancer cells.*

Cancer cell membranes manufacture abnormal chemicals which help them to spread into normal tissue by damaging the connective tissue framework of the body, using up nutrients the body needs and making new blood vessels. Their chemicals cause destruction of tissue in many ways. DEFENCE SYSTEMS AGAINST CANCER depend on the health of the Immune System based in the liver, spleen, thymus, lymph glands, endocrine systems and brain. Toxins are excreted by the excretory systems of kidneys, liver, bowel, lungs and skin. The immune system has strong connections with the rest of the body, mind and spirit.

The Cilento Survival Plan intervenes in many of these areas to reverse the harmful changes.

21 THE CELL DIAGRAM

The initiating and precipitating stages of cancer formation

If you look at the cell diagram on the colour pages the discoveries about how cancer starts, which we have discussed, will become more apparent.

Briefly, in the first diagram of the cell, *the nucleus*—the computer or cell organiser—is intact and surrounded by potassium ions. The *cell membrane*, made of a lipid/protein combination, is also intact, containing ample protection by vitamins A, C and E and the trace mineral selenium, which works with vitamin E. There is a repellant electromagnetic charge on the cell surface and sodium ions are kept outside the cell. This is a *normal cell*—the membrane is selective, allowing in only what is needed for metabolism and letting out its manufactured or waste products.

In the second diagram, degenerative changes are starting. There is stress; adrenal hormones are robbing the cell of some of its potassium and vitamins A, C and E. This cell has lost its electromagnetic charge and is at risk of invasion. Sodium ions can make their way through the damaged, 'leaky' cell membrane and disrupt the working of the nucleus. This initiating stage, caused by the sequence discussed already, may last for years, causing impaired energy levels but no actual disease.

The precipitating or final stage, in which cancerous growth is usually triggered, happens between six months and two years *before* some symptom is noticed. It is thought that the known life cycle of the cancer organism reaches a stage of development at which it is capable of invading the nucleus. This is the stage at which it may make 'growth hormone' or gonadotrophin.

The changes making a normal cell into a stressed cell

Stage A

The *normal cell* has an exterior cell membrane protecting it from invasion by viruses, germs and chemical toxins.

It contains two layers of lipids with protective vitamins A and E and protein molecules attached to sugars (saccharides)

The cell body is made of cytoplasm containing defensive peptides, vitamin C and many other raw materials. The nuclear membrane, containing potassium, protects the nucleus—the genetic working centre of the cell, made up of DNA protein in forty-six chromosomes composed of hundreds of genes.

Each molecule of the cell carries an electric charge, collectively making tiny magnetic charges on the cell membrane which repel invaders by contact inhibition and allow only selected substances to enter the cell.

Stage B

1 The cell membrane loses vitamins A and E through stress.
2 The cell membrane is fed the wrong lipids.
3 The cell becomes deficient in vitamin C.
4 The nuclear membrane loses potassium.

Stage C

1 The electromagnetic charge is lost from cell membrane.
2 The contact inhibitor is lost.
3 Sodium and other molecules enter the cytoplasm through a leaky membrane.
4 The chromosomes start the cell's dividing cycle.

As a result:

- The cytoplasm loses defending peptides and enzymes.
- Sugars, lipids and protein molecules change.
- The oxygen/energy cycle is impaired.
- The chromosomes are separating.

Stage D
1 Toxic substances enter the nucleus and change some genes to oncogenes.
2 The cell metabolism becomes so altered that it is now a non-functional, stressed cell in which genes are vulnerable.
3 Cell Division is in C2 phase.

This marks the end of the initiating stage, which may remain quiescent for years.

Stage E
1 The somatides, the cell-wall-deficient organisms of the cancer organism with growth-hormone-manufacturing pattern inherent in their DNA, enter the stressed cell through a leaky cell membrane.

Stage F
1 The somatides combine with the oncogenes, reprogramming them to make a factory for growth hormone-like chorio gonadotrophin (HCG). (See page 228).
2 The chromosomes are concentrating into two new cells.

Stage G
Already damaged genes—oncogenes, are susceptible to reprogramming by the cancer organism, so making a factory for growth hormone and unrestrained replication in a cell that has lost its contact inhibition.
1 Cancer cells form factories for out-of-control growth. This marks the end of the precipitating stage.
2 The *cancer cell membranes* make poly saccharides, enzymes and peptides, (cancer antigens, markers, HCG, hyduronidase, etc) that are thought to enhance their capacity to travel in the blood stream and lymphatics.
3 *The liver* makes substances that react against cancer cells such as tumor-necrosis factor, immunoglobulins, interferons, leukotrienes, colony-stimulating factor, etc, which are concerned in the T and B cells' attack (see page 140).

Say: *Every day and every way I get better and better.*

Recognition and destruction of cancer cells
(See also pages 168-181)

1. *Stem cells* from the bone marrow and blood, under the influence of hormones, peptides and enzymes, vitamins and minerals.

2. *Migrate* for further manufacture (a) to spleen and liver to make B lymphocytes; (b) to thymus, spleen and lymph nodes to make T lymphocytes.

3. *T cells* become differentiated into T helper cells, monocytes suppressor T cells, granulocytes and others not shown.
   B cells become differentiated into plasma cells and memory cells.
   Macrophages are made in the liver, probably from precursor stem cells which can also change to activated natural killers when given the message to attack cancer cells.

Part Six

SIDETRACKED

22   NO VACCINE AVAILABLE

While I was staying with Dr Virginia Livingston (in July 1987) she allowed me free use of her large library and gave me permission to photocopy whatever interested me for research.

One night I started reading a book by Kiichiro Hasumi, *Cancer Has Been Conquered*. The work this researcher had done absolutely fascinated me, even though I did not agree with all of his dietary ideas. I started to copy the part about diet and was in the process of scanning other parts when there was a call from the huge balustraded stairway. The housekeeper was making her way down, thinking I was in trouble or that we had burglars. I looked at my watch—it was 2.30 a.m.! I allayed her fears and went to bed, determined to finish my photocopying the next night.

At breakfast next day Dr Livingston asked me what I had been reading that was so exciting that I needed to be up till all hours. I described the fascinating book by Auguste Villequez with its beautiful time-lapse photographs of the cancer organism life cycle, shown under the dark-field microscope. She said that was her favourite rare book, out of print now, by one of her old friends and mentors, a French researcher who spent much of his life studying the organism.

I mentioned Dr Hasumi's book too, but she dismissed it with a wave of the hand. I said nothing, determined to read more before I discussed it. When I had the opportunity to read in the library several days later, the books had been put away.

Back in Australia, going over the photocopies I had taken, I mourned having no contact address for Dr Hasumi and wrote to Maruzen Publishers to ask for further information. There was no answer. I put it out of my mind, since the vaccine from Dr Livingston's Medical Centre was still available at that time.

Six months later, circumstances were very different. The doctors at the Livingston-Wheeler Clinic were completely replaced and it became obvious that patients could not get autogenous vaccine by sending their urine over to the Clinic as they had been doing. They were told they would need to go through the whole treatment program, spending two weeks in San Diego before they were eligible to have supplies of vaccine, supplements and minerals forwarded each year. This was beyond the means of most.

I had noticed that my own autogenous vaccine was now making haemorrhagic areas when I injected it. This was also happening to some of my patients who were using their autovaccines. This suggested to me that the body was now making hypersensitivity reaction to the antigen, or that it had changed with time to something less useful.

Another setback occurred because Dr Livingston's pathologist friend had sold his laboratory. He had been making part of the ingredients in her program, under her licence. Now I was told that the new owners were not manufacturing her patented products.

Dr Owen Wheeler, Dr Livingston's husband, had been very ill while I was staying with her. He had congestive heart failure, among other severe medical problems. They were a devoted couple and she had to spend more and more time nurturing him and less and less time at the clinic. This took its toll in many ways. Not long after I returned home, I learnt that Dr Wheeler had died. Dr Livingston sold the big home and bought a smaller place near her doctor son in an elite closed estate.

The outcome of all this change was that most of my patients ran out of the Livingston vaccine. It seemed to have been holding cancer in check because metastases (secondaries) then started to recur in some patients.

Who will make a vaccine?

I was desperate to find a new source of autogenous vaccine—my patients needed it. I was able to contact a Doctor X in Sydney who had been making the autogenous vaccine in tiny quantities for his patients for some years. He had originally spent a month visiting the San Diego laboratory in 1982. His persistence and dedication was rewarded when Dr Livingston allowed him to make

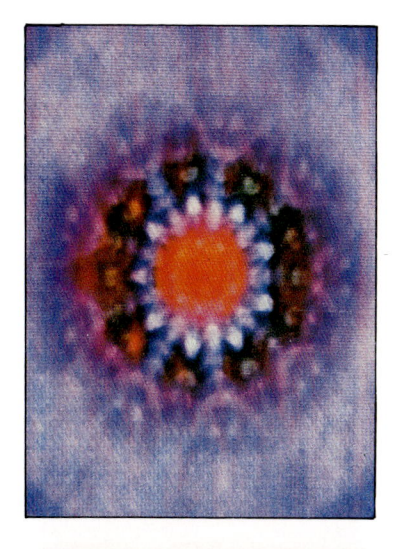

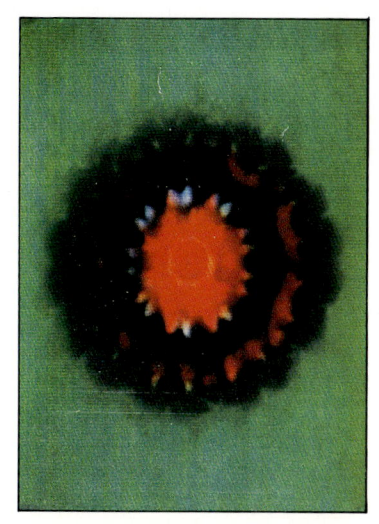

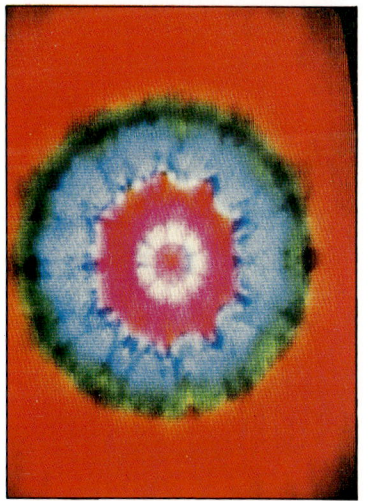

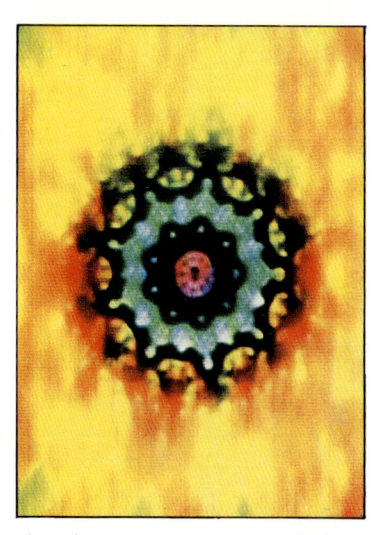

The mandala is a symbolic design used to focus concentration during meditation. The word has sacred significance for Buddhists and Hindus. The design can be any symmetrical shape, but the concentric circular form signifies a macrocosm, drawing the mind into the infinity of the universe.

Concentration on colours, which are all light vibrations of course, intensifies the depth of meditation. Each colour, having its own cosmic force and meaning, promotes different individual response in the viewer who is concentrating on it. Choose the one that appeals to you most. It can provide a constant focus (or mantra) for calming the mind, healing the body and reviving the spirit.

CHANGES MAKING A NORMAL CELL INTO A CANCER CELL

(see pages 194-5 for a description of stages A to G.)

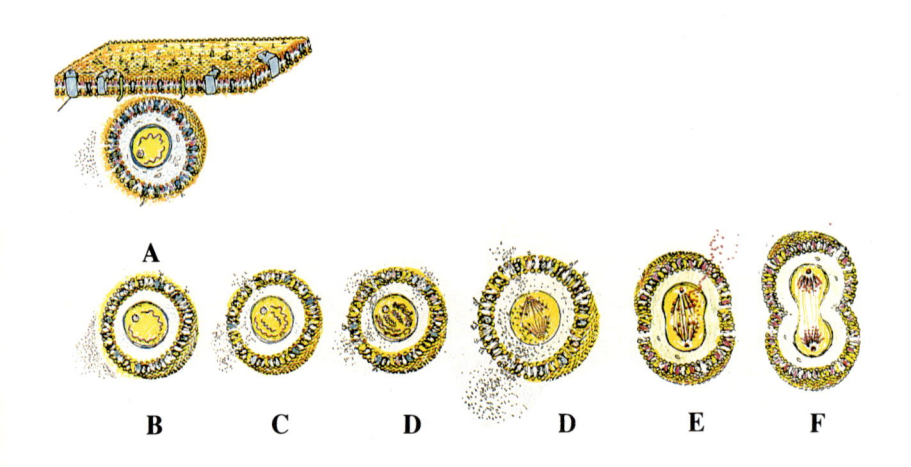

A B C D D E F

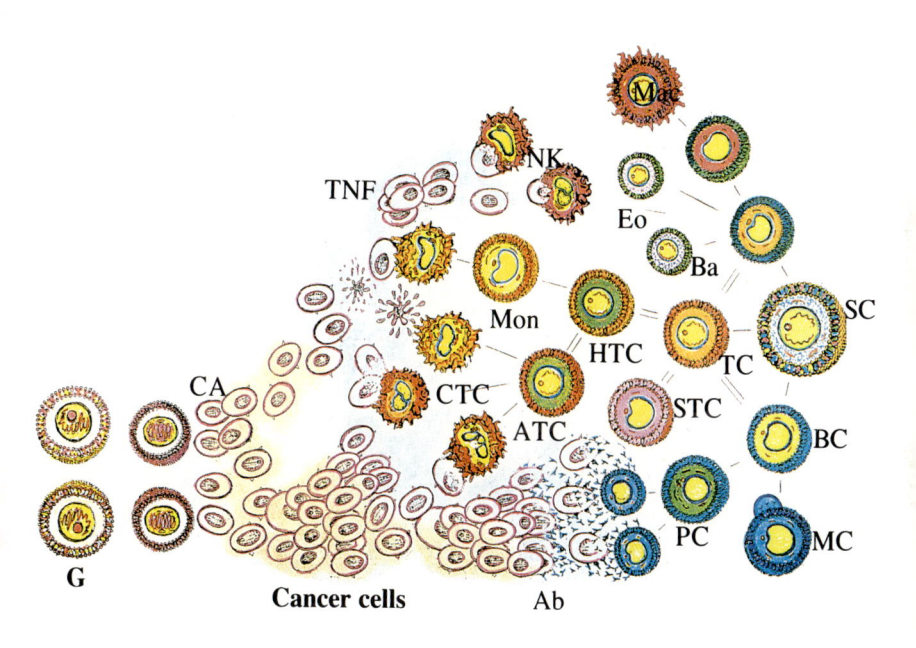

Mac = macrophage
NK = natural killer
Eo = Eosinophil
Ba = Basophil
Mon = monoctye
ATC = Activated T lymphocyte
CTC = Cytoloxic T lymphocyte
STC = Suppressor T cell
TC = T cell
HTC = Helper T cell

SC = Stem cell
BC = B Cell
MC = memory cell
PC = Plasma cell
Ab = antibody
CNDO = Cell wall deficient form of the cancer organism
TNF = Tumor-necrosis factor
CA = Cancer antigen

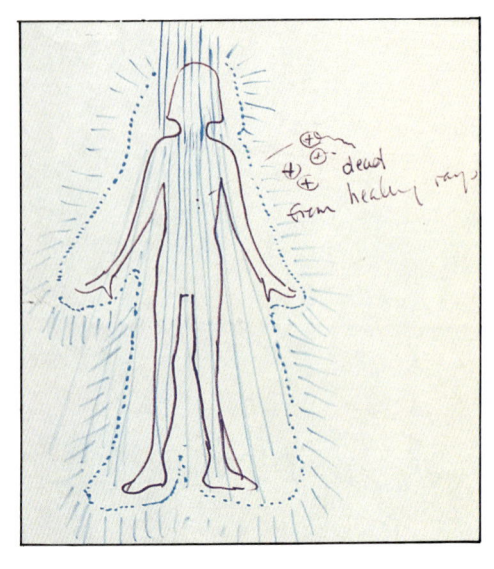

1. Denise

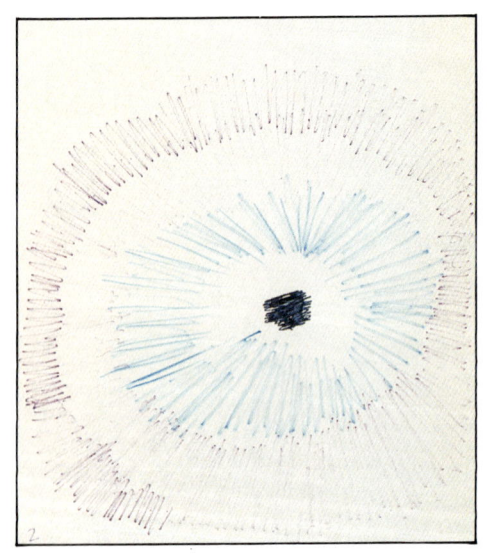

2. Marg

In drawings 1 and 2 the patients have chosen the same sort of ethereal colours, blue and mauve. Blue and mauve represent healing rays, here killing or shrinking the cancer. Both showed the cancer as black. In Drawing 1, Denise showed her breast cancer dead as two tiny black dots.

In drawing 2 the rays have not yet shrunk the cancer away—but it will disappear, Marg noted. So the rays were not actually in touch with the cancer. And so it was; she was battling it but not quite there.

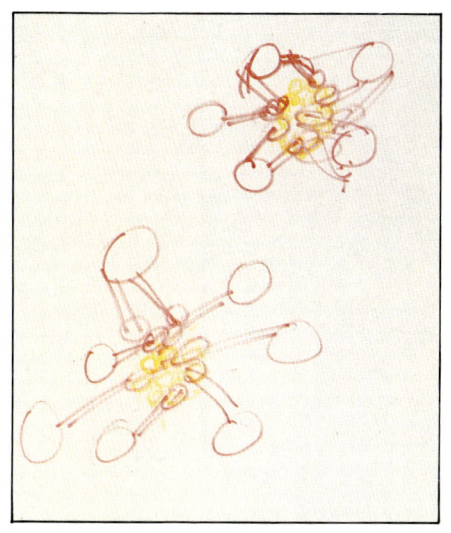

3. Lyn

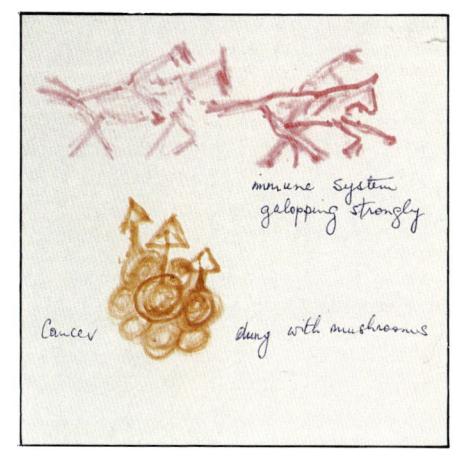

immune system galopping strongly

Cancer   *dung with mushrooms*

4. Anna

In drawings 3 and 4 the patients chose vibrant red as the active immune system. Notice how forceful the white cells are in drawing 3, engulfing the weak yellow cells. You can see them Pow! and Zap! Many people put those words in their pictures but this is pure graphic art—showing us without words.

In drawing 4 Anna, who is a horse lover, sees her immune system as horses, strong and active at first, then a little weaker. The horses are galloping right past the cancer dung which is left behind to grow fulsome and strong, without being attacked at all. That is how it was. The weekly tests were negative, showing a weak immune system, while the cancer markers were getting more and more positive. The primary cancer was never found—only the mushrooming secondaries.

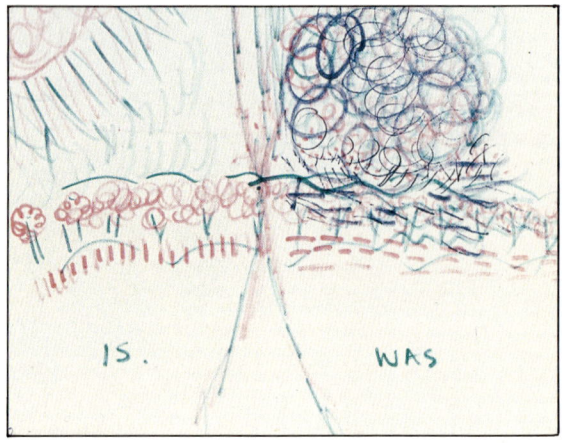

5. Willie

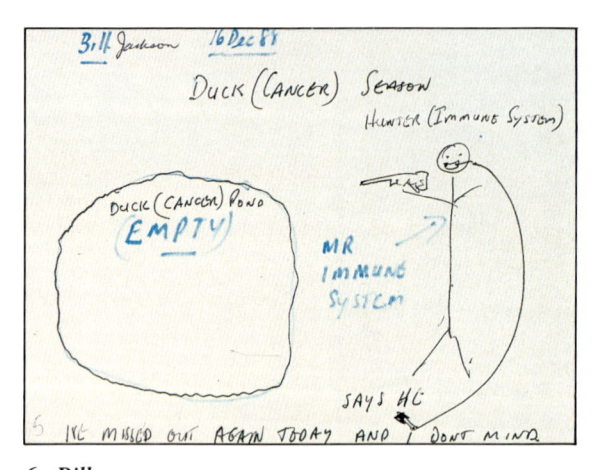

6. Bill

      In drawings 5 and 6 Willie and Bill are expressing cancers that they have overcome. In 5, Willie showed how her cancer was ominous, like a tangled black growth destroying her garden of flowers in the bowel wall. On the is side the immune system pours down like the bright sun rays to make the garden glow in happy colours of pink and green again—there is no cancer growth now.
      In drawing 6 Bill has used words to aid his graphic presentation of Mr Immune System, the hunter, aiming his gun to kill any cancer that lurks in the duck (cancer) pond. It is empty! 'I've missed out again today and I don't mind,' Mr Immune System says.

Notice how very actively the immune system is represented in these first six drawings. Now contrast drawings 7 and 8, in which no immune system is represented at all.

Both these people had suffered dreadful setbacks in their lives which pulled down their self-confidence to a low ebb and filled them with fear of the future. The development of cancer had fulfilled their worst fears and now cancer dominates the scene or their picture of life. By the central position on the paper and the absence of a base line, you can see this. It is clear that the future is 'up in the air'. There is no firm belief in recovery because there is no immune system in the picture.

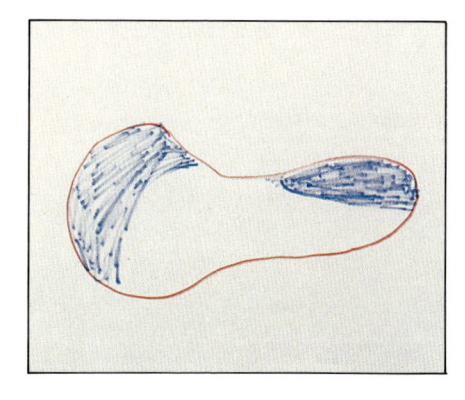

7. Ada

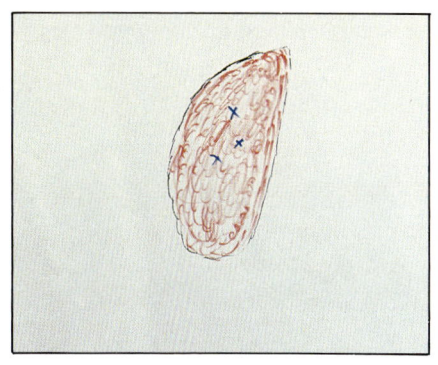

8. Fred

In drawing 7, Ada shows how her anger makes a wall to contain her cancer. In fact she did very bravely encapsulate her liver tumors by sticking rigidly to her program for a time. Two car accidents and the burglary of her home were the final blows that caused them to break out and kill her.

In drawing 8 Fred surrounded his right lung with tentative feathery lines, suggesting that he was uncertain about his ability to contain the cancer that he placed so accurately. In fact, unchallenged by his immune system, it did grow out of the lung lining to kill him eventually.

All these courageous people fought, in their own ways, to overcome the disease of the body that is so intricately bound up with the mind and emotions. The drawings can reveal the unconscious state of the body, mind and feelings long before the future outcome unfolds.

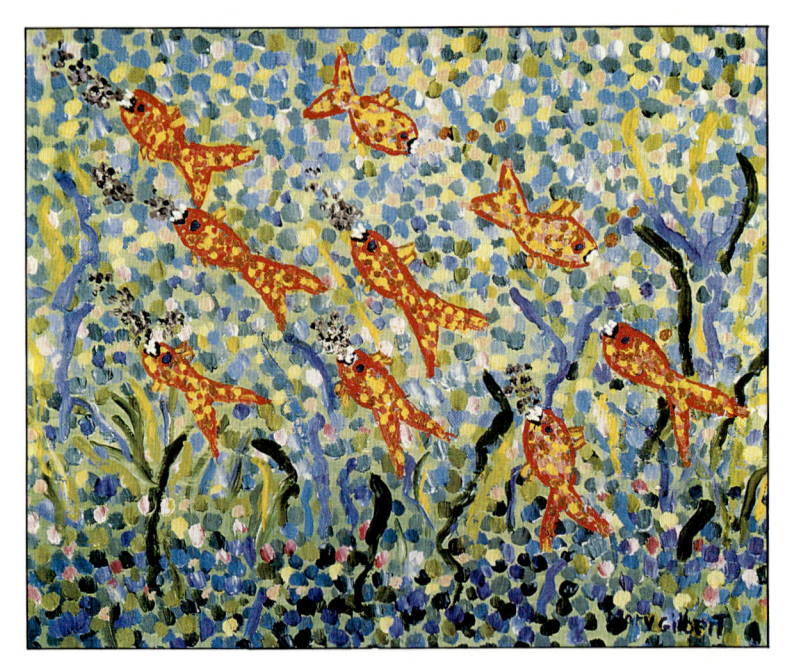

Mary has shown the gold fish (the immune system) as very healthy, in a healthy body of green and blue, gobbling up the grey cancer cells.

his version of her vaccine in his laboratory, as long as he promised that he would make it only for his own patients. Since he belonged to the same church she trusted him, and with good reason—he never broke his word.

I referred patients to him with an introductory letter asking if he would accept them for treatment. He then grew the organism from their urine to make a vaccine, which might take from six to eight weeks to prepare. The cost was a fraction of what it would have been to go to San Diego. There was enough for a year and the Customs Department was not involved.

For a short time this worked well enough and we were very grateful. Then Dr X was called to Hong Kong. I hastened down to Sydney in November 1988, determined to find out how to make the vaccine myself.

Dr X is a very serious and religious young man, who was deeply embarrassed to inform me that he had promised Dr Livingston that he would never teach anyone to make her vaccine without her permission.

I wrote to her explaining my position and virtually begging her to let Dr X teach me. She did not answer. I learnt that she was recovering from her husband's death and was now busy having a swimming pool built in her new house. She was also considering marrying again, at 81 years. Friends in San Diego suggested that I contact her pathologist friend and ask him to make vaccine for me, but in consideration of the kindness and trust Dr Livingston had shown me. I declined to do this, since it might have breached her patents.

I thought of a young medical technologist, Sandra, whose mother I had treated nutritionally for cancer four years earlier. I thought maybe she could tell me what I would need and how much it would cost to set up a laboratory in Brisbane myself.

I knew it was useless asking the commercial pathologists to make the vaccine. I had made several attempts to interest them by giving lectures to their top bacteriologists in the past. At one meeting, only a handful of the forty invited came. Only ten doctors even deigned to look through the dark-field microscope at the live

Say: *Every day and every way I get more confident.*

organisms on the slide. At that time, in 1985, their answer was decidedly *no*.

One deputy head of a pathology laboratory confided to me some months later at a party that he would have been only too pleased to make the vaccine but that it was impractical. First, he said, the laboratory would have to pay a royalty to Dr Livingston and secondly, to set up the machinery would cost a lot of money, when I would be the only person to request it on prescription. And who would pay for it? It was out of the question . . . far too costly and, most important of all, the laboratory would get a bad name for making a product 'like that'. Meaning no doubt, one that did not have the sanction of a research grant or peer approval.

I understood and did not ask again.

Sandra and I had several long talks and I visited the laboratory where she worked. The array of equipment looked formidably expensive to me, and so it was. I lent Sandra the compendium of papers on the vaccine and its manufacture. After reading them, she phoned me saying she was very sorry but setting up to make such a vaccine safely, making sure it was prepared, killed and sterilised properly, was not in her power.

Sandra was very sorry she could not help me and my patients in our search because her own mother, who had cancer, had been persuaded to stop my diet, supplements and meditation by an oncologist who had zealously given her chemotherapy. It has made the poor lady's life miserable and she had lost a tremendous amount of weight. She died on 5 December 1988, soon after my talk with Sandra.

In the meantime a letter arrived from Dr X, as a farewell on his way to Hong Kong, enclosing a copy of his promissory letter to Dr Livingston. He said he had written to her and she had said that she would rather take her vaccine patents to the grave than share them with a backyard laboratory. So that was the end of that. Later on I was to realise, when investigating the complicated processes necessary to make a successful vaccine, just how naive I had been. The regulations about manufacture of vaccines, I discovered, state that it is necessary to have a government-licensed laboratory before any vaccine of any type can be made at all.

Taking the road to Japan

In April 1989, when I was studying my notes from the USA trips of 1987, a bunch of photocopies fell out of the book, and what should be on the back of one page but the address of Dr Kiichiro Hasumi's clinic in Japan!

Immediately I wrote to Tokyo explaining how I had managed to read some of the book *Cancer Has Been Conquered* two years earlier and asking for information about the vaccine. I also asked for permission to visit the Immunology Institute in July 1989. Within two weeks I received a reply telling me that Dr Hasumi Senior had died in the summer of 1988, but that his son, Dr Ken-ichiro Hasumi, would be pleased to see me in Tokyo. I was to come early in July as he was giving a paper at the international Immunology convention in Berlin in early August.

Books and correspondence were, as ever, coming to me from all directions, I was in the process of evaluating several products that had been used against cancer with very promising results, such as Professor Kazuhiko's Asai's germanium trials in Tokyo and Dr Hans Neiper's electromagnetic field therapy in Hanover, Germany. I had to put all this into abeyance, meantime, to study as much as I could about other vaccines. I had to go back to the famous English man, Dr Jenner, the Frenchman Antoine Bechamp, the Italian Carla Fonti and dozens of others. I had no idea what I was looking for, whether the book by Hasumi was still in print or what it contained, or whether Dr Ken Hasumi could speak English.

Preparing myself for possible imports from Japan, I rang the various departments concerned with customs, health, therapeutic products and quarantine to acquaint myself with the laws regarding these. It was also necessary to install a fax machine since our phone calls proved to be hampered by language difficulties and letters were too slow.

On applying for a visa to Japan, I was shocked to find it refused. I had written in the application that my reason for going to Japan was to visit a laboratory and have meetings with other doctors. I was asked to supply copies of all correspondence between the

Say: *I learn to dispel fear.*

parties concerned. Perhaps this is general business or diplomatic procedure, but I felt rather alarmed. I chose several letters from both sides and put in another application stating that I was going to Japan to a convention and for a holiday. That week turned out to be a most exciting and interesting adventure.

Since there is only one hour's difference between Brisbane and Tokyo times and I was travelling overnight, there was no jetlag on the nine-hour flight.

Dr Ken Hasumi met me at Narita Airport and we talked all the way to my hotel, or rather I talked. Having realised that he was sometimes not replying, I said, 'Am I speaking too fast?' I was, and also using some colloquialisms that would be impossible for a non-Australian to understand. It was just excitement. Once I slowed down, we communicated very well.

He had made out an itinerary for me with his newest secretary as guide. Miss Sudo spoke English and came to collect me from the hotel each day. We spent much time with dictionaries, pen and paper, but it was all fun. Part of the time we toured the sights, shops, temples and gardens of Tokyo, but I also had the opportunity to visit both the Shukokai Institute and Clinic.

I was honoured by three magnificent Japanese dinners where I met the staff of the institute and the business manager of a new hospital which Dr Hasumi was building in another part of Tokyo. One dinner was at the beautiful wooden Inn of Lake Hakone. The building was centuries old with a delightful garden on the lake shore, in view of Mt Fujiyama.

The food was very different from what I eat at home. I managed my chopsticks well, I was assured, but on two occasions I was gently told that what I had carefully picked up to taste was part of the table decoration! Everything was delicately and artistically arranged and prepared.

Dr Hasumi gave me his father's book to read—that is, to *finish* reading—before I went to the institute. This was just as well, since the processes used in making the various vaccines are extremely complicated. Testing for product control must go on with every process so that all the stringent requirements are met.

Miss Sudo and I travelled on the train to the institute and walked from the station through a suburb that was old and closely settled in parts. It was good to see that allotments here and there were neatly planted with corn, beans and other vegetables, even in a city holding as many people as the whole of Australia!

The Shukokai Institute was built by Dr Hasumi Senior many years ago. Most of his research had been done there. Dr Ken was apologetic because the stairs and walls were workworn. It is not the look of a place but the good purpose it has served and is serving that is important to me, I told him.

The huge and beautifully kept library was fascinating. Books have been a lifelong passion with me, as they must have been for his father. There were his own medical records, articles and journals from many countries, a collection of fifty years. Text books on surgery, anatomy, medicine, endocrinology, epidemiology and immunology—everything, mostly in English, German and Japanese. I asked for a photocopy of a recent work of cancer markers to help me understand more about the pathology of the cancer cell and its relationship to the systemic physiology of the body.

I found that, just as I had been doing, the institute also uses the Purified Protein Derivative or Mantoux reaction to monitor the state of sensitivity of the reticulo-endothelial system.

As I was shown through the various sections of the building, I became more and more amazed at the complexity and ingenuity of the manufacturing processes. Everything was checked, recorded and rechecked. The white-coated staff, from office boys to MDs, were busy but courteous. The huge electron microscope, one of the first to be installed in Japan, was still there. It took up a whole room.

'My father was able to identify and photograph the cancer viruses in animals and humans with this machine,' Dr Hasumi told me. He showed me some of the original photographs from 1947.

It could be appropriate here to discuss the life and work of this man who contributed so much to our knowledge, working alone, as most dedicated researchers do, with boundless determination and conviction, in spite of his colleagues' disbelief.

Say: *I give out love and harmony.*

Who was Dr Kiichiro Hasumi?

Dr Kiichiro Hasumi was born in Japan in 1904 and graduated from Chiba Medical College in 1927. His first postgraduate training was in surgery.

In 1931, while working under the leadership of Professor Seo at Chiba University Hospital, he helped in the development of new surgical procedures for treating cancer of the oesophagus. He was then given the task of seeking out all the written work on cancer from all over the world. This gave him the opportunity to study cancer from many different points of view.

Of particular interest to him was the work of the American, Dr Francis P. Rous, who discovered in 1909 the infectivity of sarcomas in hens' eggs (see page 169). Dr Hasumi thought that human cancer might also be contagious under some conditions.

Rous said that the infestation was caused by an invisible 'agens' and was the first to prove this in an experiment. This agens (virus) was later photographed through an electron microscope by another American, Dr W. Ray Bryan. He even succeeded in measuring its size and found its diameter to be 89 millimicrons. The theory that the pathogen of the Rous cancer was a virus was thus substantiated for the first time.

When he made his discovery in 1909, Rous was thirty years old. However, his road to recognition was very rough, and it was not until fifty-seven years later, in 1966, that this vital piece of research became known to the general public. In that year Rous received the Nobel Prize for his discovery of the infectiousness of the Rous sarcoma. He was then 87 years old.

For half a century the medical world refused to acknowledge the Rous sarcoma virus theory. However, during this period his theory was reinforced by such discoveries as that of John Bittner, who in 1936 at the Jackson Institute in Mayne, showed that mammary cancer in rats is caused by a virus. Following this, various animal cancers were shown to be virus induced.

In any discussion of the human cancer virus the struggles of Dr Gye of the Royal Cancer Institute in England must be remembered. Gye thought, as Rous did, that cancer in humans must be caused by unseen viruses. He took human cancer tissue, ground it and passed it through a porcelain filter to isolate the virus.

The same idea occurred to Dr Hasumi in 1931, just as he was

becoming very involved in cancer research. For some years he worked exclusively with viruses causing animal cancers.

In 1937 he was studying the work of Russian scientist Mikhail S. Tswett, who was separating the alpha and beta chlorophyll by a method of column chromatography. Dr Hasumi realised that he might be able to adapt this method for isolating separate viruses. Tswett was using potato starch as his absorbent. Dr Hasumi tried purified kaolin—and it worked. This was a tremendous breakthrough. For the first time, different strains of virus could be separated and identified. After two years of careful research, Dr Hasumi succeeded in isolating animal cancer viruses in 1939. He went on to work with human cancer.

In February 1947, he succeeded in isolating the pure human cancer virus.

He photographed it repeatedly through the electron microscope and proved beyond any doubt that it was indeed the virus which he found in every human cancer tissue and verified by standard tests known internationally by pathologists.

This was only the beginning. When working on cancer in animals (the lethal equine anaemia virus) he had found that horses he had vaccinated with the killer virus did not get the disease. Of more importance still was the discovery that those animals which had already contracted the disease could sometimes recover if they could be stimulated to make the antibody against it by injection of the dead virus. If the organism was from an animal's own body, the results were even better.

Thus the use of autogenous vaccines in Japan was originated. The next step was to use a similar protocol for human cancer.

Dr Hasumi devoted the rest of his life to the perfection of his immunological control and treatment of human cancer. There were many difficulties. To overcome them he used careful recording and scientific study of all cases he treated. One of the main drawbacks in the use of his vaccines was that a patient was often so ill when he or she came to him that the immune system needed stimulation and desensitisation before it would react to a vaccine of any sort.

Say: | *Love and harmony come back to me.* |

He grew and preserved more than eight laboratory strains of human cancer which he used to test the sensitivity and manufacturing ability of the patient's antibody-making systems.

The Purified Protein Derivative

The Purified Protein Derivative (PPD) or Mantoux test is still a reliable method of testing the activity of the immune system. We in the Western world should all be resistant to tuberculin, a toxin of the tuberculosis organism. Children are tested in high school in Australia, and if the Mantoux is negative, they are vaccinated with the Bacillus Calmette-Guérin (BCG), an attenuated form of the Mycobacterium tuberculosis or Tubercule bacillus (TB).

Kiichiro Hasumi believed that the human cancer organism was a virus which he isolated in 1947.

In his book* Dr Hasumi states:

The pathogen of cancer is a virus. Viruses are found everywhere on earth. They may even exist on other planets. And of course they exist in vast multitudes inside the human body. When a virus becomes active under special conditions, a disease is the result.

A virus possesses characteristics which prevent it being killed even by boiling or burning. This puts it beyond the understanding of modern pathology which considers that viral diseases can be cured by killing the virus in the same way as a cell or a bacterium can be killed. Furthermore, since viruses are the smallest of microorganisms, with diameters between 10 and 300 millimicrons, their presence cannot be detected with the ordinary optical microscopes used in modern medicine. To detect viruses an electron microscope is needed.

A Vaccine must fulfil conditions

There are no means other than vaccines to combat viral diseases. This is particularly true for a systemic disease such as cancer. *A vaccine must fulfil certain essential conditions* and I will set these out in the following paragraphs.

---

* *Cancer has been conquered*, Maruzan Publications, Tokyo, 1980.

Firstly there is the question of the type of virus involved. As stated above, unless the immunogens—that is the vaccine—are of the same type as the immunogens of the disease, the vaccine is quite useless. Analogically it is like a duplicate key, which will not open the lock unless it is identical to the original key.

The second condition is that only a purified virus taken from the patient's body can be used to create the autogenous vaccine. Human cancer cannot be transferred to animals, nor is it possible to introduce a (patient's) cancer into an animal and use this to create a vaccine (for that patient).

Then we come to the question of hypersensitive antigens. The human cancer virus consists of 80 per cent immunising antigens and 20 per cent hypersensitive antigens. Careful consideration must therefore be given to the frequency of inoculations.

The ideal vaccine is one that completely fulfils these requirements, and it is worth noting that such vaccines display great effectiveness, not only in prevention but also in treatment.

In the past, vaccines could be used prophylactically and, even then, they were not effective against cancer, but only against phlogotic (inflammatory) diseases. The reason for this was that the viruses were cultured in the organs of animals and vaccines used still included heterogenous proteins. Continued administration in this form was dangerous because of the risk of death from shock.

However, the cancer vaccine which I have researched and developed is produced from viruses which have undergone pure isolation. It contains no harmful heterogenous protein. Continued administration is therefore possible, and it is possible by means of vaccination to cause the proliferation of antibodies and eliminate the virus.

Patients who come to me are initially given vaccine injections every five days. Frequent blood tests are made during this time. This is because the results of these tests provide a barometer of the patient's physical condition.

Wherever the cancer virus penetrates, the antibodies created by the vaccine attack and destroy it.

Say: *I love to eat and drink what makes me well.*

There is another question which demands consideration when using vaccine therapy. This is the fact that viruses mutate. Just as insect pests in farm crops develop resistance to insecticides, and stronger and stronger types appear, so mutations occur in the genes of the cancer virus as a result of various factors in the environment.

When this happens, existing immune bodies become ineffective, so at least once a year, or depending on the condition, every two or three months if possible, the patient's virus should be tested and if the slightest mutation has occurred the old vaccine must at once be replaced with a new autovaccine capable of responding to the new virus (strain).

Because vaccine therapy is an immunotherapy, the patient needs to be strong. Cancer patients suffer from anaemia . . . so their vitality must be built up with nutrients and injections.

The importance of pure separation

The reason that no one accepts that human cancer is caused by a pathogenic virus is that pure isolation of the virus is extremely difficult.

There are two methods of pure isolation of viruses. One method involved ultrafiltrate from the patient's urine (cell-less filtrate) through a Millipore collodium membrane. When electricity is discharged into the collodium of the filter, the sparks emitted cause the size of the pores to change according to the voltage used. It is possible to isolate different-sized viruses according to the size of the pores in millimicrons when the liquid is filtered.

The other method is to filter ultrafiltrate of the patient's urine, using chromatography.

An electron microscope is used to confirm and measure the size of the viruses thus isolated, if further inspection is carried out using an infra-red spectroscopic analyser, it becomes possible to distinguish each virus and tell whether it is that of Japanese encephalitis or cancer, etc. This method can only be carried out at my laboratory.

The successful mass-immunisation of Japan's worst cancer village

As I have already stated, the cancer vaccine produced as a result of my research has been used successfully, however, to gain acceptance in the medical world data from open experiments is necessary. I made considerable efforts to assemble corroborative data, and fortunately in 1961 I was blessed with an opportunity. I was asked to undertake a full three-year mass-inoculation experiment, starting from the summer of that year, in Heguri Village, Ikoma District, Nara Prefecture. This village was said to have the highest cancer rate in Japan, with one person in three dying of cancer. However, the cause of death was often shown on death certificates as being some other disease, out of a dislike for the word 'cancer', so the village office statistics, which were based on these registrations, were unreliable.

Then the mayor of the village took the lead in setting up a cancer-prevention committee. Their first action was to have blood tests carried out on 500 volunteers above the age of forty. Two hundred and fifty volunteers were chosen and inoculation with vaccines began. The vaccines were injected hyperdermically and it was decided to inoculate five times a month at five-day intervals, to be continued over a period of three years.

The results to December 1963 show that 116 subjects dropped out, leaving 134 who faithfully underwent the inoculations. Not one case of cancer appeared among those who went through the full three years' injections. Among those who were not inoculated at all there were fourteen cases and among the dropouts there were three.

Dr Hasumi developed his own meticulous tests for cancer diagnosis and staging. In his treatment of more than 140 000 people with his vaccines over a period of thirty-one years, he had remarkable success and accumulated a huge amount of data on the immunological treatment of cancer. His two sons are doctors in Tokyo. One, a neurologist, has not much interest in carrying on his father's work, however his younger son, Ken-icho, has followed in his footsteps, being first a successful surgeon.

When Kiichiro Hasumi died in 1988, Ken-icho took over the arduous task of running the institute, laboratory and clinic that his father had set up and where people were treated so successfully for so many years.

Say: | *I choose the positive path.* |

No wonder the steps and passageways of the institute and clinic have been well used over the last forty years or more. The 1989 International Directory of Cancer Institutions sanctioned by WHO has the Shukokai Clinic listed as having 51 115 patients with 3756 new patients and 32 760 out-patient consultations annually. There are sections for surgery and research as well as for cancer treatment, rehabilitation and palliative care.

I was overjoyed to have the opportunity of visiting and communicating with people who were using the treatment methods I trusted. Dr Ken Hasumi discussed the treatments he was now using, not only from his father but also in relation to new methods of cancer control with radium and chemotherapy.

Learning in Japan

On a memorable day I went with Miss Sudo to the Shukokai Clinic in Asagaya, another part of Tokyo. The buildings were old and crowded with patients in all stages of clinical procedure. Some were having blood and urine tests, some were undressing, being examined, dressing, waiting for their medication and appointment, in lines or just sitting patiently waiting.

Dr Hasumi was very, very, busy. He usually had four doctors working with him, but one was away. I didn't want to be a nuisance so I just 'sat in' with him quietly, trying to be inconspicuous and not ask too many questions.

There were all sorts of people from all walks of life. The nurses were neat, efficient, orderly and unsmiling, which I think is the Japanese way. Special help was given unobtrusively to young mothers with children and to the elderly. Whenever possible, Dr Hasumi explained a little of what he was doing, in English.

He explained that he and the nursing staff gave new patients careful instructions on diet, hygiene, their vaccines and injection procedure. They returned for blood tests and review every eight weeks, or sooner if needed. He had a referral system like our own for surgery, radiation or chemotherapy if necessary, although often it was not. Many people he saw recovered because, *unlike* my patients, most came *before* they were terminally ill, and so had a much better chance of recovery.

Many doctors all over Japan and hundreds from all over the world send patients to Dr Hasumi. He was arranging to stop off in Italy, after giving his paper in Germany, to see a doctor who wanted to discuss the success rate he had in treating more than 500 patients with the Hasumi vaccines.

The Clinic finished late but we met in the doctor's room to discuss the work. I was shown the ampoules the patient took home and injected every five days, and the progress cards recording, in special hieroglyphics, everything that occurred.

He offered to give me some vaccine to take home, but I declined in the light of our customs and health restrictions, about which I will have more to say.

However, I asked to take home twenty copies of the book *Cancer Has Been Conquered*, since my patients would want to read it to learn about the program in more detail than I could ever give them, before making a choice of therapy. (Books are not a prohibited import into Australia.)

On the weekend we went to Lake Hakone. I was surprised at the cost of travelling. The roads are excellently maintained and so they should be—there is a toll to be paid on every section, even in the huge city of Tokyo itself. Dr Hasumi is a charming host and Miss Sudo was there to help me understand what to do at every turn—taking shoes off and on, the procedure to adopt when having a boiling hot public bath, the way to put on a kimono, sash and jacket, and all those little niceties that make our Australian way of life seem so different—maybe rather brash, casual and disorganised by comparison.

The dinner was superb, dozens of delicately prepared and served courses, each with its own decor and elegant dishes. Nothing was hurried. We had our own suite and servants who transformed the main room into a bed chamber for the girls, with comfortable futons on the floor. Dr Hasumi had his own room where, if he wished, he could have had another boiling bath and massage.

In the early morning bitter green tea and pickled plums were served on the verandah overlooking the delightful azalea gardens, with snow-capped Fuji just visible between the mountains across the lake.

Say: | *I throw away gloom and doom.*

Later we browsed through the village shops on the lake shore, buying craft trinkets for the family. We went up to the top of a mountain on the cable car and walked to an austerely colourful shrine where the fortuneteller's paper message, translated by Miss Sudo, said that I would have a long and happy life. It didn't say anything about patience or patients, but I suppose that was part of it.

We took many photographs of each other and the view, which clouded towards the time I was to leave. Dr Hasumi drove me to the airport in the rain with my twenty books, full of hope that my patients would have a new source of autogenous vaccine to help their recovery.

23 OBTAINING AUTOVACCINES

When I returned from Japan, it seemed that patients who were suitable for a vaccine came to me 'out of the blue'. As with all therapies, there are criteria to be fulfilled. Not every new cancer patient will benefit.

Those who will *not* benefit are:

- Those who have multiple peritoneal metastases and fluid in the abdomen.
- Those with more than 6000 rads of radium or radioactive therapy.
- Those having certain types of chemotherapy.
- Those with certain types of aggressive cancer, such as mesothelioma.
- Those who are on large doses of other drugs.
- Those whose immune system is so weakened they do not react to the Purified Protein Derivative.
- Those who do not believe they would recover—or do not want to try.
- Those who think other therapies have done it all, and that the new little lump will go away.

Permits to import biological products

Two patients who read Dr Hasumi's book desperately wanted the vaccine. A professor (H) with bowel and liver cancer and a nurse (W) with breast and bone cancer were the first to receive their permits for importing autogenous vaccine and were making their way to Japan.

Then Dr Hasumi faxed that it was not necessary for the next patient, Doug to come over to Japan. To send 5 ml of serum (with the requisite papers) was enough to make a vaccine for the first four months. Finding a laboratory that would spin down 5 ml of serum from the patient's blood for this purpose was the next task.

None of the pathologists contacted were happy about doing it, for fear of ridicule by their peers. After some phone calls, I found one who would do it as a special favour. For a patient living in the country to arrange the customs agent, packing and papers, even with my participation, was quite a feat.

Worst of all was the paperwork and confusion in getting the vaccine back into the country after it was made from the patient's serum, but without the patient accompanying it.

After some weeks delay Doug received from Canberra his permit to import autovaccine and sent his serum off. Even before his vaccine arrived back, I had a letter from the Health Department in Canberra asking for details of its manufacture. I had already phoned the heads of three departments and thought everything was in order. In fact, six more patients had sent in their applications for permits. I sent a letter explaining what I could about the process, with excerpts from the book.

In the meantime, H and W came back from Japan with their four months supply of the first vaccine of their programs, saying that they had left their urine samples for the next year's supply of autogenous vaccine to be made from the organism in it and sent to Australia when it was ready.

Doug's vaccine came through the post, duly inspected and passed. I was hopeful. We were all saying our prayers.

One of my patients, Jodie from a country town, who had been keeping her lymphoma under control with my program and a laboratory vaccine—'purified antigen'—from Dr Livingston, had now run out of her supply. No more was forthcoming from San Diego and she was keen to get some from Japan because her lumps were starting to recur. I sent her the book to read.

Her husband was a Bachelor of Science and the head of a government department in that area. He didn't read the book because he considered it to be unscientific. Jodie, who was anxious and assertive by this time, thought she should get her permit straight away and not have to wait six weeks like everyone else—even if he didn't approve. She browbeat her husband into phoning his contacts in Canberra instead of going through the channels I had already opened in the four departments involved in issuing permits to import biological products.

He was sceptical about her treatment with me even though, until now, it had kept her well for over four years. The first I knew about his attitude was the arrival of a FAX from him saying permits were no longer available until I had fulfilled the two years of clinical trials of a substance that is unknown to the Health Department officials. He evidently did not read the small print. This refers to substances that are made 'not of self'. It does *not* apply to vaccine of the patient's *own-self*, made strictly under sterile conditions and not containing any external substances except a recognised and approved preservative.

But the damage was done. He had stirred up all the departments by his irrelevant and angry questions. No one was going to take the responsibility for giving his wife a permit.

I received a haughty FAX from Jodie saying that Canberra was not cooperating. Then, promptly, each of the six people who had applied for permits received a letter from the department saying that no permits were to be issued at all. I received a letter, too, saying that since the department was not familiar with this vaccine, it could not be imported.

I telephoned around the four departments involved again, but was passed from one extension to another until I realised I was being given the 'run around'. The people I wanted to speak to were out, on holiday or at a conference, etc, etc.

Eventually, a little letter came from a very helpful man in the quarantine department, telling me that if people went to Japan and had their vaccines made from their own organism while under treatment with it, they could bring their own autogenous vaccines back with them if they declared it to customs on re-entry as personal medication from me, which it would be.

So there was a legal way. We followed this plan for years, until the law changed in 1991.

Jodie moved to another city when her husband was promoted. Unfortunately the cancer was widespread when I heard from her last. She had given up the nutritional program and meditation. Thus seven terminally ill people had been denied their last chance of alleviation or remission.

When rules and regulations are changed, when replacements are

Say: *I ward off danger by planning.*

made in the public servants at the top of the four departments involved, when a new law is made and implemented, then the carefully made steps in obtaining a permit, sending urine to Japan and having the autovaccine made and returning it to the patient come unstuck. Then patients run out of vaccine or cannot get a permit or have the sample undelivered at one end of its journey or another.

There have been frustrating and difficult times in 1985, 1987, 1989 and 1991. It is no use placing blame, I just have to find the hold up and reorganise the people concerned by going through the necessary form-signing step by step and giving out written notes to remind patients of the times and procedures so it all runs smoothly.

Apart from the trouble with Jodie, only once have autogenous vaccines been held up by medical harassment. This was in February 1991 when the Therapeutic Goods Act was finally being implemented after two years of discussion with alternative therapy societies about its regulations. A number of patients were told they would not be granted permits through the Drug Evaluation Branch. I was informed by letter too, eventually, that I was not allowed to prescribe the vaccine for my patients. No explanation was given.

After many unanswered letters to the department and several prolonged phone calls to Canberra, where I was given the usual run around, I finally found the doctor concerned in the hold up.

When we finally met on the telephone he fired an abusive barrage accusing me of being an unqualified quack, using unorthodox and untried treatment, promising cures to dying patients, stopping them from having the proper treatments, charging huge prices for starving them, and so on. I didn't respond to any of these false and distressing attacks. Everything he said was patently untrue. I had nothing to hide and no need to justify myself. So I just listened until he had finished and then asked him when my patients could expect to receive permits to receive back from Japan the vaccines for stimulating their immune system which had been made from *their own organisms*, not from another animal. A carefully worded but generally accusing letter followed, but none of the request forms.

It was not until the irate husband of a patient wrote to this doctor, threatening to expose him on the media, and enclosing my photos of Dr Hasumi's new forty-eight-bed research hospital and his entry in the World Health Organisation approved International Directory of Cancer Institutes and Organisations (UICC Geneva 1990) that another member of the Drug Evaluation Branch finally pieced together the new procedure for the granting of permits to import biological products. This was done by the good offices of a patient who is also the president of the Leukaemia Foundation for Children. It took seven months of negotiation to overcome this problem, during which time many patients had to interrupt their program or wait for it to begin. For some it was too late.

Over that time I was so disheartened I often thought I would give up medicine. I was past retirement age anyway. What always brought me back to the front line was the dedication of the patients who had proved that the Survival Plan worked—also, if I retired, ignorant people who had power over so many lives could again block the progress of successful treatments. 'Don't let your vision of the future be clouded by those who have none'. That is the affirmation which helped.

International Union Against Cancer

The International Union Against Cancer (UICC) is devoted exclusively to all aspects of the worldwide fight against cancer. Its objectives are to advance scientific and medical knowledge in research, diagnosis, treatment and prevention of cancer, and to promote all other aspects of the campaign against cancer throughout the world. Particular emphasis is placed on professional and public education.

Founded in 1933, the UICC is a non-governmental, independent association of more than 250 member organisations in over 80 countries. Members are voluntary cancer leagues and societies, cancer research and/or treatment centres and in some countries ministries of health.

The UICC is non-profit and non-sectarian. Its headquarters are in Geneva, Switzerland. It creates and carries out programs around the world in collaboration with hundreds of volunteer

Say: *I change my thoughts to change my life.*

experts. Supported by membership dues, national subscriptions, grants and donations, its annual budget is about USD 2.5 million.

The UICC is governed by its members which meet in General Assembly every four years. Its elected Council and Executive Committee are responsible for program structure and implementation.

The UICC organises an International Cancer Congress every four years as well as annual symposia, workshops and training courses. It publishes the *International Journal of Cancer* (monthly), the *UICC Cancer Magazine* (quarterly), the *International Calendar of Meetings on Cancer* (bi-annually) and a number of technical reports, textbooks and manuals.

24 MORE PIONEERS WITH VACCINES

Here are brief notes about some of the pioneers who have successfully used bacterial antigens to stimulate antibodies against the cancer organism.

Drs Stevan and Marco Durovic

These doctors used isolates from the serum of horses infected with the organism 'actinomyces bovus'. This was called 'Krebiosen' and gave immunisation against Progenitor cryptocides, which is of the same family. It was effective against cancer.

Andrew C. Ivy MD

A noted scientist, Dr Ivy made clinical trials of this serum (Krebiosen) and, finding it effective, used it in several forms—as 'Carcolan' and 'Compound G'. Millions of dollars were spent in law suits fighting opposition to his therapy. Ivy won the right to continue using this serum, with the help of a great number of recovered patients who were willing to testify in court. The Ivy Cancer Research Foundation is now administered by Z. Godlowski MD. PhD, who continues the research also using nutritional and enzymatic therapies.

A. Bonifacio MD

He made an anti-cancer serum from the intestinal villi of goats. It was effective in treating human cancer.

William Merbyn Crofton MD, Thomas J. Glover, Thomas Deaken and M.J. Scott MD

All used microbial antigens made from the organisms in the patient's own tumor or body fluids to produce antibodies against their own cancer. These were true autogenous vaccines. William Crofton, an Irish surgeon, believed that the virus was a filterable, sporelike phase of a bacterium (see page 175).

Eleanor Alexander-Jackson MD

A noted research bacteriologist, Eleanor Alexander-Jackson had breast cancer many years ago. She studied the Rous sarcoma virus and the tubercule bacillus extensively, finding and developing special media for growing the pleomorphic forms of these organisms. She worked intermittently over extensive periods but in collaboration with Dr Virginia Livingston, Dr Irene Corey Diller and others. She made an autogenous vaccine herself which cured her own breast cancer.

The following quote from *The Cancer Microbe* by Alan Cantwell tells about the momentous discoveries of three courageous women, Eleanor Alexander-Jackson, Virginia Wuertele Caspe Livingston and Irene Corey Diller.

> 'While Eleanor was busy at Cornell University, Virginia was seeking financial support to open a laboratory for cancer microbe research. Grants were obtained from The American Cancer Society, The Damon Runyon Fund, Abbott Laboratories, and others. On June 2 1949, the laboratory opened at the Presbyterian Hospital in Newark, New Jersey. Virginia was made director.
>
> 'The years 1949-1953 were highly productive for cancer microbe research. Eleanor carefully pondered whether to leave Cornell and join the Newark lab. Finally the lure of working with the cancer microbe was overwhelming. In 1951 Eleanor began commuting from her Manhattan apartment to Newark. Virginia knew how to detect the hidden killer in cancer. The key was the acid-fast stain which made the hidden cancer microbe visible. Eleanor knew every guise of the microbe, and how it survived and multiplied inside the body. The two women were determined to prove that the cancer microbe *caused* cancer (and was not just a universal contaminant).
>
> 'Shortly after the lab opened, Virginia read an article in *Life* magazine about Irene Diller PhD, a researcher in the Department of Chemotherapy at the Institute for Cancer Research in Philadelphia. Irene was an expert cytologist, a cell specialist who studied the effects of anti-cancer drugs on cancer cells in animals. One day she noticed a peculiar fungus-like filament sticking out of a cancer cell. She then observed the same phenomenon in other types of cancer cells. Irene began to culture cancer tumors

and grew strange-looking microbes. She reported these microbiological findings at a meeting of the American Association for the Advancement of Science; and *Time* and *Life* magazines picked up the story.

'Virginia and Eleanor met Irene and told her about the cancer microbe and its fungal forms, and how the acid-fast stain was the key to its identification. Virginia, Eleanor and Irene formed a professional association which lasted until Irene's death in 1988, at the age of eighty-eight. Eleanor affectionately termed their trio 'The Three Musketeers of Cancer Research'.

'Irene's speciality was experimenting with mice and rats which were genetically inbred for cancer research. After learning about the cancer microbe, she began testing thousands of animals for cancer microbe infection. By injecting young, male, albino mice with cancer microbes she doubled the rate of cancer in the mice.

'The Three Musketeers' proved 'Koch's postulates' with the cancer microbe. The microbe was cultured from cancer tumors and from the blood. When injected into animals it produced cancer, and the cancer microbe was recultured from the tumors of the animals.

'The animal experiments proved that the cancer microbe caused cancer. Virginia and Eleanor envisioned a vaccine that could be used against the cancer microbe. They began experiments to test a vaccine. The trio was closing in on the biggest medical mystery of the twentieth century, and powerful people in the cancer establishment were taking careful note of their research. The three women were headed for big trouble.

'Nineteen fifty-three was a momentous year for Virginia and Eleanor. In June the Newark lab. team presented their cancer research at an exhibit at the American Medical Association meeting, held at the Waldorf-Astoria Hotel in New York City. RCA generously lent an electron microscope which televised the 'live' cancer microbe to the audience. Roy Allen's beautiful color microphotographs and James Hillier's spectacular electron microscopic photographs were the hit of the AMA convention.

Say: *I give thanks for what I have.*

Immediately, the dark forces went into action against the women. According to Virginia's autobiography (*Cancer: A New Breakthrough*), Virginia and Eleanor had made enemies in the highest echelons of cancer research. The big boys in the medical establishment knew the identification of a cancer microbe could destroy millions of dollars worth of cancer research. The microbe and its implications were a serious threat to the pharmaceutical industry and the cancer research establishment. The discovery of an infectious agent in cancer would rock the scientific world and threaten the multibillion cancer treatment industry. A 'cause' and a vaccine 'cure' for cancer would be financially disastrous for the biomedical business world.

Pressure was put on the press to kill the cancer microbe story. As a result, there was a press black-out of the exhibit at the AMA convention.

In September, 1953, Virginia and Eleanor presented papers at the Sixth International Conference for Microbiology in Rome. The conference was a great success and the two women met other European scientists who had also studied the cancer microbe.

While they vacationed in Europe, their enemies succeeded in pulling grant money away from the Newark lab., forcing its closure. Without money, there could be no cancer microbe research. And without research the new cancer breakthrough would die a natural death.

Disheartened, disillusioned, and totally defeated, Virginia moved to California. Eleanor got a job with a private firm. Things were never quite the same again, although the two women were hardly finished. In the 1960s, Eleanor secured a grant from the National Institutes of Health to study the Rous sarcoma virus, a virus that causes sarcoma cancer in chickens. Eleanor proved the Rous virus is actually a filterable form of the cancer microbe. Using cancer bacteria cultured from Rous virus-infected chicken sarcoma tumors, Eleanor made an anti-cancer tumor vaccine. Amazingly, her vaccine protected healthy chickens against Rous sarcoma disease! As usual, Eleanor's research was ignored because none of the virologists wanted to believe that the Rous virus originated from a bacterium.

Florence Seibert

In the 1960s another distinguished woman scientist joined the cancer microbe trio.

Florence Seibert (1897-90) is the noted biochemist who developed the Purified Protein Derivative (PPD) test, a diagnostic skin test for tuberculosis. The National Tuberculosis Association in America awarded her the prized Trudeau Medal for this notable development in 1938. In the 1960s, after her retirement, she took up the research into the pleomorphic organism which she isolated from every piece of tumor and from every leukaemic blood specimen she studied. Her painstaking work convinced her that the filterable form of the organism which, unlike other forms, could be grown on artificial media, was a virus. In the description of her search in her autobiography, *Pebbles on the Hill of Science*, Seibert questions why virologists still refuse to recognise that many bacteria are pleomorphic and that viruses are their filterable form.

Personally I believe we are in the 'age of the viruses', simply because the constant bombardment of our bacterial flora with multiple antibiotic warheads has driven germs into their viral forms. Human kind is hurtling towards decimation and maybe genocide by the scientific and commercial worlds' refusal to recognise what terrible destruction they are wreaking on the everchanging natural order. Vested interests are waging war against nature and, as always, the innocent and the ignorant suffer.

Virginia Livingston

Virginia Wuerthele Caspe Livingston M.D. researched and used a vaccine made from the cancer organism for many years, with thousands of patients from many countries. She used a specific nutritional method, organ extracts, megavitamin and mineral therapy in conjunction with other modalities. Her research started with scleroderma in 1956 and, in co-operation with other scientists, she rediscovered the life history of the cancer organism, so confirming the work of previous researchers. She named it 'Progenitor cryptocides' in 1970 and classified it as one of the actino-mycetales family, closely related to scleroderma, tuberculosis and leprosy. She

Say: | *I let things happen in their own time.*

added new discoveries of her own, proving in her research that Progenitor cryptocides, under certain conditions made a growth hormone that stimulated cancer cell growth.

Her work has been verified by other researchers but ignored or denigrated by the medical establishment. In 1989, at a time when she was in poor health, the Food and Drugs Administration raided her laboratory, confiscated the spleen extract she was using and prohibited her from making autogenous vaccines from organisms in the patient's own urine. Their action was highly illegal.

Even though she regained the authority to make vaccines, it was a final blow. She died of heart failure in June 1990. I think of her as an intuitive genius whose discoveries have added to scientific knowledge and helped humanity.

Chisato Maruyama

Chisato Maruyama used a serum made in 1944 from the human *antibodies* to the tubercule bacillus, instead of BCG, which is a live vaccine made from cattle. It has had some effect in stimulating the immune system in humans but, like some others made by animals, it is not specific for the cancer organisms. It is often successful in stimulating the immune system to fight cancer.

Kiichiro Hasumi

Dr Hasumi first isolated the cancer organism from human tumours in 1947 and photographed it by electron microscope. His autogenous vaccine, made from the organism in the patient's urine, is still made in Tokyo and used all over the world with success, particularly in the early stages of the disease. The adjuvant he developed is helpful on its own and also reduces sensitivity to the antigen. He discovered that the cancer organism mutates after about ten months and so avoids the antibodies made against it. This has explained why vaccines lose their effectiveness after a time and must be remade.

Joseph Issels

Dr Issels has used autogenous vaccines successfully for years. He also uses laetrile, diet and hydrotherapy in his clinic in Germany. He has now retired but his clinic still functions.

Phillipina Hartman

Dr Hartman used sterilised tumour sediment to produce antibodies in guinea pigs. Their serum, used as an antigen, caused tumour regression in humans.

Celia Culver-Evans

Dr Evans, of London, England, used a system based on Virginia Livingston's method and vaccines with great success.

Royal Rife

Royal Rife, with his wonderful 'light' microscope of the 1930s, showed two forms of the cancer organism, which he named 'BX virus' and 'BY virus'. He found also the electromagnetic light frequencies that killed them. He called this frequency the Mortal Oscillary Rate (MOR) and found that it was specific for each organism. He demonstrated this to many scientists before his five precious microscopes were destroyed by hired vandals. Doctors fought over using his discoveries which treated cancer effectively. He was a brilliant scientist and uninterested in treatments or monetary gain. (See Clara Fonti, page 177 and Gaston Naessens and Robert Lincoln, below).

Gaston Naessens

Dr Naessens is a French biologist who made a revolutionary microscope called the 'Somatoscope' in the 1950s. This is similar in some ways to the revolutionary microscopes made in the 1930s by Royal Rife, which first identified the life and death of the two variants of the cancer organism, which he called X and Y. Gaston Naessens, like Rife, encountered great opposition from jealous and unbelieving peer groups. He now lives in Canada where he no longer makes his successful anticancer vaccines. They were especially successful for treating leukaemia, as many recovered patients would have testified, if they had not been excluded from his trial.

Research with Naessens' microscope reconfirms what previous scientists had found not just from its recognition of cell-wall-deficient organisms (CWDOs) but because it demonstrates that their cell division can be initiated by micro-organisms within the body, given

Say: *I relish this very moment.*

a suitable internal environment (see page 195). This is verified by Virginia Livingston's discovery that a growth hormone (similar to chorio gonadotrophin) is made by the cancer organism.

More and more scientists are now substantiating Naessens' work, regardless of the controversies among the ignorant.

Franz Gerlach

In 1948 Dr Gerlach published a magnificently illustrated monograph describing his long-term observations, and those of other investigators, of micro-organisms associated with cancer in people and animals. From more than a thousand samples of tumour tissue, blood and ascitic fluids of cancerous patients and tumour-bearing animals, he cultured pleomorphic, filter-passing organisms which he designated as 'micromyces blastogenes'. One of the stages in the life cycle resembles mycoplasma. The morphology of the isolated organism of different media is illustrated in the plates in this monograph, as well as the intracellular forms in various tissues of experimental animals injected with the tumour isolates. The organism was highly pleomorphic, and the life cycle stages are similar in most respects to those described by Glover and many others.

Several thousand mice, hundreds of rats, and lesser numbers of guinea pigs, rabbits and chicks were injected with 'pure' cultures from human carcinomas, sarcomas and brain tumours. Ascitic (cancerous) fluids were produced in many of these experimental animals. The organisms could be recultured from these, so fulfilling Koch's postulates (see page 223).

In a later publication Gerlach uses a different name for the organism, calling it '*micromyces universalis innatus*'. Because of the definite mycelial stages in the life history, Gerlach regarded the organism as a micro-fungus. The ability of the organism to pass through a Seitz filter signified that it was possibly a virus. In 1952 Gerlach briefly reviewed studies in viruses over the preceding forty years and came to the conclusion that the (micromyces) present in all kinds of malignant tissue is not the only cause of cancer, but a latent parasite which may at any time, under the stress of auxillary factors, acquire pathogenic properties leading to the development not only of cancer, but of other diseases as well (see diagram on page 175).

Robert E. Lincoln

Dr Lincoln, a respected and inventive physician of Massachusetts, succeeded in isolating two pure strains of very virulent haemolytic streptococcus, alpha and beta, which he found in the *sinus passage* of chronically ill patients. These germs, he reported, were hosts for the perpetuation and multiplication of *two distinct and related viruses which he also isolated*: the alpha virus (on 5 June 1946) and the beta (on 24 November 1946). Of these Doctor Lincoln wrote: 'Each host germ has one, and only one, particular strain of virus as a partner. These viruses use their respective germ as a refuge in which to live and grow when they are not in contact with and destroying specific body tissue cells which they prefer, just as all disease-causing germs and viruses show a marked choice for certain specific tissues.'

This is reminiscent of earlier work by Royal Rife, who called the organisms he found X and Y viruses.

Robert Lincoln used a vaccine made of killed germs of the staphylococcus family in a serum which he called 'Staphage Lysate' (SPL). It stimulates the immune system to fight infection without using antibiotics and was useful in controlling cancer. The Food and Drug Administration in the USA has banned the sale of this useful and harmless product since 1977. It is no longer available in Australia either. *Staphage lysate* is a potent stimulant of the immune system, especially of T lymphocytes, Interferons and Interleukin 1, the precursor of Interleukin 11. SPL can be used as a skin test of cellular immunity because most people should have a positive reaction to it. It is still available in Mexico and has been sold as a therapy to control staphylococcal infections and to stimulate the immune system to control sinusitis, arthritis, Crohns disease, multiple sclerosis, allergies, herpes, warts and cancer. Although it often causes strong skin reactions, with inflammation and tenderness, when given by injection, it can also be taken orally or by inhalation.

Since the American Cancer Society listed SPL as unproven it has been used only surreptitiously in the USA but reports of clinical use are still appearing in articles written by practitioners for

Say: *I expect to enjoy tomorrow.*

pharmacological, immunological, dermatological, vitamin and other research societies in Japan, mostly with English translations.

John E. Gregory

Dr Gregory, of Pasadena, defined cancer as 'an infectious disease in which the infecting organism is a cancer virus, which sensitises cells to grow invasively and metastasise when stimulated by chemicals, irritants or excess hormones. An overwhelming infection may produce the disease.' On the basis of animal experiments, Doctor Gregory found that the cancer virus develops an enzyme which he identified as chymotrypsin. In 1952, at his own expense, he developed a serum he called 'gregomycin' and another 'antivin'. He used these sera, combined with a high-fruit and no-meat, no-fat diet, to help many recover from cancer.

William B. Coley

Dr Coley, of New York City, was a well-respected orthopaedic surgeon who noticed that some of his patients with cancer recovered after suffering severe fever from the highly dangerous and infectious skin disease, erysipelas. Between 1891 and his death in 1936, he was actively seeking organisms whose toxins would create fevers that could heal the body. He stated in 1893 that microbes or viruses were the origin of sarcomatous and carcinomatous changes in the body and he followed this over the years by clinical evidence. He used the mixed bacterial vaccines from bacilli, especially *streptococcus pyogenes* and *serratia narcescens*, to stimulate the immune system in most degenerative diseases, including cancer. Sixteen or more different preparations of the vaccines called 'Mixed Bacterial Toxins' (M.B.T.) or 'Coleys Toxins' have been available since 1893 and are used extensively in Europe. Coley's daughter, Dr Helen Coley Nauts, has spent more than forty years assembling scientific books, papers, abstracts and histories to substantiate the use of this method. The making and sale of these vaccines was banned in the USA by the Food and Drug Administration in 1977 and are unavailable in Australia also.

Helen Coley Nauts

In 1988, after reading *Cancer Blackout* by Nat Morris, I wrote to Dr Helen Coley Nauts, the main organiser and the founder of the New York Cancer Institute. No address was given, so in the hope of finding out more about her father and his important work, I just sent the letter, with a prayer, to her name as president of the New York Cancer Institute, New York City. It was delivered without a hitch and I received back a very encouraging letter and two of the many excellent monographs from her exhaustive research into all aspects of cancer. Dr Coley Nauts is keeping important discoveries alive and available to all interested people by documenting work from all over the world in these monographs.

Dr Will Coley's therapy was treated as a personal whim by the American Medical Association since it could not be discredited. His beliefs about the origin of cancer were ignored. Here he expressed his disappointment:

> Why is it that so many of the great cancer research institutions of the world give this question of the parasitic origin of cancer practically no attention today? It is because no young man entering the field of cancer research feels that he can afford to run the risk of an unsympathetic and often antagonistic attitude on the part of professors of pathology who repeatedly tell him that the whole matter has been definitely settled and that cancer cannot possibly be of germ origin ... I urge once more that we look upon the theory of a microbic cause of cancer not as a closed chapter, but as one that deserves sympathetic study. Every encouragement should be given to workers in this field.

Unfortunately most of the workers in these fields of research have been silenced, one by one. This happens when the research develops to the stage where patients who have recovered from cancer want to tell the world, when the researcher becomes a proselytiser or when established medical prestige or interests are threatened. Professor Hans Selye says: 'Great progress can be made only by ideas very different from those generally accepted at the time. Unfortunately, it is literally true that the more someone sticks out his neck above the masses the more he is likely to attract the eyes of snipers.'

Since the AIDS epidemic there has been a huge impetus to research microbiology and the immune system. This may, perhaps, turn round

Say: | *I always have more assets than liabilities.*

some of the negative influences in a great concerted need to overcome the modern killer epidemics. It will be too late, however, to repair the injustice done to those researchers into the cancer organism, people of intuitive genius and constant dedication such as Royal Rife, Gaston Naessens, William Koch, Lawrence Burton, Andrew Ivy and many others.

The candida spore controversy

In 1987 I showed the film I made of the organism in blood at the home of Dr Livingston, at an evening with Dr Joseph Issels. In one part of the film I said that candida spores and the spore-form of Progenitor cryptocides were different. He questioned this statement. 'How do you know this is so? Have you grown them in the laboratory?' he asked. I had to admit that I had not and that I could very easily be mistaken since I was only going by hearsay from people who had no specialised knowledge.

I remembered then a young doctor, Phillip Hoekstra, who studied under Professor Lida Mattmann at Wayne State University. She is a leading research microbiologist who has written many important papers on cell-wall-deficient organisms (CWDOs) or pseudo-pneumonia-like organisms (PPLOs). She has isolated these organisms in many degenerative diseases (see page 173).

In a seminar on cancer arranged by Dr Livingston at San Diego in 1985, I witnessed personally the anger and vehemence of scientific dispute. Dr Mattman was a scheduled speaker who gave an excellent presentation. Phillip Hoekstra was not listed on the program, but followed Dr Mattman with the excuse of showing his collection of slides. They were beautiful slides showing the granules in what he said was a platelet aggregation, transforming into mycelial threads and hyphae, which he said were forms of candida.

Dr Livingston leapt to her feet and rushed to the daïs, shouting angrily that what he called platelet aggregation was in fact a 'cotton ball' and that the change was into the mycelial form of Progenitor cryptocides, not candida. It would seem, from the ideas of Nello Mori, Joseph Issels, Bechamp, von Brehmer, Royal Rife, Mattman, Hoekstra and others, that the cancer organism is indeed part of the life cycle of a ubiquitous substance that may be the most pleomorphic of all organisms. New-age bacteriology is going step by step along the path of discovery started by Bechamp and Wilhelm Reich; the discovery that:

> All matter is one: it is the arrangement of matter by external forces that work upon it at a particular time that make it into the more or less stable substances that we can recognise and categorise.

Anyway, Dr Livingston was very angry. She refused to let Phillip Hoekstra speak another word and, though he continued to show the rest of his slides in silence, she held Dr Mattmann responsible for allowing her protegé to gate-crash the seminar.

In 1989 I attended a seminar in Manly, Sydney, where Phillip Hoekstra was the main speaker. He was brought to Australia by the Haemaview organisation, which sells a microscope system and a method of examining blood, alive, under the dark-field microscope. This firm had been selling Phillip Hoekstra's handbook, in which claims were made about the diagnosis, by dark-field slide of blood, of vitamin and mineral deficiencies and some grave illnesses. The method has great value in helping therapists recognise problems from a single drop of blood.

We learnt that government health authorities had notified the Haemaview sellers that this program was unacceptable, since not only doctors and pharmacists, but also people with no scientific training were buying microscopes, going through the course of instruction, diagnosing disease and charging patients.

The seminar was a revision of the whole program so we were advised that no 'diagnosis' was to be given on the results of the blood examination in future.

Phillip Hoekstra emphasised particularly that we should overlook the organisms seen under the microscope. He stated emphatically, many times, that there was no such thing as a cancer organism, that the Progenitor cryptocides was a sham, something made up by a mad old lady who 'ripped off' unwitting cancer victims. It was a familiar story. He obviously had not studied the work of the hundreds of other researchers whose similar observations had led to the making of useful vaccines in the past.

Say: *I focus on my assets comfortably.*

I was most impressed, nevertheless, by this young man's knowledge of blood cytology and was glad to have learned so much from his handbook. I felt that his remarks about the Progenitor cryptocides organism were not wholly of his own choosing. This was because he mentioned several times that his friend and mentor was Dr Vincent Herbert, a leading figure in the California-based 'antiquackery' society, with firm affiliations with the American Medical Association, the Food and Drugs Administration and multinational pharmaceutical companies. It was almost sentence-by-sentence the same spiel I have heard from members of this organisation against anything these people believe might threaten established medicine.

We are on the brink

At the end of the last century an Australian enthusiast, Lawrence Hargrave, spent many years making planes that did not fly. He knew he was on the right track—they *almost* flew. Although he had boundless enthusiasm and dedication, he didn't have enough information about what others were discovering. It was the Wright brothers who finally used his vast practical experience to put the missing pieces of the jigsaw together.

This is how we are in our knowledge of cancer—on the brink. We are in the middle of a scientific explosion. In every field large leaps forward are being made. The most intricate workings of nature are being dissected. The structure, function and chemistry of each part of a cell is being studied intensively. Thousands of new facts are reported daily. In 1953, when Frances Crick and James Watson were unravelling the structure of the DNA molecule, it was thought that they had discovered the very essence of life—while in other fields scientists were dreaming of, and then proving the existence of, quarks and black holes.

Always the dream came first: the feeling, the idea, the intuition, the conviction. These attributes of 'super mind' or 'super self', as Ian Watson has named it, are the essence that spurs the seekers on, often in the face of opposition.

The Legionnaire's bacillus was sitting there before our eyes on countless slides before it was discovered. Could it be that it is the same with this organism, that because of strong prejudice it has not been studied seriously for years? Could it just be that this *is* the cell-wall-deficient organism that is the trigger for cancer?

Who is looking for a growth hormone in the chemical life history of this organism? Who is looking for the organism, live or dead, at all? Who would fund such research? Who would publish the findings of such research? Who would dare to believe, when the full force of the 'cancer machine' could be against such discoveries?

Information is there in the work of the scientists I have discussed and probably in that of others I have not yet studied. The most important answers to many questions still asked about cancer could already be there before us.

Say: *Mistakes are opportunities to learn.*

//Part Seven

GOING IN THE RIGHT DIRECTION

25 RECOVERY, REMISSION OR RECURRENCE

None of my search would mean anything without the long-term recoveries from cancer of many of my patients, all of whom have had treatments based on healing body, mind and spirit, and incorporating the right food with supplements of vitamins, minerals, herbs and immune stimulating agents. Stress control for the mind and spirit, with an emphasis on positive enjoyment of life, meditation, prayer and revival of the natural healing spirit we all possess, are essential ingredients too.

Don't lose sight of the philosophy on which this method is founded. It is not alternative, but basic. It follows physiological and ethical medicine principles and so should be implemented as soon as a diagnosis of cancer is made or even suspected.

Most of my patients are having or have had various other treatments, such as operations, radium or chemotherapy. Many come when these have failed, as was discussed in the first part of this book. The Cilento Survival Plan works best in the early stages of the disease but it can also be successful in advanced cases, as some of the following histories will show. *All patients improve* on the program and some can get it all together to recover. Now read these case histories and see if they strike some chords in your own situation.

All the people in these case studies have given me permission to use their experiences for the teaching of others. Where possible the real name has been used and is written in full. For those who wished to preserve anonymity, the name, place, occupation and identifying factors in the history have been changed. These are designated by a fictitious first name only.

26 CASE 1: BRUCE HUXLEY—CHRONDROFIBROSARCOMA

Bruce, who conquered sarcoma of the hip, first came to see me on 26 September 1987. His family doctor had found a hard lump on his right hip bone while investigating a football injury, on 7 August 1987.

He was referred to a surgeon specialist who found nothing by needle biopsy so on 20 August he operated and took a biopsy. This proved the lump to be a malignant chondro-sarcoma Stage 2—in other words, a cancer of the hip that was still growing—outwards. A barium enema and further x-rays showed that the tumour was growing out 1 centimetre into the pelvis from the junction of the two hip bones. The general surgeon referred Bruce to an orthopaedic surgeon and they operated together on 30 September 1987.

Bruce took the precaution of giving six bags of his own blood to the hospital before the operation, since he did not want to have blood from anyone else. His own blood was used to transfuse him during and after the operation. With the problem we have had in Australia of people contracting AIDS from transfusions before the tests for it were available, we all thought this was a good safeguard.

Causative factors

Why did this seemingly healthy young man of thirty-two get cancer of the cartilage in his hipbones? Below are some of the factors which militated against him, but they are in chronological sequence, not in order of importance.

1 *Genetic Predisposition.*
   Bruce's maternal great aunt had cancer of the bowel. His father's great uncle had cancer of the lip and jaw and his cousin had

cancer of the stomach. This does not imply that cancer is inherited. What is important about it is the fact that the patterns of how we absorb, use and excrete the vitamins and minerals we take in our food and drink *are* inherited. Bruce had a possible predisposing cancer pattern from both sides—but only if lifestyle factors were also against him.

2 *Antibiotics.*
In his teens, Bruce suffered from acne, that sapper of youthful self-esteem, and he had taken antibiotics for many years until he 'grew out of it'. He still had a few scars from the deep-seated cysts. Taken without vitamin supplements over a long period, some antibiotics can damage the future immune response of the liver.

3 *Working with computers.*
Bruce is a talented computer programmer. When he first came he had been working eighty hours a week for the last two years in front of a visual display terminal, building up his own computer company.

The electro-magnetic emanations from a visual display terminal are the only vibrations, I am told, that cannot be stopped by anything. If you read books by Dr John Ott and other specialists in the vibration field (see page 245) you may understand it. I don't, really! I just know that there is a great world of uneasiness about emanations from VDTs, television sets, fluorescent lights, microwave ovens, alpha, beta and gamma x-rays and geophysical lines of electro-magnetic energy of all types. We just don't know enough about them.

In the *International Journal of Biosocial Research*, Volume 8 1986, John Ott describes an experiment he did in his laboratory on 'Effects of Radiation from Visual Display Terminals on Bean Plants' which showed how dangerous emanations from VDTs can be.

In any case Bruce's skill with computers was his life's work and he was hardly going to give it up because I said so.

Say: | *I throw away resentment—so love enters my life.*

4 *Sunglasses.*
Bruce also wore sunglasses most of the time he was away from his machines because his eyes were sensitive to glare, so the change in his light absorption spectrum was further deranged. This led, without any doubt at all, to severe deficiencies in calcium and carotene—both of which have proved to be protective against some forms of cancer.

5 *Diet.*
Another factor was the food that Bruce consumed. He lived alone so ate out much of the time, since he was not dedicated to cooking. He was a food illiterate, especially addicted to sugar and fried food, and he ate what he fancied.

6 *Alcohol.*
He also drank alcohol as spirits, and he told me he was in the habit of drinking three or four beers to get to sleep at night.

7 *Smoking.*
Bruce was a smoker. Without the deficiences in vitamins A, C and E caused by tobacco, he may have managed.

8 *Sport trauma.*
Bruce was also a very keen sportsman. Here was the precipitating factor. The first seven factors were the initiators of genetic damage within the cell nucleus but it was the trauma of constant running that caused the change in growth factor.

His sports were swimming, walking, running, cycling, football and golf. Using up his vitamins and minerals in constant exercise and not replenishing them with suitable food caused a deficit that gave no raw products to mend the small but multiple microscopic wear-and-tear areas in the softer parts of his bones and cartilage. Mending traumatised areas needs new growth and the growth went out of control.

All the people I have seen with the rarer sarcomatous changes—fibrosarcoma, neurofibrosarcoma, osteogenic sarcoma, leimyosarcoma, desmoid fibromatosis—have been athletes, of one sort or another, pursuing their sports with fervour.

Bruce was due to have his operation four days after I first saw him. His parents came with him to the interview because they were long-time acquaintances of mine and wanted to help their only son all they could. I felt that Bruce was coming to see me just to humour them—he felt that the operation was going to fix everything.

He returned two months later, on 28 November, in a blasé mood. He was still smoking and drinking, but said that he had 'cut it down'. He was staying with his parents, who were encouraging him to eat what was on my food plan, but I sensed that he was not pleased about it. His parents were providing the supplements for him. He said his other doctors were pleased with his progress and they thought diet and supplements were a complete waste of money.

Bruce was still sitting in front of a VDT all day, too, and intended to go back to work in four to six weeks. On the strength of that, and because his blood was still not up to par, I gave him the strongest free radical scavenger, 'Germanium', and some extra vitamin C as ascorbate by mouth.

On 15 February 1988, his mother phoned to tell me he was in pain again and that a CT (Computerised Tomography) scan had shown that the tumour was growing again. His surgeon scraped the bone and a biopsy proved it was new cancerous tissue.

This time Bruce came to an assessment in a more interested mood and we went through the causes more thoroughly. I got him a book, *A Cancer Therapy* by Dr Max Gerson, asked him to read it, and suggested he start on the Gerson program right away. But he was not ready to do that—not until the wound refused to heal in spite of the antibiotics his surgeon gave him. He gave up smoking and drinking alcohol then.

On March 1988 Bruce started the program with the help of his parents. They had all read the book and proceeded to work out a very comprehensive régime. Bruce recorded everything in his log book, especially his healing reactions, his weight and temperature. He never missed his check-up appointments.

Healing reactions

In the Gerson Therapy regime there are eleven juices of raw fruit and vegetables, two include raw calf's liver juice. It also includes 'Hippocrates' cooked vegetable soup twice daily, oatmeal porridge,

> Say: *In times of adversity—I win.*

mineral supplements and much more. All these must be prepared as described in the textbook. The aim is to make the chemical milieu of the body uninviting for cancer growth so that many cancer cells die. The toxins from their decomposition cause reactions in the body that can have most unpleasant effects on the liver, often for two or three days at a time. Some people, not prepared to put up with these 'flare ups', as some call them, give up the Gerson Therapy as too hard. That is why I prefer to call them *healing reactions*, a more positive term. *Enemas*, especially coffee enemas, also help the liver to discharge the bile which has become loaded with these toxic products.

The severity and length of healing reactions gradually decrease as the cancer comes under control. There are longer times between them as health returns.

Bruce is a methodical, intelligent man, keen to perfect everything he takes on. It was the same with the program. Once he started, he was so keen that I had trouble holding him back from trying every new thing he discovered in his reading—pawpaw leaf juice, wheatgrass juice and everything that was available. Some herbs and immune stimulators fit in with the Gerson program and some do not. We had long discussions, and sometimes arguments, about what was possible and Bruce tried and did it all. He also told his orthopaedic surgeon what he was doing. This time he was not put down or shaken by the negative response.

By 3 June 1988 Bruce was moving back to his own house and the biopsy wound was healing at last. Tinea in the groin and dermatitis of the hands, which he had for years, had now cleared up and he started feeling well between the healing reactions.

By 3 August 1988, Bruce's orthopaedic surgeon said his x-ray showed no cancer, only healing bone. The surgeon told him to go on doing what he was doing, even though he didn't agree with it.

Then, on 2 December 1988, the x-ray showed all clear!

We started to ease down from the strict to the modified Gerson therapy. Bruce had to be restrained from taking up his walking and golf in the old competitive manner. He had found that meditation was helpful for him, especially during the quiet times when he had to relax for the coffee enemas. Now he was ceasing those enemas he knew he must try to hold himself back from doing too much. Even so, he was soon walking some 60 kilometres a week again

> **Pawpaw leaf juice**
> This old folk remedy for cancer control probably contains trypsin.
>
> Use only stainless steel or enamel saucepans without chips to make this decoction.
>
> 1 Take 6 medium-sized pawpaw leaves (not new or very old leaves).
> 2 Wash leaves and partly dry them. Cut them up as you would cabbage and put in saucepan with 3 pints of water.
> 3 Bring to the boil and then simmer without the lid until water is reduced by half.
> 4 Strain and bottle in a glass container (no plastic must be used). It will keep in the refrigerator for 3 to 4 days. Discard if it becomes cloudy.
>
> Take half a glass (50 mls) three times daily. It may be added to your other juices.

and constantly at the VDT. His dermatitis returned and he gave up his long fast walks.

It will be difficult for Bruce to learn new ways because the emanations from the machine he uses tend to make him restless and impatient. Still, life goes on and he will do his best to stick to the guidelines he has learned, especially if it means he reaches the class of a Gerson 'exceptional survivor' (of five years) in a few years time.

His recovery illustrates many points made before, doesn't it?

The effects of vibrations, light and x-rays

You may think my concern about the visual display terminals is a bit far-fetched until you read the following excerpts from the work of the expert in this field, Dr John Ott. I have quoted it *in toto* because of its extreme importance for our future.

Say: | *I am now courageous and strong.*

The quote is from 'Effect of Colour and Light', *International Journal of Biosocial Research*, Vol 11, 1989, p. 145.

> As shown clearly in the microscopic time-lapse pictures of the activity of the white blood cells contained in the videotape of my complete lecture program entitled 'The Effects of Artificial Light on Human Health and Behaviour', presented on October 27, 1988 to the School of Architecture at Lawrence Technical University, Southfield, Michigan, these microscopic time-lapse pictures strongly indicate that certain specific electric frequencies and wavelengths of light, especially in the ultraviolet, literally switch on or off the activity of the white blood cells and functioning of the immune system. This could therefore explain what appears to be a massive, rapid killing off of all the T4 cells.

And again, from 'Effect of Radiation from VDTs on Bean Plants' in the same journal!

> Radiation generated by either the TV sets or V.D.Ts theoretically could penetrate wooden partitions and influence the polarity of the ions in the air inside closed-in bedrooms. Rather minor variations in the normal range of intensities of different narrow bands of wavelengths within the total electromagnetic spectrum that take place during the normal daytime period from sunrise to sunset will influence both the normal pattern of the streaming of the chloroplasts in the cells of *Elodea* grass and also the pigment granules in the pigment epithelial cells of the retina of the eye. This, in turn, affects the continuing pattern of growth or control of future development of the cells in an abnormal way. It changes the normal growth response to an abnormal growth response or development. Cancer, as one example, is often referred to as an abnormal growth wherein the individual cells are growing wild or out of control. I see this as an overall different approach to the study of exposure to low levels of radiation that do not produce signs of immediate cell damage as caused by higher doses of radiation.'

There is so much we need to learn about the long-term effects on our health of our new-found machines.

27 CASE 2: IAN WHITMEE- BLADDER CANCER

Ian Whitmee has recovered from invasive cancer of the bladder. Ian consulted me first on 30 September 1985, while he was a caretaker at a local caravan park. He and his wife Pat really lived in Adelaide, but since his retirement in 1982 they had been travelling around in their caravan. He had been a clerical worker for thirty-four years before retirement, working under fluorescent lights in air conditioning. He drank very little alcohol but smoked thirty or forty cigarettes daily, right up to the time he came to the Kelvin Grove course in October, 1985.

Ian also had a sweet tooth and loved fried foods and his serum cholesterol level had been high for years. In 1971 he had a coronary heart turn and changed his diet somewhat but still smoked tobacco. He had opted for early retirement because of stress in the job. He was often tired and sleepy.

Since their seven children had all grown up and left home, Ian and Pat made caravanning their life. In the preparatory questionnaire, he noted his interests as reading, people, TV, walking, fishing, travelling and doing crossword puzzles to keep the mind active.

After suffering frequency and painful passing of urine for months, in March 1982 he went to a doctor who did an intravenous pyelogram and found prostate enlargement. He was advised to cut out fruit juices and cordials but no other treatment was suggested. He started painlessly passing blood in his urine on 4 September 1985. A naturopath gave him vitamin C and Barley Green powder and sent him to a GP, who referred him to a urologist.

The cystoscopic examination and biopsy revealed a cancer of the bladder. The CT scan also showed enlarged lymph nodes in the right pelvis and round the aorta. The left ureter was partially blocked with cancer and it was spreading to the abdominal wall.

The letter to the radiologist from the urologist said that there was 'deeply invasive, grade 3, T-cell carcinoma in the (left) bladder wall around the ureteric orifice. Deep biopsies show tumour ++. I think he's a candidate for four weeks DXR (deep X-ray radium) before surgical removal of the bladder'.

Ian wanted more specific information before this treatment. He particularly did not want his bladder removed. The doctor said he had 'a 50 per cent chance of a total cure' with the treatment he advised, and intimated that he had a 100 per cent chance of a horrible death from cancer without it.

Ian talked to a naturopath who suggested he should discuss possibilities with me. The outcome was that he accepted 4000 rads of radium and, while recuperating for the two weeks before surgery, he read the book *A Cancer Therapy* by Max Gerson. There was a case just like his in the book. He decided to forego surgery and come with Pat to the two-week course at Kelvin Grove so that they could learn to use the Gerson Therapy at home. They started the program on 19 November 1985.

The Gerson Therapy

It was a worrying time for them—with their new-found lifestyle at stake. The number of juices and enemas in the Gerson program make it impossible to travel at the beginning, but they determined that as soon as the cancer was on the mend they would find a way to resume caravanning.

That is just what they did. At first, Ian was *not* a happy man.

'So-so', was all he could reply when I asked him how he was going. Then came the complaints—just as well to get them off his chest to me. Pat, who was his tower of strength, was sick of them.

'The food is so bland with no salt. It is uninteresting. I can't eat thick soup. I hate potatoes. I can't go out because of the juices and the enemas and the constant urine passing—in one end and out the other.

His weight went down from 63 to 61 kilograms. He could manage to hold only half the enema. Then he had two strong healing reactions in quick succession and I thought he might go off the program (see page 243). But he stuck to it with the goal of going home to Adelaide to see the children in February if they could arrange for the fresh liver drinks. I said, 'if you are well enough', and he made sure he was.

By his next visit he had improved, so off he went. The doctor in Adelaide was very pleased with his heart check-up. His energy level had increased, he had stopped snoring, his prostate problem was almost gone and he felt well between healing reactions. As we reduced the number of juices and put more food choices into the diet there were less complaints. His appetite was a problem, however. Always a small eater, he just didn't want to eat, in spite of the B_{12} injections and thyroid extract. By juggling the compounds used in the therapy, eventually we found a good equilibrium and improvement continued

He lost 6 kilograms in 6 months to March 1986 and then stabilised. Soon after returning from Adelaide, they were off again up north for the winter in the van. They had the juicer with all the 'mod cons' and aimed to buy all their fresh fruit and vegetables along the way.

On 25 July 1986, I received a troubled call from Cairns. Ian had passed some large, round worms and wanted to know what to do. After writing the dewormer prescription, we analysed that the worm eggs were probably on the organically grown vegetables they had bought along the way, distributed there in the liquid manure, mulch or raw compost from a piggery (pigs and dogs carry round worms). Ian and Pat both had to take the dewormers (vermifuges). They determined to wash the vegetables and fruit very carefully after that.

In August 1986 Pat and Ian were back and Ian was ready to prove that he was as well as he felt.

On 15 September 1986 the CT scan showed no sign of the cancer.

Say: | *I am energetic and optimistic.*

All clear

CT Scan of the Abdomen

10 mm sections have been performed before and after intravenous contrast.

Minimal residual thickening of the postero-lateral aspect of the bladder wall on the left is seen in the pre-contrast scan labelled No. 5. The bladder has otherwise *normal appearances with no filling defects* and with clear separation from surrounding structures. No enlarged lymph nodes are seen and no focal liver abnormalities are detected.

Vascular calcification, atheromatous changes at the abdominal aorta and the left renal cyst have all been previously noted.

No further abnormality is shown

By November 1986, a year after he had started the program, Ian was well. His cholesterol was normal for the first time in many years and his ugly appendectomy scar had faded and flattened. All his blood tests were normal. Pat was pleased because she had lost 6 kilograms too. Off they went to Adelaide again.

Ian returned in May 1987, not so well. He had a tummy upset, his white cell count had shot up and his serum iron had fallen. He had a 'gum boil', a silent tooth abscess, possibly on the root of an old dead tooth. A gland came up under the curve of the right lower jaw. I advised him to go to my dentist but they were off to the north again.

Infections or recurrence?

On 4 August 1987, Ian phoned from Townsville. There were three pea-sized lumps in his left groin and the lump under his right jaw was still there. He was sure he was staying on his program but Pat was laid up with a broken leg and since he had to take her place as the chief cook and bottle washer, the routine may not have been quite as consistent as it was when she was in confident charge.

Ian had stubbed his toe two weeks previously and these glands were showing the tail end of that infection, but it also showed his resistance was low. I advised him to come back to Brisbane to the oral surgeon and gave him a referral letter.

Case 2: Ian Whitmee—Bladder Cancer

A little drama followed that persuaded Ian and Pat to go back to the beginning of the Gerson program again. Because he had been so well—and flitting about—I had brought the juice schedule down, down, down to only six daily and by June 1987 I ceased the liver juice and thought one or two enemas daily would be enough. They were not.

Now the dentist was worried and sent him to the orthodontist, who thought the lump under the jaw was probably a parotid tumour. We were all 'watching it closely' but Ian didn't want to know about it and was resisting having it out for analysis. He finally agreed to have a needle biopsy so I sent him to a specialist ear, nose and throat surgeon who did this. The pathologist said cautiously that there were possibly some cancerous cells in the specimen taken from the enlarged gland, however the surgeon thought it could be cancer of the parotid and was keen to take the parotid out and do widespread biopsies. This is a quote from his report:

> 8th October 1987
> I feel that he requires pan endoscopy and multiple biopsies of his upper respiratory tract together with a right superficial parotidectomy. This is a prime site for metastases from intraoral lesions (cancers).

Ian said, 'No thanks. If there are cancer cells there, I'll heal them like I did the others.'

So on 30 October 1987, we started the whole program again in earnest and added a herbal mixture, while monitoring the size of the gland each month. On the renewed program, by 18 January 1988, it had decreased to one quarter its original size, and by 29 February it was gone.

It was not until late August 1988 that Ian had the decayed tooth removed. There was an abscess under it. (See page 118.)

On 21 October 1988, Ian was fit, energetic and enjoying life—'never felt better'. His weight had gone up to 68 kilograms. The family wanted him and Pat to come home, telling them that seven years was long enough for a holiday. They were concerned because a relative-in-law had been carried off by cancer just six months

Say: *I exercise happy thoughts.*

after he had sprayed the house heavily with dieldrin. So Pat and Ian went home to a loving family.

Lessons to learn

There are many lessons in Ian's history. Without Pat, he could never have recovered his health. They worked as a team, supporting each other, always optimistic, determined and persevering.

They proved that you can manage the therapy under all sorts of circumstances. Still, I think that moving about jeopardised the success of the program several times. Regular dental check-ups, for example, would have found the tooth that caused so much trouble.

Dr Joseph Issels will not have patients in his cancer clinic in Germany until they have passed stringent tests with his dentist. Often, a part of an old root left in the gum and not apparent except by X-ray can cause a silent abscess or low-grade infection which pumps bacteria into the draining glands and the blood stream. There is no doubt that the high white cell count and, probably, the increase in eosinophils (white cells whose presence indicates allergy) were caused by this.

Putting the chemistry of the body back in order can bring many other abnormal conditions under control. Ian demonstrated that he could reverse his prostate enlargement and at least partly heal his blocked coronary arteries and arthritis.

Even though this couple have returned to their home base, 'living happily ever after' may not be possible for Ian unless he keeps to the basic principles of the Gerson plan. His white cell count went up as soon as he stopped putting extra potassium salts into his juices. His metabolism evidently needs this when he is stressed. Every person is different.

You will have gathered how necessary it is to treat each person individually and monitor each step of the healing process. I hate to think what the outcome would have been if Ian had followed the oral surgeon's advice and undergone those surgical procedures. He is a strongly independent man and all the way along he gathered information and made his own decisions. To have surgery of that type with unchecked decay germs already rampant in his mouth and his white cells already battling could have turned the tables on him. These are lessons for us all.

Meditation and relaxation were never easy for Ian. He is a practical man, always on the go and his routine, daily walking was his meditation. Though at first he could not hold an enema for more than seven minutes, he learned to manage by relaxing at this time, just as Ian Gawler and others who have used this method, have found. This also became Ian's quiet time by himself, undisturbed.

Wheatgrass was part of Ian's green juice program almost from the start. It replaced the commercial dried 'Barley Green' powder that the naturopath had given Ian initially. Wheatgrass had to be grown in trays and juiced freshly when needed, so when Pat and Ian were travelling, the green powder was used instead.

The blessings of our society

Looking at Ian's history positively and wholistically, there are so many factors that came together from other people that made success possible—the people Ian chose to consult, the naturopath, the general practitioner, the urologist and the radiologists, with their miraculous scanning tools devised by unknown, clever people. Then there were the surgeons who did the cystoscopy and the pathologists who examined the specimen, the nurses and others who run the hospitals where these things can be done, the social system which paid for all these people and paid Ian a pension for years while he was living out his treatment—and that is what you and I pay with our taxes. It comes also from the taxes that Ian had paid for thirty-four years of his working life. Then there are all the people who gave him encouragement and help along the way, those who grew the vegetables and fruit, who made the medications, the enema apparatus and the telephones and the books for communication, and so it goes on.

Without the backing of this whole culture that we live in, this man would not have survived. In some countries, the freedom of choice that Ian had is denied. In California, for instance, he would not have been allowed *by law* to use nutritional means to bring about the regression of these cancers. Any doctors or others openly

Say: | *Knowledge dispels fear.*

advising him to use anything but surgery, radiation and chemotherapy could lose their licences to practise and be prosecuted as criminals. It is about time those laws were changed. Yet unfortunately we are following the USA in making more and more restrictions.

28 CASE 3: BELINDA-BOWEL CANCER

This patient was happy to have her case discussed for the benefit of others but she asked that I change the names, places and occupations to protect the family's privacy.

Belinda first contacted me by phone on 23 August 1985. She had had an operation on 2 July 1985, when a primary mucus-secreting malignancy of the bowel had been removed with twelve inches of her ascending colon.

The surgeon had cleverly joined up the ileum (small bowel) to the transverse colon. During the operation, he had seen more than twenty secondary cancers on the bladder, rectum, fallopian tube and uterus and all in the folds of the peritoneum lining the abdominal cavity. The tumour had started in the appendix region and had spread widely. It was secreting yellow mucus when cut, he told her, a 'Dukes D lesion'. He removed what he could but could not 'get it all'. Because it was a mucus-secreting type, chemotherapy and radium were not appropriate treatments.

The doctor said it was a lethal condition and he estimated that she had twelve to eighteen months to live. She had lost 5 kilograms in weight. Although there was nothing more he could do, he said, it was customary to have another operation, 'a second look' in about a year's time.

Belinda and her husband, Michael, had three small children aged five, four and two. She was determined not to die, saying, 'I'm not having anyone else bringing up my kids'.

Since their home was in an isolated part of the country, we discussed the best plan on the phone. At that time I was holding a regular two-week course at a lovely old home in Kelvin Grove. It was aimed at teaching people who needed it how to change their lifestyle, to heal themselves both physically and mentally. It was a most successful course from the patient's point of view, as we found when reviewing the range of subjects introduced and the number of terminally ill people who went on to recover.

The Gerson Therapy

Belinda thought she might manage the Gerson therapy with her husband's help, so I posted them the book to study carefully before making up their minds. They found grandparents to mind the children and came to the course on 9 September 1985 for two weeks.

For Belinda the program included not only the twelve juices, liver, soup, Gerson minerals and vitamins, but also the Mantoux or BCG test, spleen extract, human immunoglobulins, liver extract and wheatgrass juice.

Belinda was not at all well. She had two small nodes in the left side of the neck, cold sores on the mouth, inflammation of the abdominal scar and severe pain in the base of the right rib cage. She struggled gamely with the raw liver drinks and the enemas but at first could hold the latter for only seven to ten minutes.

Over the next six months, she kept her log book well and recorded her healing reactions, which were frequent and severe. We had to alter the medication many times to find the suitable amount of digestive enzymes, iodine solution and thyroid extract. Michael was out of work when they started the program, which was just as well. It is a full-time job to manage this therapy, even with a helper.

I was able to get him a carer's pension to ease the financial burden. With three little mouths to feed as well as all the vegetables, fruit, liver, and so on, it was expensive, even in the country.

Boredom and depression were the worst problems, especially when the healing reactions or 'flare-ups' were in progress. The lumps in the neck, the pain, the burping indigestion, the inflammation, the headaches, all receded.

By 16 December 1985, Belinda was remarkably better. She still had some symptoms but felt well and was gardening and looking after the children.

Vaccines and normal blood tests

On 10 January 1986 she started taking the Purified Universal Vaccine injections and mandelamine to get the pH of the blood right. Since she had previously been a nursing sister, she was able to give herself the shots. Little by little, we were able to add many more foods to her diet and cut the juices down to nine daily. She continued on the liver juices, enemas and supplements.

She was feeling very well by 4 March 1986. All lumps had gone and blood tests were normal.

Then on 3 May 1986, she came to see me with Michael, very worried. She was pregnant; the baby was due in December 1986. In my opinion, if she was well enough to become pregnant, she was, with care, well enough to have a baby. She and Michael wanted other opinions, of course. The surgeon was very surprised and said the colon tumour caused no hormonal difficulties—so go ahead. I phoned the Gerson hospital at La Gloria. Each of the several doctors there had different ideas, but the young couple had made up their minds anyway—for them it was a God-given child.

So nature was allowed to take its course. We went through difficulties, mainly with anaemia and varicose veins, but there was no sign of the cancer returning.

Belinda still managed the diet, which was expanded to give the baby more animal proteins as time went on. She was down to seven juices by the time Benjamin, the miracle baby, arrived on 1st December 1986.

Parents on both sides of the family helped in many ways and the Home Help service gave them a half-day domestic help once a week for a time. Belinda's father gave them a little farm as a gift. As they both love the farming life, they soon started raising pigs and calves as well as their children.

Not long after this, Belinda was put on the invalid pension and Michael relinquished the carer's pension. After so long without a regular job, he was surprised that their prayers were granted. In no time a permanent position with a government department became vacant quite near them. It included a house in a small community, where transport, swimming pool, school and companionship with other families were all available.

The family has not looked back. They have retained their own farm, which is an hour's drive away from Michael's work. Belinda still keeps the organic garden going for their needs. She comes to

Say: | *A loving heart dispels anger.*

see me once or twice a year for blood tests and nutritional and contraceptive advice. At last, she seems to have overcome her anaemia. Her energy level is excellent so she is planning to give up her 'invalid' status and return to part-time nursing eventually.

I am not keen for her to do that. It is one thing to work for yourself and family at home and quite another thing to work for somebody else, among sick people in a heavy and responsible job, with little pay and tiring hours. So often people who develop cancer have workaholic, nurturing, kind, conscientious personalities. They don't know when to stop giving out and feel guilty receiving. Belinda was quite sure she had softened these traits and had changed enough by her experiences of receiving help to stop driving herself.

She is well aware that her problems may return if she lets her lifestyle slip back into anxiety, depression, resentment and other negative ways of reacting when Michael is unhappy. He has at last asked for help in overcoming the behaviour resulting from his early difficulties in coping with the world. He talked to his doctor and has taken no alcohol now for ten years, though he did have a problem in that area too.

I hope that Belinda will teach her family to eat the way she knows will keep them healthy and never revert to old patterns.

Above all, the strong faith she has in herself and God to heal and protect will sustain her.

The stress background

Belinda and Michael had known each other only eight months when they 'had to get married'. In those days, it was not a matter of living together, which is now commonplace. Belinda was 32 years old, a trained nurse, a kind, serious-minded, conscientious and nurturing person, very practical and responsible. She had put all her energies into her work before she met Michael.

Michael was an itinerant worker, a man who couldn't stay in one place long because his low self-esteem made him suspicious of others. He was a handsome man, except for a facial birthmark which he hated. He was a strong, wiry type, an excellent worker, sought after year after year by the orchardists who employed him to pick fruit. He had been brought up very strictly in the Catholic faith, believing it was a mortal sin not to attend Mass. His Italian parents had rigid ideas, like many country folk, and being immigrants, they had worked hard all their lives to make a living in their new land.

Michael had two older brothers who helped on the farm, who had always been the preferred sons. His older sister was the one person in the family who had cared for him but at age fourteen, when he was eleven, she was killed in an accident.

Michael never recovered from his grief and anger at her death. His whole world fell apart. He became unmanageable at home. His parents scraped and saved to put him into boarding school at the age of thirteen. He brooded over this and felt it was blatant rejection by the family. He refused to study and after six months, he was expelled from school for stealing. He never returned to study. He left home and went to work with not a chip, but a log, on his shoulder.

The rough and tumble of an itinerant labourer's life never fitted him for domesticity. In response to stress, he had learnt to drink heavily. He had a foul temper and by the time he met Belinda, when he was twenty-six, he had several convictions for drink driving and assault. She did not know how violent he could be until the responsibilities of a wife and a new baby overcame him. He joined AA after a nasty domestic incident when his first son was just a few months old.

It was a terrifying shock to Belinda to find that the man she loved and had given up her career for was not able to support her, either financially or emotionally. Even though he was stern and domineering, he was kind and caring when she was pregnant. Being very strongly against contraception, they had three children very quickly. Belinda also tried to go back to night-shift nursing because Michael was out of work.

He was good but strict with the children. She could trust him there, but otherwise she felt trapped and helpless. She struggled with feelings of resentment and depression, becoming more and more tired and anaemic, putting off seeing the doctor about the pains in her abdomen.

It was not until she developed bowel obstructions and cancer

Say: | *Kindness and tolerance soften injustice.*

was diagnosed that this fiercely independent couple asked for help from their families.

Books can show the way

In hospital after the operation, and after being told she had eighteen months to live, Belinda read *You Can Conquer Cancer* by Ian Gawler. It was a revelation. She realised that there was hope if she made the commitment to change.

She wrote to Ian Gawler's patient support group and they sent her literature while she was still in hospital. My name was on the list of people who would help those who wanted to change their lifestyle. Since I was the only one anywhere near the area where they lived in New South Wales, she contacted me.

They were destitute, so her parents paid for her to come to the two-week course. Michael was not happy about this but she persuaded him to let her come and he even attended some lectures and films himself.

I remember him as quiet, troubled, distant and withdrawn, but obviously caring and concerned and doing all he could for Belinda. He was so different from his talkative Mediterranean parents. No doubt part of his disquiet was in having to accept help from his in-laws for the sake of Belinda's survival. His paranoid feelings settled on his father-in-law, a successful, stable farmer, who symbolised the superiority and authority that Michael had resented as a youth.

Belinda was close to her parents but had not been allowed to keep in contact until this crisis. The reunion with them emphasised her need to change her life.

'I realise I have to stand up to Michael for what I believe. First I have to work out just what I do believe. Being under his thumb for six years, completely immersed in the needs of babies and a husband, I seem to have lost my identity as a person', she told me when we were discussing the changes she needed to make.

She was not able to talk about Michael or her problems with the rest of the little group during the course at Kelvin Grove but she listened attentively to their discussions, so gaining confidence to express herself to me. This was a beginning. Encouraged by the others and especially by reading the chapter 'What my Cancer has done for Me' in the book *Getting Well Again* by Carl & Stephanie

Simonton, she realised that this crisis had come to her as a *survival* manifestation and 'by God I'm going to survive', she said. 'I'm not going to waste this message by giving in and letting it overcome me.' With that sort of spirit, Belinda made the remarkable recovery that everyone saw as a miracle.

Her identity as a battling cancer patient gave her new status in Michael's eyes. She saw him differently too, since by gaining a carer's pension, he had a legitimate role in nurturing her and the children. It was a long, slow series of learning experiences for them both over the next five years.

A spiritual experience

Belinda told me that her spiritual breakthrough had come when she attended a 'Healing Hands' workshop given by two priests. She felt that she had become part of universal love, which she described as the very body of Jesus. She started taking instruction in Michael's church, wanting very much to be part of the teaching her children were receiving at school and part of the strong faith that Michael was trying so hard to live by.

She feels that her healing from cancer became complete when she 'let go and let God in' during a laying on of hands. It was at that time that she felt that a load of resentment, anger and helplessness was lifted from her spirit. 'I let go the self-pity and became a much more positive person. I could believe in myself because I could reach my inner self with prayer', she told me.

Many people who heal from disease undergo a spiritual experience. No one can describe it fully; maybe it is a melding of right, left, mid and hind brain which function together when the vibrations and frequencies are in complete harmony. So often in the meditations of whatever belief system we have, it is described as a white light descending or filling the whole person and, of course, white light is the melding of all colour frequencies relating to the electromagnetic output of our brain, our aura, our life force or whatever you like to call something we all recognise as greater than our physical body.

The aim of meditation, prayer and relaxation techniques is to

Say: | *Blame and criticism have no part in my life.*

reach a state of inner consciousness of the spirit by cutting out external influences. With practice the feeling of peace and the release of tension that these methods bring about can become a habitual part of life that makes it easier to cope with the problems we all encounter.

During meditation Belinda never found as much success in visualising her immune system beating the cancer as in imagining the white light of God descending upon her during prayer. She felt a difference between her state in prayer and in meditation which most people do not recognise.

Every time I asked Belinda over the years about her meditation, she would say, 'Oh, I keep forgetting to do it, but of course I pray a lot and thank God.' To me, that is the same thing.

Everyone is different. There is no right or wrong way to worship or to meditate. It is easy and natural. It is not unusual for patients to tell me that they cannot meditate. 'I've tried, but I just can't do it. I don't know what I'm doing wrong,' they say. Other common explanations are 'I can't sit cross-legged', 'I go to sleep', 'I haven't time', or 'I can't stop my mind racing'. These would be true of any person at some time or another, yet none of them is necessarily an obstacle. It is just a matter of practising being still and positive inside, in whatever way seems right for you. Let go the self-criticism, the blaming and the need to control every moment.

There are many books written about the esoteric intricacies of various levels of meditation. Zealots consider their own routine to be the only true or right way. This could be so for them and their disciples. Schools of philosophy emphasising initiation and rituals are found in many parts of the world and human history. Some, such as Zen Buddhism, have practices which go back thousands of years and are still extant. In spite of the dogmas and hierarchies which sometimes become part of cults, and not because of them, meditation has become a much more common practice than it ever was. This is because it is a *natural* way to dissipate fear and anger. It is a physiological gift to us all if we care to use it.

The Gerson therapy doesn't suit everyone

It may seem from the previous three case studies that all the people who survived used the Gerson program. Certainly many were in that category, however, as mentioned earlier, only a selected few of more than two thousand people with cancer I have seen are able to use it. All the others have used the Cilento Survival Plan in the best form they were able to manage. Many of them also survived and continue to do so. The Cilento Survival Plan as a whole is all-embracing. It is not simply what you put in your mouth.

Below are some typical case histories of people who have recovered from terminal cancer on the Cilento Survival Plan. They are also in the category of what the American surgeon and author Bernie Seigal calls 'self-selected survivors', those who have often travelled a long distance to learn about what they need to do and have put all their energy and faith into carrying it out.

Say: | *I dwell in the house of the Lord.*

29 CASE 4: ROBERT NEVILLE —MELANOMA

Robert Neville saw me first on 14 August 1984 and allows me to use his name. He and his wife Jill owned a motel which they managed together. Rob, at 46 years, had led a very active outdoor life, particularly at waterskiing in which skill he had won State and Australian championships.

During an Easter Championship Competition in Perth in April 1984, he noticed a pinkish lump on his right shoulder. It was not sore but seemed to be growing into a blister. It was not dark like a mole, but because his skin was not the olive, tanning variety, he was concerned to have it examined by a specialist.

He went to a skin specialist who removed it in the surgery saying that because it was nothing to worry about, he would take it off neatly, leaving very little scar. When the pathology report came back, he was astounded to find that it was a type of very aggressive desmaplastic malignant melanoma.

Since the doctor had not removed it widely, there were malignant cells, unseen by the naked eye, in the skin edges where he had excised the lump. This meant that the disturbed cancerous cells would most probably grow in or near the scar while it was healing and cause a recurrence.

What had tricked the skin specialist was the fact that in this rare type of melanoma there is no pigment. It is usually mistaken for a simple papilloma, which is benign.

Rob hurried off to a general surgeon for a wide excision of the skin and flesh surrounding the area. It was necessary for the surgeon to take an area of tissue of 8 x 10 centimetres and right down to the muscle in depth. This big area can not be covered by pulling together the skin at the wound edges; it has to be grafted. This was done in May 1984 by a doctor who was very experienced in melanoma cases. He told Rob that with small melanomas, removed widely at an early stage, the chance of spread was minimal and 95 per cent of patients were alive and well five years later. But in this large, aggressive type, 95 percent of patients were dead in five years. As Rob's only chance of survival, the surgeon advised block dissection of the glands of the neck in the area to which spread might occur from the shoulder lesion. This operation was performed in June 1984, but because nerves had to be cut, numbness under the chin and on the shoulder has persisted.

Hard decisions about lifestyle

The diagnosis and subsequent operations were a dreadful blow to Rob. Having worked his way to the top of his career as a sportsman, he was now not only disfigured by a scar which had to have full thickness skin grafts as it was so large, but he was told that he must stay out of the sun forever.

When he came to see me he was depressed and worried about the future. He hated the thought of spending all his time at the motel, which had quickly become a symbol reminding him of his problem.

He had rarely been ill, except for an accident in 1980 which led him to have a lower back laminectomy operation. We began to piece together the events which could have brought about the malfunction of his immune system, the loss of his anti-cancer antibodies and the development of the malignancy.

The pattern of life changed when Rob's two children, a boy and a girl, began to work professionally at waterskiing each summer in Florida. They had always been out on the water with their father. Now they were away most of the time. He was bored, with next to nothing to do most of the time at the motel, and Jill's mother there needing attention.

These were the situational disturbances which led to an attack of thyroiditis in 1983. This is quite a rare affliction, thought to be caused by lack of immunity to the infection causing it. So the

> Say: *I am wanted; I am loved.*

stage was set for the overgrowth of cells stimulated in the skin by ultraviolet light and not controlled by the already flattened immune system.

The job was now to build the immune system up to destroy any abnormal cells. This was possible with the Cilento Survival Plan, which brought into the body a large amount of fresh, raw food and the supplementary vitamins and minerals needed to oxidise the cells and put back the pH and electrolyte balance.

Unfortunately Jill had not attended the course as a helper, so all her knowledge of the eating and foods necessary, and their preparation, came second-hand through Rob. Men who don't do their own cooking are notoriously ignorant of kitchen practice, so it was understandable that phone calls with questions and answers about what was allowable on the diet occurred. This is the best way. I would rather clear up dietary questions and answer frequent phone calls from patients than have them eating damaging substances for eight weeks before the next appointment.

It became a matter of sorting out what was suitable among ordinary restaurant-type meals. Major favourites, such as smoked ham, fried foods (especially in batter), ready-made breakfasts, sweet tinned fruits and drinks, white flour, sauces and gravies, roast pork with crackling and so on—all were gone. What was there left to eat? Bran upset Rob, as it does me, so he cut that out.

Rob found it particularly hard to meditate. He said he was so relaxed now he didn't need to. He resisted coming to the Friday group to learn more techniques. He is a very quiet, private man who does not like to show emotion. It would have been just too much. I referred him to the library at the Relaxation Centre. It was easier when his son, a wonderful athlete, came home, because he also had a strong interest in keeping his body fit through diet and fruit and vegetable juices.

I kept track of what was happening by looking at the cancer organism in Rob's blood and noting which stage of its life cycle it was going through, based on the pH.

Organisms in the blood

Rob was feeling so fit and well that by 19 March 1986 he was back skiing, but now with a heavy covering of UV cream. On a check-up later, he said that he felt well but tired. His blood tests were not as good as before. He was drinking tea, eating veal, having wine with meals and generally letting too many chemicals, bad ones, back into his body.

His dark-field blood examination showed it. I have discussed this technique, which I learned at Dr Virginia Livingston's laboratory and from studying the photographs in works by Villaquez and Glover, earlier. This was long before the 'Livecell Analysis' and 'Hemaview' people came to Australia from the USA and it is not based on the same premises. The life cycle from one stage of the organism to another can go on only at certain levels of pH. Rob's blood was showing some bad forms (see page 175) which suggested that his own antibodies against the cancer organism were waning.

We discussed going to San Diego for the making of an autogenous vaccine, but since Bob had been neglecting his B12 injections and diet, he decided just to get back into the full gamut of substances already prescribed but not taken.

When I next showed him his blood, on 22 May 1987, it was perfectly normal. The mild anaemia and allergy reactions had gone.

Relieving stress

Another crisis developed in November 1987 when Jill's mother became afflicted with Parkinson's Disease and needed special care. She had turned away from them all. Rob was anxious and depressed, waking early to worry about a little lump under the arm. To someone who has been through a cancer diagnosis, every little pain or lump can trigger anxiety about its return. Is it a recurrence?

It turned out to be adenitis from an infected cut, and tests were negative, but it gave Rob the impetus to get out of the house and start a business in what he knew best—waterskiing equipment. I gave him a mild anxiety reliever because he still could not manage meditation to release stress. He began to discuss selling the motel.

This plan finally came to fruition in November 1989, much to the couple's relief and delight. They are now building in the country away from pollution and the beck and call of other people.

Say: *In calm and trust I find my strength.*

The regular monitor every six months is still necessary, we agree. Rob keeps up his vitamin supplements because they have helped him to feel really well for the last five years, with no recurrences of this lethal type of melanoma.

Assessing treatment choices for melanoma

In this case the surgeon's and pathologist's reports were the crucial factors. The skin specialist didn't pick the lesion as serious because the pale blister-like top looked like an infection at first. A less experienced team would have left it until no surgery would have helped, lulled into a false sense of safety by the lack of melanotic (black) colour in the lesion. It was the surgeon who, after another month, acceded to Rob's wishes and sent the specimen to the pathologist.

Removing the primary cancer by surgery is very often unsuccessful in stopping the spread of aggressive cancers because it does nothing to help immunity by building up antibodies. In my opinion radium and chemotherapy are of little use for this type of cancer and pull immunity down further.

Whatever treatments are used, careful attention to nutrition and lifestyle, which we *know* to enhance the body's defences, is also necessary for making sure cancer does not recur.

Interferon and chemotherapy

Over the last five years, grants have been given to a team at one of our leading hospitals to repeat work done in America on terminally ill* melanoma patients. It includes the use of alpha interferon with chemotherapy. During that period eight people have come to me *in extremis*, in other words dying, from this combination. You could say, 'So what? they were all going to die anyhow.' This may be the information given in the textbooks but it is simply not true. My patients have shown that many of those with melanoma in a

---

* Removal by operation of the primary melanoma is the treatment of choice. It is understood that once melanoma cells have started growing elsewhere— that is, metastasised—the patient will eventually die of melanoma. There is no *orthodox* cure. This means that the person is terminally ill.

second or third stage *can survive* the five-year term that prescribes them 'cured' with the physiologically sound Survival Plan.

It is too late to try to turn round the effects of this chemotherapy when the patient, with its nausea, vomiting and other dreadful side effects, has lost 10 kilos, has a white cell count of 0.9 thousand, and is so debilitated and depressed that he or she wants to die anyway. These symptoms are not caused by the cancer but by the 'treatment'. So few people benefit from this type of chemotherapy that I believe it has no place in the useful treatment of melanoma.

All I can do for these sufferers is to try to help them manage without pain and fear in their last weeks.

My mother used to say that in the future the last forty years of cancer treatment with man-made poisions will be known as the 'age of barbarism', in which the barbarians often attacked and killed the patient, not the cancer with radium bullets and lethal chemical warfare.

Zealous family members wanted Rob to have radium treatment and chemotherapy 'to be on the safe side'. He read up about it and decided to attend our course first. *He* made an informed choice to follow the physiologically sound way.

Skin treatments

For Rob, going back to waterskiing to prove he was as skilled as ever was part of his self-esteem and self-respect. He had to do it. He found that the UV creams contained some products were very harsh and unpleasant on his skin, bringing him up in a rash, which was counterproductive. We changed to a paraamino benzoic acid (PABA) derivative, since it is a natural body product belonging to the B group and is *not* damaging, as has been suggested recently.

Rob found that this not only stopped sunburn but also helped his arthritis. In fact, I brought some back from the USA, where I was taking it for arthritis myself, and it helped tremendously. The joint discomfort took about four weeks to go away and it has not returned. The formula is:

> Say: *Forgiveness is the key to healing.*

Gluconic ester of methylated glycine (B_{15}) 50mg
Thiamine mononitrate (B_1) 50mg
Para amino benzoic acid (PABA) potassium 50mg
Para amino benzoic acid (PABA) sodium 50mg

I took this in a capsule twice a day with meals for eight weeks. By that time the arthritis in my spine and hip had stopped giving me any pain or restriction of movement at all.

Rob has been telling his children about health practices for years but they took little notice. Now, however, they are coming round to taking care since one of them started having some skin problems of his own.

Rob is not out of the woods. His skin is extremely sensitive to sunlight and still breaks out into a rash of small *basal cell carcinomas*. He has had four frozen off with dry ice by his skin specialist so far. I have found that for the little ones a weed growing in most gardens—Petty Spurge—is as effective as dry ice or laser treatment. It can be used at home and leaves less scarring.

Petty Spurge *(Euphorbia peplus)*

This plant has other common names; such as milkweed, radium plant and cancer weed.

Identification: The leaves are soft, hairless, pale green and 0.7-2.0 cm long. The lower leaves are stalked and alternate; the upper leaves are stalkless and opposite. The greenish flowers are minute, about 1-2 mm wide. Both the stems and leaves ooze milky latex when broken.

Distribution: The southern half of Australia, north to Alice Springs (NT) and Maryborough (Qld), New Zealand, Eurasia and the Mediterranean.

Uses

The genus *Euphorbia* is one of the largest of plant genera, having over 2000 species worldwide. It is a very diverse group. Poisonous latex is produced by most species. This latex corrodes animal tissues and is intensely irritating to the skin, eyes and mouth. Consequently, few animals are able to eat spurges.

The corrosive properties of spurge sap have been known to

herbalists since the time of Galen in the second century. The latex was, and still is, a well-known cure for warts, corns, callouses and sun cancers.

The white sap is applied to the sun cancer daily for from one to five days, until the cancerous area reddens, forms a scab and finally sloughs off. Because of its potency, the latex must not be allowed contact with the eyes, lips or skin adjacent to the site.

In Sydney last century Petty Spurge was used to treat what were then called rodent ulcers (sun cancers) 'by physicians of the highest standing'. Its effectiveness in modern times was reported by a dermatologist writing in the *Medical Journal of Australia* in 1976 (volume 1, page 928). He found that daily application of the latex for five days removed a basal cell carcinoma (the common form of sun cancer with raised surface and pearly edges), leaving no evidence of residual scar.

Similar plants

Scientists have tested many spurge species for their therapeutic use when the latex is applied to skin lesions. The dramatic results suggest that most plants of genus *Euphorbia* may be used as wart and skin cancer removers. In nineteenth-century England the latex of Caper Spurge (*E. lathyrus*) was often applied; and in Brisbane botanists Dr and Mrs Cribb have recently used Painted Spurge (*E. cyathophora*) with success. Australian Aborigines used several native spurges for removing warts and cancers. When the stem is broken, the white sap which emerges is carefully dabbed on to the lesion *only*, once a day for three to seven days, depending on the size and depth of the lesion. The skin cancer cells take up the alkaloid and the lesion turns red and angry, usually for a day or two, but up to a week. Then it gradually settles and a scab forms which falls off in three to six weeks, leaving clear skin. It may have to be repeated several times at intervals if the lesion is very large but it does work for basal cell carcinomas.

Note: Spurge is *not* to be used for melanomas.

Say: | *I turn scars into stars.* |

30   CASE 5: GWEN CLARK—SKIN CANCER

Gwen is a happy patient who has allowed me to discuss her treatment. Aged 61 years, Gwen has had dozens of skin cancers burnt off and cut out by specialists. She came to me on 27 August 1989 with another crop of basal cell carcinomas on her arms, legs, face and neck.

Her mother, of English and Irish descent, had skin sensitive to the sun and always wore a hat and long sleeves. Gwen spent much of her time outdoors, at the beach, playing tennis or gardening. Having her mother's skin type, Gwen started getting her skin cancers at about twenty-five years of age. Over the next thirty years of battling with them, she had many operations, many burnt off with liquid nitrogen, courses of radium, Retin A retinoin—exfoliating skin creams, chemotherapy as 5-fluorouracil, grisiofulvin—antifungals and cortisone cream.

The lesion that was now worrying her most was a deep leukoplakia of her lower lip. This had been sprayed with dry ice by a dermatologist years before but had recurred. She had seen a brother-in-law with a misshapen face from a lip operation. She did not want to have the extensive reshaping of her mouth that would be necessary with an operation if the cancer was left to grow. Her younger son had a similar cancer on his lip at age twenty-seven and the operation was disfiguring.

So Gwen wanted information about herbal treatments. First we dealt with some small cancers on her arms and legs, using Petty Spurge, the cancer weed, on some and not on others.

We also used 'Curaderm', the Devils Apple skin cancer treatment of Dr Bill Cham, for some. Both treatments were successful, but Gwen decided on the Petty Spurge for her lip since it needed no occlusive dressing. Gwen had prepared herself by having the Cilento Survival Plan juices, food plan and supplements especially for the skin.

In October 1990 she started seven days of careful application of fresh Petty Spurge juice. It stung badly from the second application for an hour or so after it was applied and the whole lip came up in a red swollen mass. It was so inflamed that she had to have liquid food to drink through a straw for three or four days at the height of the swelling, but we had carefully discussed what to expect so she persevered. Gradually the redness, soreness and exudate subsided. A large scab formed. I told her on no account to pick at it, touch it or get it wet. Finally it fell off, leaving no scar, just a clean pink dent on the lip with no sign of the cancer.

Gwen used Vitamin E cream (Vitaglow-brand—my mother's prescription) on the edges of the scab and on the scar after it fell off. Two or three times a day she patted a little over it until the scar just disappeared. I saw her nine months later and the leukoplakia had not recurred.

The substance in Petty Spurge is not just an excoriant. The alkaloid had sought out the cancer cells on the inside of the lip very deeply too, just as solasadine in Devils Apple does.

Gwen is delighted with the result and so am I. She always has a whole bed of bright green spurge growing in her garden now in case of future need.

Say: *I can achieve; I can overcome, God willing.*

31   CASE 6: LESLEY—BREAST CANCER

Lesley was aged thirty-eight when she first consulted me on 5 October 1987. She is a school teacher with a Bachelor of Science degree, so she sent me an excellent report of herself which I have had her permission to print. It puts down all the salient points of her history. Her husband Tom is a company manager, and they have two sons, at that time six and four years old.

Dear Dr Cilento,

Thank you for fitting me into your busy schedule. After hearing you speak at the C.I.S.S. Seminar, I feel you may be able to help me. I thought it might be useful to write and give you a bit of background information before my visit next Monday.

I had a lumpectomy performed on my right breast last April and am three-quarters of the way through a series of treatments involving three months adjuvant chemotherapy, five weeks radiotherapy (on the breast alone) followed by three months chemotherapy. There was no evidence of secondaries but there is a possibility of the cancer having spread on a cellular level. My hormone receptor test was negative.

I feel my problem may have begun as far back as '74 when, following my marriage, I began taking a high-dose oestrogen pill which I continued to take for seven years. During that time my breasts were quite swollen and, at times, tender. At that time I also began studying for my degree externally while teaching full time, and this involved quite a deal of stress, especially in my last year ('79) when I completed a year of university study equivalent to a full-time load and worked full time.

My teaching career extended over a period of twelve years and during that time, in my capacity as a Science teacher, I've come in contact with hundreds of chemicals. I can remember, years ago, playing with carbon tetrachloride as if it was water.

Over these years and in the years since then I have suffered from recurring monilia infections—one point that interested me in your lecture. My gynaecologist has treated me by giving me a curette and diathermia which removed the cervical erosion that apparently 'feeds' the candida organism. I have recently had a diathermia (performed by my GP) but have had other monilia (candida) infection since then.

My two boys were born in consecutive years ('81 and '82) and I can remember feeling a lump in my right breast while feeding my second boy and thinking that the milk wasn't being 'let down'. Following their births, I went back on the Pill again—this time a mini-pill which also involved some breast enlargement and the disguise of the breast lump. I stopped taking this Pill in November last year because of the monilia problem and because my breasts were becoming sore. As the hormonal swelling subsided, I was then able to feel a definite lump.

There was one other particularly traumatic year in my life, since the birth of the two boys, when three years ago my brother-in-law died a prolonged death from stomach cancer and my father died of a heart attack six months later. This left me with two small children and a grief-stricken sister and mother to try and give help and support to.

One other point mentioned in your lecture involved the relationship there may be between glandular fever and leukaemia. I know I don't have leukaemia but I had glandular fever in '64. I was fairly sick for three weeks but had no recurrences.

I would have said, before my experiences over these past few months, that I had a good diet, however I do feel that my immune system was not as effective as it could be. I seemed to catch any infection that seemed to be around at the time. I have been seeing a dietician and nutritionist who has set me straight in the food line. I'll explain more about this when I see you.

To my knowledge, there is no history of breast cancer in the

Say: | *God give me a strong body, a calm mind and a perfect spirit.*

family, although there are three other incidences of cancer that I can remember. My father's mother however, died at an early age so I have no way of judging her susceptibility.

I hope that this information may be of use to you—at least as a starting point. I'm looking forward to speaking to you on the 5th.

As time has progressed, Lesley has managed very well indeed on her chemotherapy, but there are several important lessons to learn from her history.

Factors in recovery

Thrush

First, the treatment of Lesley's constantly recurring monilia (candida or thrush) was completely inadequate and served only to make her more susceptible to it by the trauma of burning the eroded areas of the cervix *without* any concurrent use of a simple vaginal cream made with lactobacillus acidophilus yoghurt culture and vitamin C.

Certainly she still had a heavy infestation of candida when I first saw her, which was not unexpected since she was in the middle of her courses of chemotherapy (cyclophosphamide, methotrexate and 5-fluorouracil). Since these pull down the immunity to everything, including candida, she did not recover from it until she started on the systemic antifungal, amphotericin, in December 1987, after she had finished the chemotherapy in November.

Most of our consultations have been by phone, since Lesley lives in another city. It is just not so personalised talking on the phone with no eye-to-eye contact, and possibly cutting short our conversation because of cost and time.

Conviction and determination

Lesley was not convinced about my diet or supplements. She had been taught 'Science' in the teaching method which decries anything but the 'Recommended Daily Allowance' (RDA) of vitamins and minerals. She also believed the fallacies that eggs and liver were bad for you, so she was not eating them or the supplements I advised. She did manage the juices and the meditation, however.

Allergies unbalance the plan

Because of her chemotherapy and her recurrent candida, Lesley had developed reactions to certain foods which made her feel nauseous and headachy. So it was difficult for her to stay on even the anti-candida diet. Consequently her blood tests did *not* show the quick recovery from the chemotherapy that are usual for most people on the Cilento. Her haemoglobin, red and white cell counts remained low and her cholesterol, especially the LDL, was high right through 1988 and into 1989.

Travel is stressful and debilitating

On 13 February 1989 Lesley told me in a phone consultation that she had been overseas with the children for five weeks on a holiday in December and January. She could not stay on the diet or the juices over this time and was not on supplements. She developed severe pain in the jaw and had a decayed tooth out in December while away. Also travelling with two small boys was stressful, she was not meditating and she was 'churning in the stomach at night'.

Punishing perfectionism

We discussed doing a course in meditation and self-esteem to help Lesley overcome the punishing perfectionist attitudes she had. She drove herself and whipped herself by 'setting a high standard', as she called it, a standard that no one, even the best housewife and mother, could ever maintain.

Lesley promised to make time to go to a group but as she had also started work again three days a week, I felt she would shelve that priority too.

Benign cystic hyperplasia or chronic mastitis

Lesley phoned quite soon after to tell me she had 'flu' for the first time for two years and that she had just found another lump—in the *other* breast.

Say: | *Time may be the best healer.*

This was what finally convinced her that she needed the Survival Plan supplements and prescribed diet. The one she had been using from her dietician friend was completely inadequate for a hormonal disorder.

I sent her the notes I give to patients who have benign chronic mastitis (other names are lumpy breasts, fibrocystic breast disease, precancerous hormonal breast tissue disturbance) and a new meditation tape, and hoped she would use them.

On 13 September 1989 she phoned to say she was very well, that the lump had disappeared and that she was going skiing without the children. The supplements, especially the evening primrose oil and the anti-oxidants, had caused the abnormal cells to go from her breast.

This does not mean that cancer can be cured by these substances. What Lesley had was a *pre*-cancerous lump. All the chemotherapy and radium and the dietary advice of her scientifically trained dietician *did not alter the pattern of her metabolism*.

Cancer is not inherited, but patterns of absorption are

Cancer is not inherited, but the pattern of how we use the vitamins and minerals from our food is. I suspect that Lesley has a genetic predisposition to cancer, as shown by the other people in her family who developed it. Her maternal grandmother died of cancer of the uterus and her uncle of bladder cancer.

However, without the *hormone overload* of oestrogen and other synthetic hormones in the pill, taken for seven years without a break, it is possible that she could have managed the stressful life she chose to lead without the final cancerous changes. The liver makes steroid sex hormones from cholesterol under the direction of the pituitary gland and ovaries. It also breaks them down again for excretion through the kidneys.

Any infection or *chemical insult to the liver* can damage its wonderful capacity for this detoxification. The liver is the only organ of the body that we know will continually regrow and renew itself. However it can clone cells that have been damaged and are less able to perform their duties.

Glandular fever

Lesley's attack of glandular fever in 1963 undoubtedly did some damage. This virus invades the monocytes. These are cells of the immune system living in the liver and spleen, which may become inflamed and tender during the attack. The repercussions came later when the liver cells were overloaded with substances such as excess, unphysiological amounts of hormones and the many chemicals she used in the laboratory. The detoxification is not completed and substances such as oestradiol, which is a halfway product in the breakdown of oestrogen, are held in the body in much too large amounts. *Too much* oestradiol can cause disturbance of cells in the breast, uterus and ovaries, so putting these organs at risk of cancerous changes.

Since Lesley was feeding her second son at the time, it was in the breast that the first lump developed.

Other stresses

Other stresses which Lesley listed at the assessment were:

- Persistent candida infection and the immune disturbance it caused (see page 341).
- The illness of her sister's husband and the support she needed to give her sister in her grieving after he died.
- The death of her father to whom she was very close.
- Supporting her mother in the time of her grief after her father's death.
- Her perfectionist personality, which caused her to drive herself continuously, not only at home in her management as a wife, mother and homemaker, but also in her work as a student and science teacher.

For each person with cancer, I try to help them make an analysis of the factors precipitating the condition. It is hardly possible to stop the cancer without understanding the long-term processes that promote the original cell damage in the cells' defences and then

Say: | *I let fear go to let love in.* |

the precipitating factors that promote the actual change to uncontrolled, cancerous growth. All destructive factors must be considered and managed, if at all possible. No one factor causes cancer—no one factor will cure it. No one can change the past, but by changing the environment, externally and internally, much can be done to change the future.

It took two years for Lesley to believe in my program completely. After all, only five of our consultations were eye to eye, and three were by long-distance phone. Chemotherapy was most valuable to her at first. She was not prepared to take my advice about her metabolism until her sister developed precancerous mastitis and she herself found a new breast lump, which told her what was going on in spite of all her 'specialist' treatment. The role of the essential omega 3 and 6 fatty acids in the pituitary-adrenal axis, for instance, is a very well-researched subject.

Opening the mind is difficult for most people. Many of us have been brought up not to question, but to believe the textbook. To keep your notes perfectly and know what the examiner wants you to know is the easiest formula for passing examinations. We may waste a lifetime trying to be perfect in every way and learning nothing about life, enjoyment and happiness. Most of us learn most by mistakes. But for the self-critical perfectionist, mistakes tend only to depress self-esteem and raise anxiety and fear-of-failure levels, which block the lessons that could be learned.

Lesley is working very hard on all her lifestyle changes. She finds meditation 'incredibly difficult' and she tells me her diet still needs work, but she is now *enjoying* the relaxation exercises of yoga with the help of a private tutor and a group which gives her the support she needs.

Lesley had all that the best orthodox treatment plans could provide—the usual surgery, radium and chemotherapy. Althea, the subject of the next case history, rejected all treatments.

32 CASE 7: ALTHEA—BREAST CANCER

It is rare in our culture to find women who have *untreated* breast cancer. At the time of writing, one woman out of every thirteen has this disease diagnosed definitely by biopsy. Of these new cases, half will die of the disease. Overall, the survival rate has not improved over the last thirty years, in spite of all the better surgery, more sophisticated radiotherapy and chemotherapy procedures. Women who have 'the lump' diagnosed when it is in stage 1—before it has spread beyond the one primary nodule—and who have this nodule removed surgically, have the best chance.

There has been a great deal of research into the staging which categorises breast cancer types, with the aim of discovering what treatment is best, if any.

Unfortunately, most breast cancers are often not even felt as lumps at this stage. In my opinion mammograms, in spite of their current popularity, have a very limited use. Apart from delivering a rather large dose of radiation to the breast, the machine squashes the breast tissue traumatically to get the picture. Inaccuracies in the interpretation of the pictures range from 4-40 per cent of false negatives. At least in this country we still have the freedom of choice to refuse a routine mammogram as part of the diagnostic process if we don't want it.

The only way to be sure that there are cancer cells present is to see them under the pathologist's microscope. The tissue comes from a needle biopsy or a lumpectomy. A second way of making a decision is now becoming available—testing the serum for the presence of breast cancer 'marker' CA 15.3.

Cancer markers

Cancer cells make many biochemical products that can now be detected in body fluids. There is an enormous amount of literature about this subject, covering many years of research by hundreds of biochemists and immunologists all over the world. Analytical methods have shown that some cancers produce biologically specific chemicals, 'biomarkers', in a higher concentration than are present in normal body fluids. Testing these chemicals can give an indication of the growth of those specific cancer cells. Because of the multiple factors to be considered in the amazingly intricate chemistry of the body, the biomarkers are still being developed as tools of clinical diagnosis; however, they are becoming increasingly useful in monitoring the effectiveness of treatment. In the serum there are levels of many substances made by cancer cells which are present in all of us. They are simply called 'cancer antigens' (CA). Those I use most for guidance are CEA (carcinoembryionic antigen), CA15.3, CA19.9, CA125 and PSA (prostatic specific antigen). Though they are excellent sources of information, they are expensive, so Medicare is reluctant to pay for them except in the terminally ill.

If levels of CEA and CA15.3 are raised in a woman with stage 1 cancer of the breast, it has been found that she has a higher risk of having a recurrence of cancer, whether the primary cancer is removed or not.

Most people come to me when they have already had their operation and affected lymph nodes have been found—usually in the armpit. Many have had years of treatment with radium, hormones and/or chemotherapy, but the cancer has returned in the lung, bones, liver or other areas. All these people are considered to be 'terminally ill' which means that nothing medical science can do will stop the cancer from leading to eventual death. In other words, further surgery, radiation, chemotherapy and hormonal treatment are palliative not curative. The many treatment programs all aim at killing the cancer cells off to cause a remission. When the body's own defences are brought into the scene as well the usual treatments are much more effective.

The aim of the Cilento Survival Plan program is to reduce the activity of the cancer cells and enhance the power of the defender cells. The body's positive response or 'winning ways' can be monitored by the tests in conjunction with the way the person looks and feels clinically.

If every person could have these benefits as soon as cancer was diagnosed, fewer would die of the disease.

Althea's case history illustrates briefly the natural history of untreated breast cancer.

The natural history of untreated breast cancer

Because almost all women who develop breast cancer today have had some form of treatment, the only way to discover information* on the untreated condition is to study reports from long ago. The survival of 250 patients from Middlesex Hospital from 1805 to 1933 was reported in one study. Breast cancer was confirmed at autopsy in all these cases. Surgery, radiotherapy and hormone treatment had not been used for any of them. The results of this study showed the duration of life from onset of symptoms, compared with the lifespan of women during the same period of time of similar age who did not have cancer.

The mean survival time from the diagnosis of cancer was three years. 18 per cent survived five years, 3.6 per cent survived for ten years and 0.8 per cent for fifteen years. The longest duration of life after diagnosis was eighteen years three months. There is no record of nutrition or lifestyle in this study, but it does show unequivocally that breast cancer, untreated, may have a long natural history. Therapists of today should keep this in mind when weighing up the efficacy against the discomfort and side effects of their treatments.

Why do people refuse treatment?

Why do some deny they have cancer in spite of the facts? Althea hid her breast cancer until it was too late.

She came to me at the end of May, 1989, when she was aged fifty but looked ten years younger. She and her husband Matthew had two children, a boy of twenty-two and Valmai, aged twenty-one. The children had left home now. In fact, Althea was living alone for the first time in her life in her 'empty nest'.

---

* This information is taken from the *British Medical Journal* 2:1805, 1962, 'Natural History of Untreated breast Cancer', Bloom H.J.G., Richardson W. W., Harries E.J.

Say: | *I concentrate on love—and let go hate.*

Matthew had left her in 1979 for another woman, and though they went through a divorce in 1981, they could not really separate from each other. They originally ran a cattle property but when he brought his girlfriend home Althea went to live in town. He paid maintenance for her and the children, who were still studying, but he would not leave her alone. He visited her every Friday and Sunday, and would hand over the money only to *her* personally. Every second year for six years he would come back to stay for a month while his other woman went home for a holiday with her people.

The children loved the cattle station. They spent time there with their father on Saturdays and in their holidays. Althea hated disagreements and never stood up for herself. Even though the children could see what was going on, they learnt that it was no use pushing Althea to do anything about it because she just could not make a decision. *When I say no, I feel guilty*, the well-known book by Manuel J. Smith says it all for Althea.

Not long before I saw her, soon after Valmai had gone to the university to study, Althea finally summoned up enough courage to sell the house and move to another town some distance away— a good day's drive—so that Matthew could not visit as much as before. She still found it impossible to tell him to go altogether. 'I'm accustomed to him coming and going,' she said.

Althea was the oldest of four children. Her parents had a cattle property in South Australia, which was where she had met Matthew when she was twenty-one. Her father was a martinet who ruled the family with rage attacks, bad temper and verbal abuse. They were all frightened of his anger. Althea, being the eldest, had most responsibility and was manipulated by both parents and expected to slave for the family. Her mother's way out of the situation was to retire into ill health.

'She practically lived at the doctor's,' Althea said. 'I hated that. I swore I would never do that. I had my turn when I was little.'

Childhood illness

When Althea was four years old she had a chronic upper respiratory tract infection which settled in her left mastoid bone, behind the ear. She eventually had to undergo a painful operation 'to clean out the infection from the bone'. The wound had to be dressed by nurses for months before it finally healed enough to be looked after at home. Even then, the mastoid was weeping constantly until it was packed with black tar twice weekly for a long time.

At age ten she was sent to boarding school, where she had severe hay fever leading to a chronic discharge from her right ear. When she was twelve years old, she had her first antrum washout, and these continued every *week* for two years! No wonder she refused further operations when the old sinus trouble returned in 1984.

Her mother never stood up for the children or for herself. She developed breast cancer in 1970. Her husband, George, paid little attention to her illness and she died in hospital at the end of 1973, a little over three years after diagnosis. George had trouble finding and keeping people to help him work the property. The elder of Althea's two brothers stayed for a time but was dismissed for stealing from his father. Her sister and other brother had also fallen out with George. He was bombastic, dominating, unfair, unforgiving and self-righteous in his outlook, and so unpleasant that his own brothers and sisters couldn't stand him.

The tender trap of co-dependence

Althea was the only one who stood by George. He retired from the property in 1976 and when he sold it he bullied Althea into helping him move to a seaside property up the coast. Although she lived two hours drive away, he became more and more dependent on her as the years went by. She was required to go to him on one pretext or another about twice a year. Her own children disliked him and would not go. Matthew detested him and moved the family as far away as possible. Still he phoned Althea every day.

It is hard to imagine how this kind of co-dependence can develop when people are not living near each other, but old childhood patterns of obedience to and fear of his anger and disapproval remained. He reinforced her subservience by calling on her sensitivity to his loneliness and his inadequacy in the house now that his wife was gone. He was developing an enlarged prostrate gland to add to

Say: | *Love rules; always!* |

his own ill health, and the last step in his complete dominance was his financial involvement.

I surmise that the co-dependence was a big factor in the separation of Althea and Matthew. Not wishing to be under any obligation, Matthew had always refused assistance, but when the divorce came through, George made a large monetary settlement on Althea which bound her to him still more firmly and helplessly. She then had all the classical 'set-ups' that Lawrence Le Shan and many others have described as the psychological precursors of cancer development:

- A life dedicated to helping others—nurturing but not being nurtured.
- The tender trap—being trapped in an unresolvable situation that calls on a person's sensitivity, sense of duty and need for approval, and being loved only on condition that one serves.
- Helplessness—the timidity born of years of domination which means that there has never been an opportunity to develop self, one's own personality and the self-esteem that follows personal achievement.

Althea was completely acquiescing to everything anyone suggested; her defence was in passivity—she was doing nothing about it and making no decisions. This is what had happened with the cancer.

In 1983 she had a cystic ovary removed. In 1986 her periods stopped without any menopausal symptoms of discomfort, so her oestrogen level was still high. In 1987, when packing up to move after twenty-five years in the one home, she noticed a lump in the right breast. Valmai had already left home and Althea did not think about asking her son to help her move. She disregarded the lump. In November 1988 she developed a lump in the left breast and the one in the right was becoming taut and red. She told no-one, but went on making her garden and fixing up the new little house.

Was this because she feared disapproval and rejection from her father and children if she was sick like her mother? Was she fearful that she would be talked into unpleasant and painful processes in hospital because she couldn't say no? Maybe it was a throwback to her dread of being 'cooped up', as she had been as a helpless child. Althea had no explanation at all. She denied in her questionnaire that she had any anxiety or depression.

Althea felt *happy* when she came to me because I discussed telling the family about her cancer. She had hidden it from them for two years. We rehearsed the ways it could be done and what to say and she told them after the second visit.

Overcoming destructive patterns

Althea had made no attempt to read anything about cancer, although she was an avid reader. If she avoided thinking about it she would not need to make a decision to do anything. She was not clinging to hope, she just didn't want to know. Why did she come to me then? I think she came because sub-consciously she knew she would die of the disease. She told me that her mother took three years to die and, as though it was a foregone conclusion or a self-fulfilling prophecy, she thought she was on the same path. She did not want to go the way her mother had, ignored and unloved in the cold atmosphere of the hospital. Yet she had no idea how to gather the family about her because she was locked into the situation with her father that she did not recognise as abnormal. She needed more help than I could give her there.

Gaining insight can be a long, slow process and I could see her only once every eight weeks. I rang a kind colleague who, as a psychiatrist, has devoted his time to helping the terminally ill. He would be able to see her more often.

Although she was not much interested in the books on cancer I recommended, she recognised herself immediately when reading *Co-dependency No More*, an excellent book by Melody Beattie.

Althea had a wonderfully bright and cheerful nature. She was smiling even when faced with adversity, so that for a time I thought it was a false front for her anxiety. But no, Althea was genuinely delighted that she was finding reasons for her problems. The psychiatrist was helping her to recognise her own choices and make her own decisions. Yet she saw him only three times altogether.

You may think that Althea was backward and dull to have allowed

Say: | *Tolerance dispels resentment.*

a situation like hers to develop and continue for so long. But intelligence cannot be gauged on an emotional score. She was intellectually bright. The habits and attitudes of behaviour which she had developed were originally for her protection and survival in her family situation and, being established at a very early age, were not consciously re-evaluated as she grew older. She never went through a rebel stage as a teenager—a time at which old childhood patterns are usually revised in the light of new situations, more mature intellect and experience.

Each time I saw her we discussed her situation, looking not for the problems but the solutions. Her father was to have a little prostate operation and tried to persuade Althea, who was not at all well, to spend a few weeks nursing him. Instead of rushing down to his side and dropping her own program, which she would have done previously, she was able to tell him that she was not well and suggested that he could employ a nurse.

She gave him times when she would be available for phone conversations three times a week, instead of allowing the draining daily contact. To be able to make these alterations herself increased her self-esteem and she proceeded to contact Matthew, her ex-husband, whose second wife had left, and ask for his help. This was another big change. Matthew stayed with her and helped her for a time, but she sent him away when he kept pressing her to have other treatment and when he tried to renew his physical relationship. Having cancer gave her a new status, a new role and a valid reason for saying no to her father and to Matthew.

Althea had complained to me that the children had no interest in her. She began to realise that she never contacted them. They had become somewhat estranged through her own reticence in expressing her feelings to them and her pre-occupation with their grandfather. She wrote to them, now, explaining her illness and how much she needed them. One by one they visited her and started to keep in contact by phone or letter.

When Althea came to me she was terminally ill. I thought, though, that she looked well—until I saw her cancer. Her right breast was a huge purple mass that had broken through the taut skin and was oozing fluid constantly, as the mastoid in her ear and her sinuses had done when she was a child. She told me she had never been allowed to cry. Symbolically her body had always wept for her eyes.

She had several large lumps in the left breast also, not as far advanced. In spite of this, her blood tests and her general appearance were very good, she had a fair appetite and her only complaint was occasional feelings of exhaustion.

She came to the one-day course which introduced her to the Cilento way diet, meditation and visual imagery. She wrote the following about views on 'What caused the cancer?':

Factors influencing the formation of cancer for me

'Stressful situations.
Emotional divorce, hard to let go of marriage.
No time for myself.
Family difficulties.
Devoting my time to my father.
Selling house, packing up after 25 years.
Resettling in new area on my own.'

I added the following:

- Empty nest—husband and children gone.
- Meat three times a day, salted with sodium nitrate.
- Seventeen years without love.
- Mastoid always discharging, ear and sinus infections.
- One root filling giving trouble.

Making the choice to die

Althea accepted the diet and acted upon it to the level of her capability, living alone in an isolated valley 24 kilometres from town. She drove a car and did her own shopping. She found meditation and visual imagery difficult, usually drifting off to sleep with my tape at whatever time of the day she tried.

All other treatment plans I offered her she rejected. She would always listen politely and attentively, smiling, but when it came to making a move, she quietly reneged. She told me she had no intention whatever of putting herself in any doctor's hands ever again. It became increasingly plain to me that she intended to die,

Say: *The more I receive, the more I can give.*

so it was my concern to let her do that with as much dignity and freedom from discomfort as was possible. There was no malice or revenge against anyone in her choice to die. It was her chance to grow spiritually and she took it.

She tried electromagnetic field therapy briefly while Matthew was with her, but she soon gave it up. It did not help anyway. She rejected hyperthermia and any thought of radiation of chemotherapy—which would have been useless anyhow. Surgery was out of the question because the breast had no normal tissue. Any cut made in cancerous tissue will not heal and may spread the cancer.

Sometimes her condition affected other people who came in contact with her. She now told people what was wrong and usually found solace in their sympathy and concern. However, the nurse who came to give her B_{12} injections could not stand to see the right breast. It looked angry and smelt bad. She didn't have to dress it—Althea did that herself. The nurse badgered Althea to try to make her go to the radium hospital by telling her all sorts of lurid stories of the horrible death she was going to have unless she had 'orthodox treatment'. She also presumed to be a spiritual guide, exhorting her to confess her sins and ask forgiveness for all the anger and hate in her life to avoid going to hell. This upset Althea very much. I suggested she went into town to the hospital for her injections, but she finally gave them up altogether. The nurse still called and tried to interfere in a pushy way until Althea found the courage to tell the agency and ask for her to be admonished.

In fact Althea was not in much distress. She was having no pain then and never did.

About the time Althea told Matthew to go, the cancer started galloping ahead, pouring out its own toxins. Her ankles started to swell then, and it was more and more difficult for her to breathe and eat. She kept to the diet and meditation as much as possible.

Valmai came home to care for her and managed the distressing phone calls to George once a week for her. In November 1989 she was losing weight and could not walk. Her local doctor put her in hospital for x-rays and found fluid round both lungs. She refused to have it drained, although it was pressing on the heart and causing palpitations. She accepted fluid tablets which made some little difference, but she went home from hospital much the same as when she went in. She hated going to hospital because of her childhood memories.

Her son came home to see her and said he would be back for Christmas. I spoke at length to Valmai on the phone, explaining what was happening and what to expect at this stage, when the body is losing ground and the soul is crying to be free of it. We discussed many spiritual, as well as practical, aspects of dying. I knew Althea would wait for the boy to come home. She was accepting and patient. There was no pain. She died quietly with her children around her a little over three years from the time she noticed the first tumour.

Living and dying

If a person feels inside that the time has come to go, then that is his or her choice and it must be respected. The family so often tries to hold onto the loved person because of their sadness and distress. A time must come for us all. Let it be the peaceful departure in love and acceptance that it should be. The family, as much as the dying person, can make it so.

Much of my time on the telephone is spent counselling the families of people going through the dying process. We have no training nowadays in how to handle this final stage of growth in our lives since more people die in hospital than at home. In other times and places throughout human history this was not so, but now the dying are often so heavily sedated, perhaps for months, that they cannot communicate sensibly with their loved ones. Then they are taken off to an impersonal hospital ward, when they become incontinent or too difficult to manage at home because the family is fearful and helpless. Few are close to the scanty palliative care teams that do such very good work in the larger cities. Certainly preparation for going to hospital should be made, but the constant administration of heavy doses of opiates, the commonly recommended practice, is soul destroying for all concerned.

Opiates may be very helpful for severe or intractable pain, but the three-hourly regime so often recommended may be given indiscriminately when a lighter medication would be enough. Sometimes reassurance and comfort are all that is needed. Most doctors are taught that pain is a foregone conclusion before death,

Say: *I am growing.*

and most people who have never seen people die, except on television, believe this too. Many doctors, faced with a terminally ill patient, want to do something to ease the situation which they feel helpless to cure.

The Sisters of Charity and other religious groups have dedicated bands of people who do marvellous work in this field. Most cities have caring groups who will call regularly to the home of the dying. Death is not usually a painful process, unless the spirit is distressed. In my experience it is a winding down, a slow fading, a loosening of one energy after another until the final letting go. No one went to hospital for this process until hospitals became the clearing houses for the very sick. Most people who are dying prefer to stay with their loved ones and family for as long as possible.

Dos and don'ts

If you are facing this area of care, please read *Death and Dying* or *Death, the Final Stage of Growth* or any of the other excellent books by Elizabeth Kubler-Ross. *A Guide to Dying at Home*, by Deborah Duda, is very practical, and there are many others.

Those close to a dying person often feel helpless, do not know what to do, and therefore often stand round the room sobbing, rush in and out with nursing duties without speaking to or looking at the patient, or gather together, talking and laughing in an effort to be bright, but without including the patient. Some even talk as though the patient were already dead and could not hear just because his/her eyes are closed.

Do ask the dying person if there is anything you can write, phone, arrange or do that he or she cannot do because of incapacity.

Feeding the dying

In what I call the fourth stage of cancer, when the patient's metabolism is winding down to inevitable death, there is a profound loss of appetite. Very often taste has changed or is absent and it is a hard job for the carers to find something that the patient will eat. The patient may call for a favourite food but, after it has been carefully prepared, may manage only a few mouthfuls.

As the circulation and digestive processes are becoming weaker, nausea, vomiting and/or constipation may be a problem. Dehydration can follow many metabolic changes such as an increase in blood urea, blood calcium, liver enzymes and cancer toxins, and a decrease in cholesterol, iron and maybe globulins. Confusion and irritability may dismay the family.

People in this situation should not be cajoled and teased—it only distresses them. They usually refuse juices and solid foods but will take sweet, soft foods such as jelly, custard and puddings, and these are easiest to digest. Soups are useful and porridge may be taken but fried foods cannot be digested and will usually cause nausea or vomiting.

Don't keep pleading with the patient to eat just a little more of this or that. Make up only a little food at a time. Lack of appetite is not a matter of will at this stage. Just go along with what the person wants or likes. If it isn't on the diet you are using that doesn't matter now. The person may not want to eat or drink at all.

Frequent sips of water or sweetened drinks are essential to help relieve dehydration and constipation. Morphine will be prescribed by the doctor if pain is a problem. It is an extremely useful drug for some people who are dying but should *not* be used indiscriminately for everyone in this natural and usually pain-free process.

Constipation can make the patient exceedingly uncomfortable and can usually be relieved by stool softening drugs and herbals, such as Coloxyl with senna, or other proprietary preparations. Fibre and bulk producers such as psyllium seeds (Metamucil) are *not* recommended since they may swell up in an inactive bowel and cause obstruction. Occasionally an enema will be called for or impaction of faeces may need medical or nursing aid. Incontinence of the bowel or bladder may be just as distressing as constipation for the family as well as the patient. Visiting nurses may be available to help or teach the carers how to manage.

Some commercially prepared nutritive powders such as Sustagen, Ensur, Energy Shake and many others can be most useful when feeding is a difficulty.

Fluids are often called for, but a feeding cup or spoon may be needed. Even if it is only a spoonful, it may help to ease dryness of the mouth. Water or water with a teaspoon of peroxide to a ½ cup will be helpful for wiping out the mouth from time to time.

Say: *I see only the good in myself and others.*

Visitors

Don't let a whole crowd of people visit at once. Of the closest family, one or two at a time is best. If the patient is alert enough to talk and wants to, encourage it. There may be worrying problems that have not been resolved that are holding up a quiet passing. Ask if there is anything you can do. Ask if the patient wants you to just sit with him or her and maybe hold hands. He may only be able to sign 'yes' or 'no'. Some people find gentle massage soothing, others do not. It is the same with music, radio and TV. Ask and have them all handy if needed.

Stertorous breathing and Cheyne-Stokes breathing, continuously or intermittently, can go on for days, or it may be, with coma, a sign of impending death.

Coldness and blueness of the extremities is progressive before death. As the circulation is failing, a warm, not hot, water bottle may be called for, but it will have little effect now. Use a warm, light blanket over a sheet.

Plastic sheets with disposable padding and panties are helpful, if you are nursing someone who has lost bladder and bowel control.

If you are in an area where the Blue Nurses, St Lukes or other nursing teams visit, then do get in touch and ask for instruction on turning, lifting, bed bathing, injections, mouth toilet, panning and so on. These experienced, compassionate people are a Godsend at this time.

What shall I talk about?

Keep it light and simple, if that is what your patient wants. If he or she is alert enough to enjoy the family photograph album, now is a good time to go through the happy times you had together.

What dying patients want to hear is that life has been worthwhile, that they have done a good job in whatever way you can mention and that they are loved and cherished. They also want to know that those they love will not forget them. You could say: 'I always remember how good it was when we . . .' or 'We all enjoyed it when . . .'

Some patients have grown up with a great fear of death because of their religious beliefs—some still believe that hell fire and damnation await the sinful. To give peace of mind, bring the priest, minister, rabbi or holy man for blessings. If there are none in the district and if it is appropriate, read the parts of the Bible or other appropriate writing that are peaceful and full of hope; for example, the 23rd and 121st psalms, the Sermon on the Mount, or any part the patient knows.

Reading aloud, even if the patient seems to be asleep, can be enjoyable. A wave of the hand may ask you to stop. Read favourite poems and stories, maybe (for some) naughty or amusing rhymes and snippets from the paper or whatever is of interest. You don't have to talk all the time. You may go in and out of the room. This is a time that can be boring and frustrating for you and the patient, so you can expect some signs of irritability. Don't take it personally. Make sure you have something to eat and that you get a reliever to take turns with you so you have some sleep. If you are there by yourself, you may feel angry and wish it was all over. Don't feel guilty about anger. That is perfectly natural—your patient probably does too. Yet this can be a beautiful time of quiet closeness and harmony when all old hurts and worries are forgotten.

My mothers' death

At ninety-three my mother decided when she wanted to go. She was a very healthy woman until she had the devastating sadness of watching my father's health slip inexorably after he became bedridden at the age of eighty-three and could not be cared for at home. She gradually developed arthritis and a small, silent stroke upset the balance of power in her left leg muscles.

A family physician and medical journalist for sixty years of her life, her goal was, after Dad died, to survive long enough to finish writing her autobiography and see it published. Several people had attempted her biography but she had become frustrated and lost interest in their efforts because as she said, 'No one can write the way I *feel*, so I'll do it myself'.

At the age of ninety she was still writing a little every day, in spite of the fact that the cataracts which had been diagnosed several years earlier were progressing.

Say: | *When I'm in the pits—the only way to go is up.*

Each Thursday night, on my way back from a country hospital, I would call in to see her. Usually, I read what she had written so that I could cross the T's and dot the I's to make it legible for typing. Because she could not reread it, the lines of writing often crossed and there was sometimes repetition. I always had to read it back to her and if I had altered one word or the construction of one sentence, she would crossly correct me on it. Her secretary, Paula, and I were able to decipher it but, because of her frustration with it, she persuaded her ophthalmic surgeon to do a cataract operation, even though she was ninety-one! She came through it beautifully and after three months was doing her own correcting.

As her appetite failed gradually and her walks in her organic vegetable garden became less frequent, she lost weight and energy. Poor sleeping, constipation, forgetfulness, irritability and lethargy are the legacies of ageing. 'Winding down', she called it. I had to curb her tendency to make my visits an opportunity to recite grievances, anxieties and fears.

'Tell me what I can do for you and what you can do for yourself to fix it, so we can get onto talking about something pleasant', I would say to her. This cut down the habit which old or sick people can develop of dwelling endlessly on problems instead of finding solutions. The constant repetition of unpleasant symptoms serves only to perpetuate and exacerbate them. Together we would search for and decide on a solution and then discuss future plans or a happy incident of the past. Sometimes (though rarely) she took my advice.

Mother used to tell me that she was not a spiritual person—that she wished she could have the sort of simplistic faith that did not analyse and question. Yet she was one of the most spiritual and practical of people. She attended many different churches without prejudice or favour. It was her belief that service to humanity was worship and that she had been put there by God to learn to understand herself and others and to do what she could to help them heal if that was what they needed.

She encouraged me in every way to fulfil my aims, since it gave her great pleasure to see me following in her footsteps. On 13 March 1987, her ninety-third birthday, her book *My Life* was launched. We had a wonderful party. The publishers, the Lord Mayor, the Premier's wife, the heads of vitamin-making firms, all the family who were able, old friends, her specialists, church people and other well-wishers continued to pour into the house all day. The book was a great success and we were all so proud of this culmination of her work.

She had been holding on with her hypertension and heart trouble for this very time. As always, she battled over the next few months, but old age was catching up with her apace. Since she started researching nutrition in the 1930s, she had been a dedicated vitamin-taker. She rarely had any infections until the last years of her life and disliked taking any medication which her medical specialists prescribed, even after she had developed some cardiac ischaemic attacks.

During the previous four years she had had several short trips to intensive care units. She made sure that the nursing staff were extremely attentive to her, and usually stirred up the kitchen staff, too, by demanding wholemeal bread, freshly squeezed fruit juices and salads. She was used to organising her own diet as she would for one of her patients. They were glad to see her take herself home as soon as the specialist's back was turned.

However, when she did finally decide that her body was just not making the grade, she phoned the hospital one day and put herself into intensive care, much to her GP's surprise. At that time I was still in America, showing my film, but Paula told me what happened:

'Lady C. was strangely subdued; she seemed very tired. She said she thought her kidneys were packing up. After all, she was ninety-three. I suppose they were. She would know. She listened to what her body was telling her.'

Over the next two days she had a phone brought and asked Paula to come in. They talked for hours to finalise all the unfinished business. Then it was the minister's turn. He went through a little personal service with her and discussed the hymns and psalms and service she wanted at her funeral. She gave him one of the notes she had written in her own hand previously, saying she wanted no resuscitation in the event of a cerebral stroke or heart attack. Two of my brothers were away overseas and my sister, Diane, was

Say: *I persevere to reach the good goals I have set.*

travelling to Vienna on the train at the time. Mum spoke to my sister Margaret in Melbourne on the phone, and brother Carl stayed with her to talk to her during the night. She really didn't want us all to be fussing about her.

'I don't want to live in this body any longer,' she told Carl. 'It's done its best for me but it is just worn out. Nanny always said there was a Hereafter and that's where I'm going. I don't want people to be mourning and grieving. I want you all to celebrate my life by helping each other along like I did.'

It was 2.10 a.m. when I looked at my watch in the plane from Los Angeles. I had been dozing. I felt a strange sensation—unrest, agitation and relief all at the same time—an urgency to get home and a feeling that something tremendous was happening. It gave me a short period of palpitations and I couldn't get back to sleep. My sons met me in Brisbane at 3 p.m. and told me mother had died suddenly of a massive heart attack at 8.00 a.m., while I was in the air.

That is the way she wished to go—knowing she had done what she set out to do in her own way and accepting that there was nothing more that she could possibly do to patch up her old body. Her time had come and her spirit was ready to move on.

On an earlier occasion, when she was frustrated and disgruntled at feeling poorly and not having finished her book, she told me she wanted some tapes of mine to listen to, not the drugs the doctor had suggested. I brought her the Strauss Waltzes I knew she liked and a tape I made specially for her that I thought was soothing, which said in essence that she had finished her work in life. She threw the waltzes down in disgust, because with her hearing deficit the sounds of the lower register were just like discord. She handed my tape back to me saying, 'Don't leave that morbid thing here. I don't like it. I'm not finished yet you know!'

But this time she was ready to let go and, with her forthright nature, she went about it in a business-like fashion, still in control. We had the jolly but sad wake she wished us to have too, with the family gathered together relating happy and funny remembrances of her joyful life.

That is the way I want it to be with me. We can all plan our passing; this was a lesson she gave to us all. I was fearful of death, not because of pain—I had personal experience of controlling that myself—but mostly because I thought I might be helpless and not able to speak up for myself. The ultimate would be loss of dignity and self-control. After my mother went, I knew that these were groundless fears. Make your desires known, tell your loved ones what you want.

This is why, in caring for the dying, we should ask these questions that are so important for those left behind too. It is not only what is in the will but what will happen to the pot plants, the animal pets, the letters, the care of the family, the debts, the state of the finances and other important matters.

These are times to forgive old hurts and let forgiving love take the place of anger and resentment. It is the time to say 'I love you'. 'We all love you'. 'We are all proud of you.' 'I am especially proud of you.' 'You are an inspiration to me and to . . . ' 'Your body is so tired, it has been working so hard for you. You may have to let your body go but your spirit will still be here with us all. You will still be watching over us'. 'We will meet again.' You may also say, 'You are safe and loved.' It has a wonderfully calming effect.

Say: *From where I am—I can see forever.*

33 CASE 8: GERALDINE—BREAST CANCER

Geraldine, like Althea, had cancer of the left breast, but she reacted very differently and is spending her life keeping it under control. If you called Althea's story 'Dying for approval', you would call Geraldine's 'Searching for life'.

Geraldine came to see me in May 1984, from a southern capital, when she already had a two-year history of treatment.

In November 1982 she had felt a lump in her left breast. She went to her GP, who sent her for a mammogram. This was 'suspicious', so she went to a surgeon who took a biopsy. The report from the pathologist said 'Grade I Adeno-carcinoma'. The GP arranged for the mastectomy with another surgeon in another town, but Geraldine could not go through with the operation.

Why? She just didn't want to. It was her right to choose. She hated the atmosphere in the hospital, wanted time to think, was fearful of the anaesthetic and particularly apprehensive about putting herself, in a helpless state, into the care of anyone with an operating knife. I found later that these fears related back to unpleasant episodes earlier in her life.

Instead she devoured every book she could find about cancer, being most impressed with *Getting Well Again* by Carl and Stephanie Simonton, *Vitamin C Against Cancer* by Dr Herbert Newbolt, and *A Cancer Therapy* by Dr Max Gerson.

Geraldine went back to her home state and found a colon therapist who gave her five high colonic enemas* a week and a strictly

---

* High colonic enemas are used by some naturopaths to wash out faeces from the full length of the colon. It is a procedure that can be debilitating, so it is *not* recommended for people with cancer generally.

vegetarian, raw diet for two months. She lost a lot of weight and felt terrible.

'But the cancer was beating me, and I was fading away,' she told me. 'I had diarrhoea most of the time when I wasn't having bowel washouts.'

By March 1983 she had started visiting a kinesiologist who gave her vitamin A, protein and iodine. She had liver juice and also coffee enemas, instead of colonics, which helped to pick her up.

Over June, July and August 1983, she read books by Anne Wigmore, Edie May Hunzberger and Jacki Davidson and established herself again on raw food. By the end of August she was so nauseated by the thought of it that she took a month off, eating all cooked food.

It was during this month—September 1983—that she met a female doctor, whom we will call Dr May, who was supportive and sympathetic to what she was trying to do.

Dr May read the book by Dr Max Gerson and she and Geraldine together instituted as much of his therapy as they could, including the set diet with porridge, soups, liver and other juices, Lugols iodine, thymus extract, digestive enzymes, hydrochloric acid, daily enemas and so on. The breast lump reduced in size and became softer.

By November 1983, Geraldine thought she had breast cancer beaten but she was utterly exhausted doing all this herself, so she cut down on the therapy. Within a month she was just as fatigued and the lump was increasing again. This time it was painful.

Iscador

Geraldine went home to her mother where she read the book by William D. Kelley, *One Answer to Cancer*. She also learnt about the Lukas Klinic where Dr Rita Le Roi uses 'Iscador' in her program of cancer treatment. This is a natural substance—an extract of mistletoe grown mostly in France—which has been researched in the last century from folk medicine sources. It is given by subcutaneous injection at regular intervals around the tumour site. Blood must be taken and sent to a clinic in Arlesheim, Switzerland,

Say: *I am proud of the way I manage my life.*

for testing to see which type of iscador is suitable. The medication has been used constantly in Europe for many years and is available by prescription on medical benefits in most European countries, including England.

However, iscador is a prohibited import into Australia, as are so many useful and sometimes life-saving products. The range of pharmaceutical and food supplements that Australians are allowed to use is becoming more and more restricted. This is being perpetrated against the best interests of Australian people because of the rigid thinking and ignorance of those people able to influence the Commonwealth Government Health Department, the National Health and Medical Research Council (NH and MRC), the Drug Evaluation Department, the Australian Medical Association, the Pharmaceutical Association, the Therapeutic Goods Division, the Quarantine Department and the Customs Department.

Some useful substances that have been prohibited, often as a result of American influences, are iscador, amygdalin and all its derivatives, benzaldehyde, liver extract (ripason), staph. lysate, BCG, thyroid extract, comfrey, isoprinosine, germanium and hydrazine, to mention just a few.

Incredibly, many dangerous and unproven substances are being imported into Australia at the same time and are used without adequate testing in industry, agriculture and medicine. The NH and MRC admits that only 10 per cent of the thousands of new pharmaceutical products gaining access to Australia are tested here. The health authorities have publically declared that for data on efficacy, side effects and contra-indications, the word of the manufacturer of most medications is taken as true and no testing is done. That was the case with thalidomide. Yet the import of a product that has been proved elsewhere to be useful medication and may be kinder and cheaper than chemotherapy is rejected absolutely with no valid reason given and no court of appeal. The politics of drug marketing and medical fashions can be very involved and dirty, it seems.

Geraldine asked a senator she knew how to import iscador for her own use. She was directed to a well-known physician who was the director of a department at a leading hospital. He made the request for Iscador through Geraldine's GP and was able to import it for her, as her letters showed me. The iscador seemed to help, but she also followed William Kelley's regime with a fast with a large amount of magnesium sulphate initially, 'to wash out the toxins' and then a course of detoxifying juices. The pain left and she stopped the juices but continued on the iscador.

No permit allowed

When I saw her, in May 1984, she had been using iscador for about five months. She came because she had felt another lump. In fact there were two, one in the edge of the breast, and one in the left armpit. Though she was worried, all surgery, chemotherapy and radiation were rejected as out of the question. What she wanted was another prescription for iscador, as she was running out. I gave her one so that she could apply for an import permit.

We discussed going back to the Gerson Therapy but she would have to go home and settle somewhere to carry it out properly. She promised to do this and see her physician again. It seemed she had been running from pillar to post in desperation.

A fortnight later I had a letter from the Commonwealth Department of Health advising me that the medication I prescribed was a prohibited import and that Geraldine would *not* be issued with a permit. I was also told not to prescribe it in future.

Geraldine, I heard, made arrangements to bring it in illegally, because she preferred not to return to the leading physician whose standing had been sufficient to procure her permit before. I didn't see her after that first visit for fourteen months, and in that time she had really not stopped anywhere long enough to start the Gerson program again.

Geraldine never spoke about her early life. She was married to a man who had a nervous disorder. They had two children, now adults, who lived and worked in Melbourne. Geraldine's mother lived in another state and was ill with arthritis. They were not close, but Geraldine had a strong sense that it was her duty to go home and look after her mother. When she did go home they found it difficult to live together for more than a few weeks at a time because their personalities clashed.

Say: *I am contented and peaceful.*

Geraldine is a kind, very understanding and sensitive person, but also suggestible, restless and imaginative. She is an independent thinker, ready to be influenced but to evaluate each new wonder. The way she dresses expresses and also influences her mood. She may be depressed or feeling ill, but hides her feelings, wrapped in whimsical, pastel-coloured, floating clothes, or in loud, strongly colourful or feminine, flowing ones.

She had been a music teacher for many years to be a provider while the children were growing up, since her husband's earning capacity was erratic. They finally separated in about 1975, but since the children were not through their schooling, Geraldine continued to teach high school music. It paid poorly so she learned to do without many of the so-called necessities of modern living. When the children left home she gave up teaching and asked for the pension.

It was about a year later that she felt the lump in her left breast.

Comparing Althea and Geraldine

There are many similarities, but also many basic differences between Althea and Geraldine. Both women were in a menopausal stage and suffering the loss of husband and children, which is the loss of love, nurturing ability and emotional interdependence.

The loss of her home for Althea and her job for Geraldine meant a disruption of security—a subconscious feeling that could be described as helplessness and a sense of being alone in the wide world. Though both women developed cancer in the left breast, their attitudes and reactions were completely different when it came to fighting it.

Through the seven years that Geraldine kept in touch with me she went through an amazing series of experiences. She was on a never-ending search for self-expression and understanding. As she became more and more in touch with her inner self, she began to throw off the guilt and fears which had been holding her back. As children we all have psychic senses which we let atrophy with disuse because our culture demands 'left-brain' conformity.

Geraldine was slowly discarding old patterns and, just as it had with Althea, having cancer gave her a valid reason for changing her lifestyle and permission to search for answers in her quest for life.

To nurture that vital force—to find it and keep it alive—was her aim. Her life search has allowed her to explore all sorts of unusual beliefs and to throw off anxiety about money and health. Expanding her boundaries, she seeks external powers to heal her body while she heals her soul.

During the fourteen months before I saw her again (on 2 September 1985) Geraldine, in fear of the cancer spreading, went back to her GP, who sent her to a cancer unit at another hospital.

The oncologist she saw wanted to give her chemotherapy but she rejected that idea and looked elsewhere.

Ernesto Contreras in Tijuana

This time she was off to Mexico to see Dr Ernesto Contreras in Centro Medico del Mar at Playas de Tijuana.

The first time I met Dr Contreras was with my mother in 1981. He was invited to Australia on his way to the Philippines where he was to lecture to doctors and to the public. The Relaxation Centre of Queensland had invited him here to lecture on the very successful work in oncology in which he has been specialising since 1965.

My mother was eighty-seven years old when I came down from my farm in the country to take her to meet the man she had heard so much about. She had arthritis in her knees, which made it difficult to climb the stairs to the lecture room. She was also partially deaf, but she insisted on going to hear him so we sat in front.

He gave a fascinating lecture interspersed with case histories and results of his studies. Mother wanted to speak to him after the lecture but I dissuaded her, since she could hardly hear him or interpret what he was saying, although she enjoyed his charming accent. We did not stay on.

Dr Contreras invited the whole audience to inspect his clinic, but it was to be three more years before I was able to take up that invitation and visit Mexico.

The only disappointment of that evening was the fact that, of all the doctors invited, only four came: my mother, myself and two others. Dr Contreras is such a well-respected oncologist in

Say: *I forgive and accept what I cannot change.*

international medicine, we were sad that so few of our colleagues could drop their prejudices or extend the courtesy even to hear him. If he was offended he did not show it, but he said he would not visit Australia again.

The problem was that he was an advocate of laetrile, or amygdalin, which he had manufactured in his laboratory and used extensively to relieve pain in the treatment of cancer. The controversy about the efficacy of laetrile as an anti-cancer agent was still raging in America. The long investigation was raising some very nasty tactics on the part of those who were making their billions out of the cancer industry. The outcome was the banning of laetrile in all its chemical forms, in spite of the evidence of its efficacy and safety in some painful cancers. The witch hunt that followed caused many innocent therapists of all disciplines to lose their licences to practise medicine, because they had gone on prescribing a substance that they had found useful and had drawn their own conclusions about the supposed evidence against it.

So our medical flock were, as usual, too fearful of 'peer sneer' to listen to or be seen at a lecture by a visiting specialist who was to them a 'heretic'!

My mother, always ready to say what she thought, was not going to let them get away with that. She had recently retired from writing her weekly article for the *Courier Mail* and *Sunday Mail* after sixty years of medical journalism, explaining the cause and treatment of medical problems in plain language. She still commanded a huge audience with the occasional freelance story. So she wrote a letter to the editor soundly berating her chicken-livered and narrow-minded colleagues. She always loved a 'stoush', 'to stir the pot', as she called it. After all, she had made the effort to keep up to date with the latest work at her age.

My visits to Dr Contreras

I made several visits to Centro Medico del Mar later. In 1984, when I first went to the USA to see for myself what research on cancer was actually getting to the people who were ill, I made contact with Dr Contreras through his Californian information service. Most Mexican clinics have an office in Southern California, across the border, so that English-speaking enquirers can discuss their problems or make arrangements to visit. Unless you speak 'American' Spanish, this is necessary because the telephonists in that part of Mexico are very busy indeed and are, in my experience, only able to understand American English.

I made an appointment to see Dr Contreras at the clinic on his day for speaking to visitors. I took the famous San Diego trolley to the border, walking across into Mexico by the overbridge with hundreds of others. The taxis stand in the carpark waiting, but all fares are arranged through a city-appointed officer who allots you to a driver after enquiring about your destination. This overcomes the problem of travellers being beseiged by jostling drivers fighting for a fare.

As we reached the sea at Playas de Tijuana, the stadium of the bullring came into view right on the beach. Across the road was the Centro Medico del Mar where I was due to meet Dr Contreras.

The public relations officer was a beautifully presented Mexican lady who spoke perfect English. She escorted me through the three floors of the building, from the hotel rooms for patients and visitors on the top through the waiting, consulting, files and office rooms to the treatment, lecture and conference rooms on the lower floors and the cafe in the basement.

Dr Ernesto Contreras founded the clinic in 1971 and is still the director, now working with his two doctor sons, Ernesto Junior, and Francisco. The nearby hospital is available for patients who need specialised diagnostic procedures, surgery, radiation or chemotherapy.

However, the clinic is wholistic in concept. Dr Contreras told me he treats body, mind and spirit. He believes that people who develop cancer should have the immediate benefit of treatment for all areas of the body in the basic program. He uses fasting, juices, intravenous vitamin C and colonic enemas to detoxify the systems, then continues with added megavitamins and minerals, hormones and other medication when appropriate, plus laetrile (amygdalin) enemas, stress diffusion programs and a detoxification diet. He counsels patients personally, but also advises work with the psychologists at the clinic for deeper emotional problems. On

Say: *I replace hate with understanding.*

Thursday evenings he conducts a sing-along of spiritual songs at which he plays the guitar and other instruments, and on Sundays he gives the sermon in the family-orientated Roman Catholic church which he had built for the town and his patients, next to the clinic.

Although much of it is different to my way, the principles are the same. It is a very full program and has given some excellent results.

When I visited the clinic again in 1987, on a Clinics Bus Tour arranged by Frank Cousineau after the Cancer Control Society's annual seminar, there were many changes.

Dr Contreras again gave an excellent lecture to our group and invited us to visit the new buildings being constructed for the accommodation of patients coming from afar. The preformed plastic motel units, called *girandoles*, were still in use, but the new facility will be far more serviceable for more people.

Because we must all work on basic physiology to build up the body's immune defence, *many treatment diets appear similar.* This is not from copying each other. There are hundreds of thousands of chemical processes going on in the body at any one moment yet, so far, we have discovered only hundreds of them. We all work to enhance these good substances, made up of the main forty-three elements so far discovered in the body, to the best of our ability. So many physiological pathways are the same whatever therapy is used—vegetable juices, for instance.

Depending on the *further* beliefs of the therapists, many diets and supplements are different too. Dr Contreras uses the amino-acid *trypsin* and *vitamin A* in much greater doses than I do, for example. His diet differs from the Survival Plan since it contains nuts and nut milks and no dairy products.

Dr Contreras uses much more trypsin, vitamin A and food enzymes such as pepsin and bromelein because he subscribes to the trophoblastic theories of John Beard, DSc, 1858-1924 (who was for many years a Professor of Embryology at Edinburgh University) and Ernst T. Krebs, a physician from San Francisco.

The panel of doctors who, with Dr Contreras, discussed Geraldine's case advised her to have 20 milligrams of tamoxifin twice daily, and gave her a program of coffee enemas, wheatgrass juice and diet. They asked her to seek help for coming to terms with her inner self. They further advised that when the breast lump had regressed she should have a lumpectomy, following by radium-therapy. Then they said that when she had stopped the tamoxifen, she may need to have her ovaries removed.

This was a far more stringent program than the Australian doctors had suggested. She hurried back to Australia in alarm.

Geraldine was already having enemas and wheatgrass juice, and what she could take easily of my diet. She was also pursuing every self-awareness course she came across that was not too expensive, to help with her inner problems. Back in Australia, the breast lump *did reduce* with the meditation, the tamoxifen and the rest, so she decided to forego the lumpectomy and just add the radium.

Geraldine has radium

Back in her home state, Geraldine had a battery of tests which were all normal and she took it that her detoxification efforts were working. This was a great step forward for her. The oncologist then persuaded her to undergo a small series of treatments with radium in accordance with Contreras' views. The Australian doctor told her that the course of ten treatments was 'palliative'. The only hope of a '*cure*', the doctor said, was to have a simple mastectomy followed by lymph-node dissection and more radium. Actually, the fact that her cancer had already spread to the armpit meant that these measures would most likely be only 'palliative' anyway.

I know that Geraldine hated the thought of having radium. Because she was fearful and antagonistic and did not believe that it would help her she had little chance of benefit from it.

So, in August 1984, Geraldine had four treatments with radium, but her sensitive skin reacted so badly that it was discontinued. She never had the ten prescribed.

Another precursor that I give if my patients are to have radium treatment is the lesson in visualisation of the immune system shielding itself from the radium beams that then home in to zap only the destructive cancer cells.

This instruction is reinforced by listening to a very interesting tape, 'Meditation, Imagery and Cancer' by Mark Yarnell and Barbara

Say: | *A soft answer turns away anger.*

Wilkins, available from Unity Village, Missouri. On it the personal experience of this psychological protection is described.

The build-up of motivation and expectation of success has been shown time and time again to give the best therapeutic results from any treatment, whatever it is.

Barbara Wilkins, who is an American nurse, had breast cancer. After her operation she had irradiation and chemotherapy—which was the protocol used then for her stage of the disease. During the radiation she visualised the good cells having golden shields that deflected the rays onto the cancer. She came through the treatment extremely well.

Radium burns

Geraldine used vitamin E and aloe vera juice straight from the plant to help heal her radium burns. She pricked a capsule of vitamin E with a pin and squeezed out the oil onto the lesion at night. This is very good for taking the soreness out of sunburn too.

In the morning she broke a piece of green aloe leaf 2-3 centimetres long, peeled the skin off and put it through a garlic squeezer. She then applied the gluey green juice to the burnt area. At first, when it was blistered she covered it with a piece of cloth, but later she just put the juice on and let it dry there. The leaf can be crushed with a fork, cut or chopped so that juice oozes out, or it can be put in the blender. If this treatment is used as soon as the damage is done the continually weeping and red congested areas that radium causes on sensitive skin can sometimes be healed. Left untreated, these lesions can take years to heal or may never do so.

The primary tumor and axillary nodes were still there and Geraldine felt that she was losing ground.

Geraldine, the surgeon and Iscador

Since radium was unsuccessful in her experience, Geraldine thought again of lumpectomy, as Contreras had advised. She contacted her local doctor friend for a referral to the Associate Professor of Surgery, Avni Sali, at the University of Melbourne Repatriation General Hospital in Heidelberg. It was October 1984 when Geraldine had her consultation with this very practical, knowledgeable and open-minded surgeon who has brought the adjunct of peace of mind to his patients by teaching them meditation and relaxation techniques before and after operations. He thought that Geraldine had accepted surgery as the next step but, having time to consider it, she decided against it again.

After wandering here and there to stay with friends, to her country house and to her mother's home, Geraldine came back to Brisbane in late 1985. She was having iscador every second day by subcutaneous injection into the breast, but was not keeping to my schedule of juices or supplements. She had stopped the enemas and wheatgrass juice.

When I examined her, the lumps in the armpit had gone but the lump in the breast was bigger, now pulling in the nipple and causing knots of little blood vessels in the skin on the lower side of the breast. I looked at her live blood under the dark-field microscope, as I usually did when I saw her. There were bad forms, 'motile rods' and 'cotton balls', that showed she was not making antibodies against the organism and that her blood was too alkaline. We discussed again the changes that were possible in her diet and lifestyle to help her regain control. In making choices of various useful therapies, we had to take her restlessness and constant moving about in her search for self into consideration.

Geraldine, the Bhagwan and energy levels

Next time I saw Geraldine she told me that in studying yoga methods of healing she had come across the teachings of Bhagwan Maharishi Ragneesh. Having joined the Orange People, she arrived at the Friday Cancer Quality of Life Support Group in a filmy pink and orange dress with her unpronounceable new name on her introduction tag. It gave the rather staid members of the group some new vibrations to consider and they decided they liked her old name better!

She was staying in a share house with other Ragneesh devotees. She asked if she could help with gardening at the Kelvin Grove Centre some mornings. With her usual verve and conscientiousness, she put so much energy and so few fluids into this activity at the very hottest and most perspiry part of Queensland summer that

Say: *God help me to control untamed desire.*

she soon wore herself out, became dehydrated and developed cystitis. Antibiotics fixed this and also improved the pH of her blood so that, by 16 November 1985, her dark-field blood examination was clear.

I explained to Geraldine that people with cancer have a limited amount of energy because their electromagnetic fields are so out of balance and easily disturbed that they must be careful not to overdo any exercise pattern. The production of energy for exercise uses up the vital minerals and vitamins necessary for fighting the cancer, puts the Ph out of balance and may push cancer cells, with their attendant showers of free radicals and destructive toxins, into new areas via the lymphatics and blood vessels. Apart from all this, she admitted that there was some smoking going on at the house.

Geraldine and the Gerson program

Breaking up with the Ragneesh people, Geraldine felt wretched and decided to go home and try the Gerson Therapy in earnest while continuing with the iscador when she could get it. She said she had read *A Cancer Therapy* by Dr Max Gerson again. I arranged some prescriptions for things she would need.

The first healing reaction or 'flare up', when toxins are being released from the cancer breakdown, was a 'ghastly experience', as Geraldine put it. By phone I was able to tell her that the nausea, weakness, aches, pains and temperature were all part of this toxic reaction and would pass quickly if she took oatmeal, gruel, peppermint tea and enemas. Manipulating the number of juices was important, too, because she had burning lips from too much carrot, beetroot and silverbeet.

For the next six months, there were just a few phone calls and an occasional letter in times of crisis. Geraldine was going through so much in her search.

More self-awareness, magnetic therapy and crystals

During 1986 Geraldine studied with a group who had 'heart talks' and 'truth sessions' to release anxiety and old revenge patterns of the past. She also learnt 'rebirthing techniques' as she told me, 'to open up to love myself, to stand back and let go, to stop running away and inspect my feminine/masculine self. I have always resented male authority and domination', she said, 'because my brother and my father always put me down but expected me to be a fabulous achiever. I tried to do everything right so dutifully. So now I want to be myself, now I am finding out who I am.'

Geraldine also took up more study of the 'Course of Miracles', another self-awareness course, said to be written from lessons sent to a 'channel' or spiritual medium in the USA. She had undertaken this with friends in 1984 at the Relaxation Centre of Queensland in Brisbane, but there are now study groups in most Australian capitals. At this time the breast lump regressed somewhat. It was softer and smaller, and the nipple looked less retracted.

Then her mother became ill. Though Geraldine looked after her continually, they had never been very close. Her asthma returned in this frustrating situation. It became impossible to follow her own program after constant trips to take her mother for doctor, physiotherapy and x-ray visits. The cancer waxed and waned, quite definitely according to her state of mind, her diet and her detoxification program.

'When I am with mother, I have negative movies going into every cell', she said in August 1986. She was having, at that time, acupuncture and traditional Chinese herbals and also attending another orthomolecular physician in Melbourne.

On 8 April 1987 her dark-field blood examination was excellent. She was having *magnetic therapy* and wearing a coral ring and crystals. Did these help? Who knows? They certainly helped her self-esteem.

Dolphins

On 27 November 1987, I saw Geraldine looking marvellous. She had been on a trip around the east coast in a van, taking her juicer with her. She had been to Cairns, where she studied dolphins and became fascinated by their survival techniques. She followed this search for dolphins, visiting many of the wonderful white sand and surf beaches right down the coast, especially where rainforest came nearest the sea. She was studying rebirthing which she said put

Say: *I look forward with hope and courage.*

her in touch with some of her other reincarnations and that there was an affinity in the past with dolphins.

In that year (1987) she met a gentle, sensitive Aboriginal man, Burnam Burnam, at the Relaxation Centre. He has written a beautiful book following his study of the myths and legends of his race. He discussed with Geraldine the specially close tie of ESP between the Aboriginal and the dolphin in the tribes of the east coast of Australia. She made contact with other Aboriginals in North Australia and, in July 1987, travelled to Arnhem Land.

The last contact I had with Geraldine was when she came back with jaundice from an Aboriginal camp where she had stayed for three weeks. She feared she might have a secondary cancer in the liver, so I arranged for some tests to be done. However she left no forwarding address and the test results never arrived, so I didn't know whether it was the relatively harmless hepatitis A virus carried by water, flies, fingers, cups and cutlery, the much more serious Hepatitis B virus, carried in body fluids, or the end of the road, liver metastases from the cancer. I hoped and prayed it was the first.

Then Geraldine came to Brisbane, in March 1990 to lecture about dolphins. She was very well, so we decided that she must have had hepatitis A, a mild case. She is now writing a book about her personal experiences.

Vis medicatrix naturae, the healing force

So, what has Geraldine taught us in her long and courageous tussle with breast cancer? Was cancer visited on this kind, infinitely sensitive and aware person so that her spirit could escape from the bondage of her early upbringing—just as in the case of Althea who took a different path? The tenacity, sense of wonderment and *joie de vivre* which Geraldine brought to all her journeys into new fields would certainly fulfil my mother's criteria when she would say, as I do, to a patient, 'Leave no stone unturned'.

Geraldine was, and probably still is, in search of the *Vis medicatrix naturae*, the healing power of nature which has been recognised as the healing force throughout history. As the greatest surgeon of the Renaissance, Ambrose Paré, stated of his own skills, 'I treat, God cures'.

We heal ourselves through the spiritual perfection that is within each of us, if only we can toss away the burden under which faith in our God-given power lies hidden. Put it this way: the best that the doctor or anyone else can do is to help get rid of these burdens so that the patient's own miraculous processes can restore the natural order and balance to the body, mind and soul.

In 400 B.,C. Hippocrates, the great physician and father of medicine, recognised that disease was not just the symptoms of poor health, but also the effort or energy the body put out to re-establish order and function from a disturbed electromagnetic equilibrium; the healing power is an attribute of life itself. It is the **VITAL FORCE**.

Here is some of the correspondence from Geraldine which kept me in touch with her program from afar.

Old Years Day 85

Dear Ruth

Thank you for being there and for being such a special, inspiring person. I hated to phone you, but feel relieved that there is an answer to my tiredness.

Happy New Year! Now that I've landed for a while I can write.

Mum's been fantastic and supportive, and the vegies are bouncing out of gardens all around. Best I've ever tasted. Lips and skin are calming down. I think I got too excited over the carrots!

As Beata* writes, one's life closes in, and mine did before two years ago, and instead of staying in, I burst out. Still I suppose I needed this long journey to work out just what is effective. Twelve juices are more powerful than four!

The healing people I met in Brisbane seemed to come to me and I'm meditating whenever I can. To know that love comes from within is the greatest lesson I've learnt in the three years and I need to re-affirm that often.

---

* Beata Bishop, author of *A Time to Heal*.

Say: | The body may die—the spirit still lives.

I loved my work at the Centre, and felt we were a good team.

Xmas with the boy was great and he fiddled with a turkey, and even made me some juices. (Xmas was the climax of that first great flare up—I could hardly believe it was happening to me).

So I'll see you some time at the end of January.

We're breaking routine on Thursday and going to one of my favourite places for a picnic.

Fondest love for '86—Geraldine

*   *   *

4 p.m. Friday 24 January 1986

Dear Ruth

Good to hear your voice this morning. You made me think and my realisation now is that I am an excellent grower of a tumor!

Trying not to panic. Certainly will not tell Mum. But I think the overdose of Lugols and thyroid combined have made the tumor take off! This accounts for the curry *smell I've had the last few days. The swelling is the tumor.*

Mum's out at present so I tried to call you but forgot you are at the Centre.

Well I've panicked before. That's not much of a choice. So I'll diligently get on with coffee enemas to clear the body and maybe not have Lugols tomorrow.

I also have woken up the last two nights, although I've slept very soundly before.

*Lots of Love
Geraldine*

*   *   *

Feb 23rd 1986

Dear Ruth,

It's five weeks since I spoke to you, and progress has been slow.

As the tumor went down a little, I seemed to get asthma wheeziness again, and especially at night, so I'd hop out of bed and have an enema, thinking that the wheeziness was connected with toxins floating in the body.

Gerson does say asthma is relieved, and of course I wondered why it was coming back, especially as in Brisbane, in about November, it went away and I stopped taking Nuelin twice a day. The asthma's comings and goings have intrigued me, even before cancer diagnosis in Nov. 82. Asthma started in 1978, lasted 3 years until just before onset of cancer, and then returned Dec. 1984 when the tumor regressed after radiation, with wheatgrass and iscador.

Liver juice intake has fluctuated I think mainly because I got tired of searching for fresh liver (just why can't we freeze it for 2-3 days? Vit. C diminishes?) Mother also has been in pain for the last three weeks, and I've been the chauffeur nearly every day—Doctor, physio, doctor, physio, x-ray, osteoporosis and a visit to the orthopaedic surgeon this coming week.

So with a large depression engulfing me—(why am I not improving?)—I examined the pieces again.

Potassium nil for last three weeks. I've been waiting for the local chemist to expedite bulk quantities of acetate, gluconate and phosphate. Finally I've ordered a small one from the city.

Liver now three times daily. Wheatgrass now three times daily.

I'd been drinking wheatgrass, 2 oz x 3, all along, but on its own it wasn't having the magical effect it's had previously. So now after four days of three liver juices daily, echoes in both armpits and left breast have gone, energy has risen, and I think tumor shrinking.

Still four enemas daily.

Added to this list of woes was my unfortunate eating of a poisoned apple. The Snow White saga is too long to tell, but it was Triquot* for blackberries and twitch, and after two days of multi-juices and six to seven enemas, I survived. That's when I started the liver properly again.

---

* Triquot is a poison used by some apple orchardists against pests.

Say: | *I persist until I succeed.* |

Skin crystallisation on the hands and face. Skin cancers started immediately.

I can only hope I have enough iodine in my system and vegies and liver to do the rest.

I'd like very much to be seeing you soon, but feel I must hang on here for the old lady's sake for a few more weeks.

Whilst here I've managed to help my Aboriginal friends organise quotes for 1000 cassettes, and an application to the Arts Board for a grant, and that's been some light relief. (An old tape from 1968 sealers' dance tunes.)

I don't think I could really live with my mother for ever, unless I had my own living quarters, as she leads such a different lifestyle from mine. And at the moment, the pressure of my own survival is enough for me to take.

However I've found that loving and hugging her have really helped both of us in our relating.

So this is to let you know that I'm still journeying on. It's strange that, unlike Beata, I've never been able to get friends or relations to read books about cancer to help me in any way. It's as if I have to learn and research every piece independently to be my own textbook. Still meditating as often as possible.

What would Dr Gerson and Dr Ruth suggest now, eh?
Love and peace and hope to see you soon,

Geraldine.
I had to take a Nuelin last night and again today.

*　　　　*　　　　*

Mar 12th 1986

Dear Ruth,
Feeling great and full of life!
I'm flying to Brisbane next Monday, 17 March, and I hope I may see you during the week. Please ask Faye to write me in the book!

I suppose I'd really like to see my blood if that's possible.

Looking forward to seeing you so much.

Fondest love, peace,

Geraldine.

34 CASE 9: MEGAN McNICHOL— MELANOMA

One of the most dramatic remissions for cancer was in a patient of mine who went, on my advice, to the Livingston Medical Clinic in San Diego. Megan McNichol has allowed me to use her name and history because she wants people to know that reversal of an aggressive, lethal cancer is possible. To change a lifestyle is difficult— but if you really want to recover from malignant melanoma, it can be done.

I was giving a lecture to some people at the raw food Hippocrates Clinic in the hinterland of the Queensland Gold Coast when I met Megan. She and her fiancé came to me after the lecture and asked my advice about where to go for further treatment, since she had just had a recurrence of malignant melanoma in her neck after her fourth operation. I told them it was illegal to give them advice on medical treatments publicly. Though I had been talking about nutrition and stress control to prevent cancer, these are not considered 'medical treatments'. Megan therefore decided to make an appointment. She and her fiancé were planning to marry in one month's time.

I saw Megan with her mother in my consulting room on 7 February 1987. She told me the following relevant facts:

- She had had a large malignant melanoma removed from her neck in August 1985.
- She had been using an *oral contraceptive* for two years previously and was continuing to use it.
- In January 1986 proven *german measles* (Rubella) developed, even though she had overcome that virus many years before. It rarely recurs.
- In 1986 she developed *thrush* (monilia or candida) in January, March and June and it was treated by the wholly inadequate cream-for-five-days method.

- By November 1986 another cancerous melanoma had grown in a lymph gland on her neck, so she had extensive surgery—a block dissection of the lymph glands of the left side of the neck.
- Within two months there was a lump on the right side also; the disease was extremely aggressive. CT scans were done to make sure it had not travelled to the brain. They proved negative. Another specialist in melanoma was consulted and told her just to have the lumps taken out whenever they came. So the one on the right side of the neck had been removed just ten days before I saw Megan.

After going through my usual descriptions of how and why cancer started and the diet I advised, I discussed with them the seriousness of the situation. Melanoma seems to travel upwards in the body. It was obvious that the immune system had stopped making adequate antibodies not only against the rubella virus, but also against the cancer. With nothing to stop cancer cells moving through the lymphatic and circulatory system, and with Megan's stressful lifestyle, it was rushing ahead—literally. The head, especially the brain, would be the next port of call.

UV radiation is one of the original stimulators of the melanomatous cancer change, so radium is not a useful remedy against melanoma, although it is sometimes used. Chemotherapy for melanoma, in my experience of terminally ill patients, has been a dismal failure. Interferon had been used only recently in Australia—the grant was given by drug manufacturers for the use of chemotherapy with it. Maybe there are some successes, but all patients I had seen had come to me dying after that experimental treatment had failed.

I had seen only three people who had completely recovered from melanoma when it had reached its aggressive, 'terminal' stage like Megan's. Two were patients I met in Dr Livingston's clinic in San Diego, who were six and seven years free of the disease respectively, and one was my own patient, Tom (see his history on page 339). whose secondary cancer was in the groin and pelvis and had been in remission on the Cilento Survival Plan for two years—not really long enough to be considered. Also, the Cilento Survival Plan worked very slowly for melanoma without the vaccines which were then unavailable to us in Australia. So I thought immunotherapy with vaccines at San Diego was the best course.

The Livingston Medical Clinic

Having discussed the program in San Diego in detail, I gave Megan, for the meantime, my dietary program, the meditation tape and the supplements for the Survival Plan. I also lent her the VHS videotapes I had bought in the USA, 'The Livingston Medical Clinic', 'Dr Virginia Livingston', 'Laboratory' and 'The Immunology of Cancer', to help her decide. I thought it would be best for Megan to postpone her marriage until after she had the treatment but she was adamant that marriage came first, whatever her decision about going to San Diego would be.

Shortly afterwards, her father came to have a talk about Megan's future. He took her to several other doctors while she was making up her mind, including a well-known Sydney oncologist. All this took several months.

On 3 April 1987, Megan returned after a check-up with her local doctor. There were four more lumps around the scar on the right side of her neck, going upwards. She had been 'slack' with the juices, she said, only managing two or three daily at the most, for the last two months. She wasn't taking many of the supplements either.

We looked at Megan's live blood under my dark-field microscope. There were 'motile rods' and 'cotton balls', target cells, many L forms, Heinz-Erlich bodies, spheroplasts and mesosomes—it was the life story of the Progenitor cryptocides under one coverslip from a thin spread of blood no bigger than a one-cent piece. Some of these forms of the organism showed that Megan had no immunity against it. I urged her to go as soon as possible.

Her mother had seen the video films and decided to go with her to San Diego. On 13 April 1987 they had received the Immunology Clinic brochure and I gave them a letter to Dr Virginia and the address, also, of Charlotte Gerson, in case they wished to visit her. They had read the books by Beata Bishop and Jacki Davidson, and were now convinced that there were better ways than radiation and chemotherapy to treat this illness if survival, not palliation, was the goal.

Back from the Livingston Medical Clinic, Megan came to see me on 5 May 1987 with the fully documented follow-up treatment

Say: *I change my thoughts—and I change my life.*

from staff physician, Dr C.E. Holmes Jr. She was unable to see Dr Virginia, but was most impressed by the friendly, caring atmosphere and thoroughness in treatment at the Clinic. Especially useful were her sessions with the nutritionists, who explained in great detail the use of the foods and supplements, and why she should continue these for at least five years.

Lifestyle changes

Now was the time to discuss future lifestyles. Megan lived on a large grazing property not far from Toowoomba, a city on the Darling Downs in Queensland, a great pastoral and agricultural area. She came from a family of horse-lovers and an interest in bloodstock and horse racing were integral parts of her life. At twenty-eight years old she had proved herself to be a competent stud manager. She spent most of the daylight hours outside in the sunlight, though sunbathing on the beach had never interested her.

Now she must wear long-sleeved, all-cotton shirts and slacks, sun-cream for face and hands and a broad-brimmed hat so that there was complete cover, especially for her head and neck, even in our hot summer.

It was *not* advisable for her to wear sunglasses, however, since we know from the work of Dr John Ott that full spectrum daylight is necessary, through the pupil, for health.

Megan was about to marry now, but the steroid formulations of oral contraceptives would be harmful to her because they damaged the hormone metabolism. She had trouble for years with hormone imbalance—mainly with cystic ovaries indicating that there was abnormal metabolism of her steroid hormones and essential fatty acids. This is one of the factors in cell membrane changes that can allow cancer to occur. So we discussed other more physiological contraceptive methods.

The diet and supplements were not going to be too difficult, and since Megan was familiar with injection techniques for her horses, it was no problem to administer her own injections of vitamin B12, augmented purified antigen, purified antigen, immuno-globulin and autogenous vaccine, in the doses and at the times prescribed by Dr Dan Magtira at the San Diego clinic. She went to her local doctor for intravenous vitamin C and B6 three times a week, and to have her many blood and urine tests done every fortnight and, later, every month.

Purified Protein Derivative tests and BCG

Another part of the schedule was the testing of her immunocompetency by the PPD (Mantoux) test each month. If the test was negative she was to have a BCG vaccination repeated until it 'took', that is, until the body reacted to the BCG by inflammation, crusting and scab formation similar to that which we experience from a smallpox vaccination, but less severe.

Here was a problem. BCG is made by our Commonwealth Serum Laboratory (CSL), but is not available for my use except for immunising people against tuberculosis. I had some frustrating exchanges with the head of the Queensland branch of the CSL department, where this product is manufactured, when I tried to implement the Livingston immunology program in 1985. He simply refused to sell it to me.

So, we were unlikely to obtain BCG here. As it turned out, however, Megan's local GP was able to buy it from the CSL by saying nothing about how he was using it.

In all, Megan was taking seventy tablets a day. Many were the same vitamins and minerals as I had given her previously, but the Livingston program gives them all separately; for instance, the B vitamins are given one by one, not in the compound capsule that I use. The diet is somewhat different from the Survival Plan since Dr Virginia was of the Adventist faith and no animal food is allowed. Megan wondered how she would manage this since she had been a heavy meat eater.

There is some evidence, not yet proven, that 1-phenylalanine, one of the essential amino acids occurring among other foods in red meat, encourages the formation of melanin (black material) and the melanotic (black) tumours. On the strength of this some therapists prohibit *all* foods containing phenylalanine. I do not find their arguments convincing because:

Say: | *I count my blessings.*

1 Megan's tumours were *not* black melanomas. They were 'amelanotic' in spite of the fact that she ate much meat.
2 We need this amino acid in every cell of our body. It is one of the eight *essential* amino acids that we cannot manufacture from food. There are hundreds, maybe thousands, of amino acids which all have their different properties and uses. One of those, present in red muscle meat, may be a growth promoter that encourages the growth of cancer, but it is not known which one it is.
3 Some of the peptides, the smallest molecules derived from amino acids, are essential for the inhibition of cancer cell growth. Antineoplastins are made by the body from some proteins.

Removing the last lump

Megan managed the program very well and, to everyone's great delight, five of her six tumours disappeared within the first six months. The big one on her left shoulder just would not regress—it was very much like the one that Beata Bishop discusses in her history.

Every six months Megan went back to San Diego to have it checked. In January 1988 Dr Dan Magtira injected it with purified antigen but it still did not regress so, eventually, in June 1988, she persuaded him to let her have it removed. She had the operation done by a Sydney oncologist under local anaesthetic so she could see what it was like inside.

Just as with Beata's case, it was like a cyst. There was a thick fibrous outer wall containing dead grey necrotic tumour, but right in the centre there was a little bit of tissue like grains of red sand which, under the microscope, proved to be malignant melanoma cells. The cancer was there, but *the body had walled it off*. Megan was very relieved and even more determined to stay on her program religiously.

When I phoned her three years after out first meeting, she had no recurrence and was 'going great guns, lots of energy', as she said. She certainly sounded vibrant.

Some of her many tablets and injections had been reduced but she was still sending her urine to San Diego every six months for the making of new supplies of autogenous vaccine from the organism in it. She has not needed a BCG vaccine for eighteen months now because her immune system is working, as shown by a positive PPD every two months.

How long does this treatment go on? There is no generalisation; each patient is different. Forever could be the answer, or maybe for five or ten years more. Who can say? Learning to control the stresses of life is part of the answer too. Megan does her meditation and visualisation regularly. I didn't ask her if she still uses my tapes. She doesn't need to now, I should think.

I asked her if she considered this constant treatment a hassle now she is working with her horses again. She laughed. 'Better than being dead!' she said.

Healing attitudes

There are several points to discuss in Megan's history. Firstly, because I have detailed three recovered cases of melanoma it may seem that it is an easy cancer to overcome. It is not. I have seen dozens of others who did not survive, for many and complicated reasons.

Some just came too late, when they were dying with the overload of the toxins this cancer makes and the effects of the malnutrition it causes by stealing the food the body needs. Coupled with these are the after-effects of the treatments that have been tried in a vain hope of stopping the melanoma with radiation and/or chemotherapy.

Secondly, it can be seen that there's not just one treatment program but several that work, all based on giving careful attention to the needs of the body and mind in diet, meditation, supplements and support at home. Whatever else helps, these are imperative.

Thirdly, the three healing attitudes prevailed:

- **Belief** in the therapy;
- **faith** in the self, the doctor and the positive outcome; and
- **determination** to win and keep on winning.

Melanoma can apparently be cured, with no sign of illness for years, and then can come back when the resistance is lowered by stress of some sort. Remember that there may be those live cells walled off in a cystic lump.

Say: *Mind plans the way—God directs the steps.*

Case commentary: Stephanie

I had a dear friend, Stephanie, who was my playmate when we were children. We worked together for a time and remained close friends as adults. She had a melanoma on her calf which was first removed and then widely excised, right down to the muscles, in a two-stage operation. This was followed by skin grafts to the denuded area. She and her family had forgotten all about it when, eight years later, she suddenly had a series of epileptic seizures and died of a huge brain metastasis. I was helpless and devastated. There was nothing I could have done; it happened so suddenly. I didn't know anything about nutrition and stress control at that time. Now I make very sure that patients realise that it is adopting a new lifestyle—for ever—and a new way of thinking about life that counts.

Cancer formation and spread

Though people are becoming more knowledgeable about cancer there is still much misinformation, causing confusion and anger.

Many people blame the surgeon when the cancer they thought was completely removed recurs. This follows the belief that cancer is a lump and all that needs to be done is to remove the lump to cure the cancer. A surgeon may often reinforce this erroneous belief by saying to the patient, 'You are lucky, you don't have anything to worry about now—I got it all!'

Consider these facts about cancer formation and spread:

1 *The climate of the body* which allowed the cancer to grow has not been changed at all. All the same chemistry applies, except that it becomes worse for the short time during the stress of the anaesthetic and operation. The eye can see only the grossest lesions, the pathologists sees only what the surgeon removed, the blood reveals only what was in the sample taken, the scans, x-rays and other wonderful diagnostic aids we have still show only a very small part of the picture, limited by the technique.

   Now you know the changes that precede the formation of cancer, you can see that many areas of living need to be re-examined and changed to stop the disease.

2 *Multiple primary cancers.* Some cancer can occur in several different areas simultaneously. Think of skin cancer—not just

'sunspots' but basal cell and squamous cell carcinomas. The doctor may remove two or three at the same session. The environment of the body, with the skin as the target organ for stressed cells, was ripe for the cancers to form—more will form unless the lifestyle, and with it the chemistry, changes drastically.

3 *Habits of spreading.* Cancer cells of different tissues behave differently:
   (a) *Local spread* describes the cancer that causes symptoms by growing bigger and bigger in the area it started—such as in the brain.
   (b) *Spread by lymphatics.* Cancer cells can be carried by the lymph to the collection points for poisons called lymph nodes (glands) which drain the area near the primary cancer—breast cancer often metastasises to the lymph nodes in the armpit, for instance.
   (c) *Spread by the blood.* Cancer cells can be carried in the blood to distant areas where they may be caught up and lodge in a small blood vessel to grow and cause a new, secondary cancer. This way bowel cancer may spread to the liver, for instance.

There is a *time lapse* for these changes to occur, depending on many factors such as the stage the cancer has reached before it was causing symptoms and was discovered. Don't ever forget that it also depends on the *climate of the body and mind.* All treatment of whatever kind is aimed at stopping the spread of cancer.

Our job is to keep the climate right so that cancer cells will not grow.

It is a very widespread belief that 'an operation will let the air into the cancer and make it spread'. I have known fearful people to use this idea as an excuse to do nothing about a cancer until it has reached an advanced stage when no treatment can possibly turn it around. *Fear and ignorance cost lives.*

It is *not* 'letting the air in' that does damage, it is doing invasive surgical or cutting procedures when the body and mind are not prepared to heal.

Say: | *Laughter is the very best medicine.*

All procedures should be preceded by a build-up of healing and resistance factors through supernutrition and supplements.

Even without medical supervision intelligent and caring people do this anyway. It goes back to folklore to take the right food and herbs when preparing for a physical or mental challenge.

Urea and Dr Danopoulos

One of the treatments that I investigated through Megan's visit to the Livingston Medical Clinic was the use of urea. She told me that it was being used but I had never heard of it as an internal medicine, so when I visited the Clinic in July 1987, I asked Dr Bill Forster about it.

The original research into using urea was done by a Greek physician, E.V. Danopoulos, Professor of Internal Medicine in Athens from 1954 to 1971. On 10 March 1987 he sent a long letter to Mr Norman Dacey in Ireland, who wanted to write a book about urea. The letter is too long to quote here, but it gives the essence of his life time of research and observation on the successful treatment of cancer patients with urea. His early experiences showed that human urine has anticancer properties. After many years of testing every substance excreted in urine he found in 1969 that the useful substance was a nontoxic crystaloid product of protein amino acid excretion: urea.

Professor Danopoulos was very sceptical at first, but after using urea to treat several liver cancer patients, who recovered, he was surprised to find it truly was the potent antimalignant agent he had long sought. Subsequently many other inoperable and advanced cancers were arrested by urea treatment.

He found that high concentrations were needed, 45 grams daily, in six divided doses, for forty days, then reducing to 20 grams daily, as a maintenance dose, for two years. This regime has a pronounced effect in stopping metastatic spread of cancer, no matter from which cell source it arises. He has successfully treated adenocarcinomas, sarcomas, malignant melanomas, basal and squamos cell carcinomas and a variety of other tumors.

His first results were published in the British medical journal, the *Lancet*, in 1974. These articles were on the treatment of external cancers of the lip, skin, conjunctiva and cornea and were written in conjunction with his daughter, Dr I. Danopoulos, who is a dermatologist. He was at that time a member of the Board of Trustees of the Hellenic Anticancer Institute which also runs a hospital, so he was able to teach and collaborate with a number of doctors in his research there. However, the opposition and harassment started with the publication of his papers about successful treatment with urea, a common and cheap substance.

Other doctors in the USA, Germany, Scotland and elsewhere are now using his discoveries, but Dr Danopoulos lost his position on the Board and has now retired from medical practice.

When Dr Virginia Livingston suffered similar humiliating harassment in the USA in 1987, she decided to visit Professor Danopoulos in Athens. She had been using urea in the treatment of inoperable cancers of the uterus, colon, rectum, liver and breast after reading his articles. She died of a heart attack while in Athens pursuing her lifelong goal of winning agaipst cancer. Her doctors at the Livingston Medical Clinic still use urea successfully in the treatment of selected cancer cases, I believe.

I thought urea might act similarly to the chemotherapy hydroxyurea, which is being used by our own oncologists particularly for brain and blood cancers, but which has far greater side effects.

I have been loath to use urea because there is so little information about it yet and I do not use my patients as guinea pigs. It would be good to see some grants given to physicians here to research it, but since it is a natural substance, not a drug, and since it is cheap, I would be very surprised if a drug firm (the usual backer) would put up the money to investigate something that would bring in a minimal financial return. 'Orphan' medications are those that cannot be patented because they occur naturally. No-one will 'own' them because they will not be profitable. Lithium carbonate, urea and epsom salts, for instance, are all useful but not promoted. Vitamin C was in the same bracket but some enterprising chemists found a way to alter the molecular structure a little, call it something else and patent it, and were able to promote it at three times the price.

Elsewhere I have mentioned the laws relating to treatment. Here

Say: *I look forward with hope.*

is the place to discuss its economics. There are some patients who are caught in a trap—*they can't afford to have treatment*. When I am assessing which method is possible for the person who comes to me for advice, there are many factors to take into account.

Set-backs to cancer recovery

Location

People living in the outback who can't get down to the city won't be able to have the surgical procedures, the radium treatments and the chemotherapy, all of which need supervision. Nor can they have the blood tests, the hospitalisation—all that wonderful help that this country has provided free to those who can't afford to pay. We, the taxpayers, pay for those who can no longer work. In Australia, the social services and the hospitals provide an astonishingly complete care. But if the patients are stuck out in the bush, isolated by poor roads, with no transport and non-supportive or no family, there is just no way they can carry out a complicated treatment. All I can do is to talk to them on the phone.

Availability of medication and dietary aids

Both these factors are closely allied to location. Some people are just too far away from centres and towns to have fresh fruit and vegetables. Fresh liver is out of the question for many, so it is useless to prescribe it. This is why we have to stock all the supplements which we can send to patients by mail. Also in my cookbook are notes on how to grow sprouts and wheat-grass for homegrown greens.

Money

This is the key to recovery for many, unfortunately. For those who can afford to pay for vaccines from San Diego or Japan, for the first time and then maybe every six to twelve months, these immunology methods are available. To others they are not. We need to have acceptance and manufacture of these curative substances in Australia. *There are no pathologists here that I have contacted who will make autogenous vaccine.*

Some cannot afford to buy the supplementary vitamins, though ours are so discounted that they pay less than in the shops for them.

I supply them in order to make sure that patients use the right ones and the ones I know are the purest and best, not because I make any money at all out of carrying this stock.

It is incongruous that some drugs, which may or may not be helpful, may have damaging side effects and cost the taxpayers of this country billions of dollars, are practically free on the health scheme and through the hospitals. Yet vitamins and minerals, which are not only preventative but curative of some of the chronic degenerative diseases, are becoming exorbitantly expensive and out of reach for some people. That is, of course, the way some drug manufacturers want it to be. Medical schools and medical power groups put down, denigrate, disallow and smash confidence in natural ways of healing with God-given herbs and substances harmless to the body. There is little money for the greedy and no prestige for the proud in Nature's way.

Avoiding destructive treatments

The following case histories are just two representing patients who have been advised to have extensive destructive treatment after discovery by surgical biopsy of life-threatening cancer. Many people who have been feeling just a little below par but not in pain or discomfort will strenuously decline such treatment. The inner self tells them there are non-destructive ways even though they have read nothing about it. They seek knowledge. Where are they to go for information? To the plethora of books about diets for natural healing—which mostly disagree over major points? It is all so confusing. Some say eat garlic, some say it is poisonous; some say use coffee enemas, some say high colonics; some say fast, some say don't; and what about cold-pressed oil and carrot juice; and so the list goes on.

I can advise only what I know works for certain situations. Everything I teach has been researched before me, studied in practice with people, not rats, and found to work in the healing program for some. I am beginning to know which patients will benefit most from what non-invasive immunity-building methods. Each person has an individual program.

Say: *I release the past and enjoy today.*

35 CASE 10: NANCY—RECTAL CANCER

Nancy was born in Germany fifty-three years before I first saw her on 4 October 1986. In May 1986 she had had trouble passing motions and felt a lump inside her rectum. This was not bleeding but it was increasing in size. She went to her local GP, who arranged a barium enema and x-rays. This revealed the tumour so he referred her to a surgeon who removed a rectal polyp on 15 September 1986.

The pathology report described it as an aggressive adenocarcinoma which had not yet penetrated the bowel wall. The surgeon wanted to remove the rectum and give her a colostomy—that is, bring the bowel opening out into a bag higher up the colon. In that position in the bowel the secondary (metastatic) spread of the cancer is by the haemorrhoidal veins directly to the liver. Metastases in the liver are classed in the textbooks as invariably fatal. The method used in the attempt to prolong life in these terminally ill patients is to give chemotherapy—usually 5-fluoro-uracil. Nancy refused a colostomy so the surgeon did a local operation and told her he had 'got it all'. He advised local treatment of the area with radium 'to mop up any cells that had already got away'. This should be followed, he emphasised, by chemotherapy to make sure that any cells already in the liver were destroyed. If there was the slightest trouble a colostomy was a necessity, he told her.

Nancy had been feeling very tired, in a stressful period of overwork in caretaking a motel which she and her husband ran. Now that the operation had given her a reason for decreasing her work load and looking after herself, she felt better.

The prospects the surgeon had described alarmed her, but being a forthright, intelligent person, she wanted to know more before submitting herself to the debilitating effects of further treatment which would be destructive to the immune system. She wanted instruction from me because she was not going to have 'a bag of faeces to carry round for the rest of my life', as she said. She came to the fortnight course at Kelvin Grove, starting on 6 October 1986.

Most of her tests—the full blood count, liver, kidneys, pancreas and electrolytes—were normal. None of the cancer markers were abnormal. Her serum cholesterol, however, was strongly elevated, especially the low-density lipid (LDL) which is the one suspected of causing blockages in the arteries which lead to strokes and heart attacks. She said this was a familial (inherited) condition; that her cholesterol had been high for a long time whenever it was tested. She had an underactive thyroid (also familial) and took thyroxine as a daily replacement. The conditions were related.

Nancy was overweight in the evenly distributed, athletic fashion of the adrenal type of weight gain. She had a red 'butterfly' rash across her nose and cheeks, and also dry scaly red areas on her outer calves. She had always found it very difficult to stick to a diet because she loved all types of food, fried foods and sweet things particularly. She had never been really motivated to change. Now, however, change was a much more serious matter.

Other associated factors found during the assessment were a workaholic, assertive nature coupled with strong feelings of frustration in the home environment. Also she had a hypersensitive reaction to fungal elements of Candida in the bowel. This skin test hypersensitivity was not showing up as itching round the anus, but as gas, bloating, and irregular bowel habits—but more of this later.

All these areas needed attention to put the body, mind and spirit back in balance.

We started with the Cilento Survival Plan diet with its five fresh and raw juices, salads, soups, cooked vegetables, protein foods and supplements to suit her condition.

In six weeks she lost 8 kilos and felt a great deal better in energy level, although weight loss is *not* the aim of this diet—it advises what to eat, not how much.

Nancy found that meditation was a problem with her busy schedule at home, where she was always at everyone's beck and call. By

Say: | *Laughter makes my soul sing.*

going to Bert Weir's 'Centre Within' weekend at the Relaxation Centre she gave herself permission to expand her own interests without feeling guilty. She joined a positive support group in the far North Queensland area where she lived, and took a short holiday in Sydney to visit a friend in need. She also gave herself time to meditate daily.

Supplements became a problem. Nancy does not like to take tablets. We cut them down to a minimum but continued the injectables. She found fresh, unfrozen liver difficult to obtain so we eliminated that too. She suspected that in her case it might be contributing to her high serum cholesterol. The propensity to make more of the dangerous low-density lipid cholesterol instead of the harmless high-density lipid in liver metabolism is associated with eating saturated fat in large amounts, obesity with hypothyroidism and taking thyroxine only as a replacement for the full complement of hormones that the thyroid should be making. Unfortunately synthetic thyroxine is all that is obtainable in this country. The amount taken daily is crucial to the proper functioning of the putuitary gland also, since this tiny gland in the base of the brain stops making thyroid stimulating hormone (TSH) if the dose of thyroxine is incorrect.

High cholesterol: which type?

In fact, taking liver cooked as food, raw in a drink or as an injectable extract makes no difference to serum cholesterol in the vast majority of people. This has been proved by the administration of these substances and the careful recording of serum levels every eight weeks in thousands of my patients over the last nine years.

Stress, on the other hand, makes a tremendous difference to the way the liver metabolises cholesterol in making the many products, such as sex hormones, for which it is the basic ingredient.

Nancy's cholesterol level, which was 9.2 millemoles per litre when she arrived in October 1986, dropped down to 6.6 in the first six weeks of the program. However, it then started to rise and fluctuate again, always with the LDL too high. She realised then that it was not fluctuating with the diet but with the stress level.

One of Nancy's ongoing stresses was the relationship with her husband Hank. He is as dour and uncommunicative as Nancy is outgoing and optimistic. In his best moods he is a hard-working man, particularly clever with practical things. But in his cycles of depression he would become withdrawn, suspicious and lethargic, almost to the state of paranoid delusion. He had been suicidal several times. Nancy was at the end of her tether when he was depressed.

I questioned Hank closely about his depression and found it was episodic and severe, coming on suddenly without any apparent cause. He had found that he could keep it at a manageable level by strenuous sustained exercise; cycling was his lifesaver. Exercise had no lasting effect, however, but at least it gave him some relief from the agony.

Since Hank was against doctors generally, averse to injections and drugs and took any tablets reluctantly, I did not refer him to a psychiatrist, but gave him vitamins and mineral supplements and advised him to see his good local GP, whom he trusted, for antidepressant prescriptions. Together with the supplements these were very effective and with his cycling, he can now recognise the beginning of a 'downer' and take steps to rectify his chemistry before his mood becomes too paranoid and out of kilter for him to comply with any advice from anyone, particularly Nancy.

It is not all medication and supplements that help. Understanding, coupled with a plan of action, is necessary too. Here is the instruction sheet I gave Hank.

This home situation seems to make its impact on Nancy's liver metabolism. Her serum cholesterol rises and falls with her tension. She has found meditation difficult even after her intensive ten-day seminar with Ian Gawler's group at the Living Centre in Melbourne.

Nevertheless, Nancy enjoyed the course and for a while was practising assiduously. When anyone says to me, 'I've been naughty. I've not been doing it as often as I should; then I know they have not really understood the purpose of meditation. When it becomes part of your life, you don't forget it and don't have to say 'I should' or 'I must', or think you are a naughty child. I don't ever forget it because nothing goes as well without it.

Anyway, Nancy lost contact at the end of 1987. Living so far away we were relying on telephone consultations but then she forgot to telephone, or forgot to have her blood test, without which the

Say: *It is not too late to follow my dream.*

> ### Overcoming anxiety, depression and negative feelings
> - **Do** relaxation techniques, meditation or prayer learnt at your yoga group or Tai Chi, or go to one of Bert Weir's 'Centre Within' courses.
> - **Say** your affirmations to push out negative thoughts.
> - **Phone** friends to talk about happy things. Communicate!
> - **Exercise** with pleasure to use up angry chemicals—walking, swimming, tennis, etc. (but no jarring exercise if you have cancer).
> - **Play** music—waltzes and happy tunes, not blues or hard rock. Play an instrument if you can, or sing.
> - **Play** games, write, crochet, knit, draw or do some other creative thing to use the right brain.
> - **Do something to help others** with your church or other group (not to wallow in negative thoughts).
> - **Do not** go to bed and be sorry for yourself.

consultation is not complete. It was two years later, at the end of 1989, that we met again. I was giving a talk in North Queensland on 'Living well in a polluted environment'. She came to the workshop, looking fit but a little worried.

One of her aunts had developed terminal lung cancer recently and the doctor, discovering that Nancy had been considered for a colostomy, was demanding with dire threats that she have an immediate colonoscopy and also a regular one each year. Nancy was confused and fearful. She admitted that she felt so well that she had drifted away from her program of diet, supplements and meditation to some extent.

We did all the old blood tests again and some for new cancer markers. Everything proved to be in good order. She was relieved, but the new crisis helped her to get into the program properly again. She decided to play some new meditation and music tapes daily and to reinstitute her system of exercise, eating and taking the right supplements.

I have no doubt that, if she continues to do this, the cancer will not recur.

Domestic brawling

One of the unpleasant pitfalls which Nancy, Hank and I discussed together was the destructiveness of domestic brawling. I don't mean physical violence, I mean the verbal sniping and put-downs that some couples use to hurt and possibly destroy each other.

This kind of unrest is basically a self-hate projected onto the nearest, dearest and most vulnerable person.

We discussed a program of learning to love 'self' as a first step in constructive communication. They are both working on this with the help of the old classic, *Psychocybernetics* by Maxwell Maltz, and *Love is Letting Go of Fear*, by Gerry Jampolsky. Other wonderful books which we would all enjoy are *Pulling Your Own Strings, I'm OK, You're OK* and *Your Erroneous Zones* by Wayne Dyer. There are many*.

The most destructive ploy of all in domestic relationships is to tear down the combatant's life-saving defence by throwing in, sneeringly, in the heat of an argument such comments as: 'Why don't you go and meditate, you need it', or 'What you need is your pills, you haven't been popping them lately.'

These remarks can break down and negate the coping system so carefully built up by undermining it with negative, angry and resentful power remarks.

So, what do you do if confronted with such remarks? Just walk away. Don't hand over your energy to the other person. Don't listen. Don't argue. Don't justify yourself. Don't put in the smart rejoinder.

---

* Dr Wayne W. Dyer *Pulling Your own Strings*, Aron Books, New York, 1978, and *Your Erroneous Zones*, Aron Books, New York, 1976; Thomas A. Harris, MD, *I'm OK, You're OK*, Pan Books, London, 1973; Maxwell Maltz, MD, *Psychocybernetics*, Pocket Books, New York, 1967.

Say: | *It takes adversity to reveal genius.*

Just walk away and simmer down in private. Talk it out to yourself, exercise it out, write it all down—but don't send it—make a tape of what you think about the situation if you like—but don't send that either.

Use any way you can of expressing your anger in a form that doesn't hurt yourself or anyone else—however much you may want to at the time! Remember the wise saying of Seneca, 'the best cure for anger is delay'.

Anger is a survival emotion that is often roused for a useful purpose. However, we all have to learn to control it and harness that energy for a good and preferably constructive outcome or solution, rather than letting it overcome reason and become a destructive habit for manipulating others.

Cold climate skin

One further factor that needs comment in Nancy's history is her skin. Coming from a cold climate with little sunshine to the very hottest part of the Sunshine State, her sensitive skin never adapted to the climate. She was always red in the face on a hot day and her sandy complexion had started to develop small basal cell carcinomas in the five years before she grew the serious cancerous tumour.

The local GP inspected her skin regularly and burnt off the little carcinomas with dry ice whenever new ones became evident. Nancy needed to wear a big hat, long sleeves and UV blocking sunscreen whenever she went out. This was a nuisance because she liked to play tennis. She often forgot her sun things, which could have dire consequences, as it did for our next case. One cancer does not preclude the formation of another of a different type at the same time.

36 CASE 11: TOM-MELANOMA

Tom was thirty-eight years old when I saw him first on 1 May 1986. He says it was by accident, but personally I don't believe so. He was in Brisbane seeing a doctor about his asthma when he mentioned to another patient in the waiting room that he was just recovering from a second operation for cancer. The other patient suggested he get in touch with me and, since we had just had a cancellation when he phoned, he came along that very day.

When I heard his history I encouraged him to come to a two-week course before returning home to the country. Although the operation had been a success, nothing at all had been done to stop a recurrence.

Tom had a malignant melanoma removed from his left ankle by his GP in November 1981. This was followed by a wider and deeper excision by a general surgeon in the same month in 1981. 'We got it all', the surgeon said.

Tom's mother is subject to skin cancer of the basal-cell carcinoma variety, and his father has moles. Two paternal uncles died of malignant melanoma, and a maternal cousin had a malignant melanoma removed from his back in 1984. So there is genetic predisposition on both sides of his family to cancer disturbances of the skin.

Tom discovered a painless lump in his left groin in March 1986. His GP thought it was a gland from an infection somewhere and gave him antibiotics at first. This made no difference at all to the lump and since he had no infections anyway, Tom was concerned and asked to be sent to a specialist surgeon. On 26 March 1986, the surgeon performed a block dissection of the glands in Tom's left groin. This means he took out all the lymph nodes that drained lymph fluid from that leg. Two of the nodes were filled with cancerous melanoma cells. This surgeon also said that he 'got it all'.

As far as surgeons can see, that is a valid remark, and it is the conviction that cutting out what you can see will cure the cancer that keeps surgeons keen on perfecting techniques for doing just that. When a secondary cancer appears in a distant part of the body the doctor usually tells the patient that 'a few cells had already got away into the blood stream—they can take up residence anywhere'.

Unfortunately this simplistic view used to absolve the surgeon from any further responsibility or advice to the patient. Today more and more doctors are coming to realise, by reading the mountain of evidence available, that cancer is *not* a localised disease but a systemic one—that means that it is a manifestation of the poor condition of the whole body. Strong antibodies against cancer made by active cells of the immune system protect those of us who do not have the disease. When there are too few of these cells, or they are not in good condition, they fail to make these protective substances.

Causative factors

There are possibly hundreds of factors involved in the breakdown of immunity and the formation of the free radicals that can precipitate the final cancerous changes in cells. We are slowly discovering more and more of them. Some factors now being studied more intensively are the individual differences in absorption and use of nutrients from food needed by the immune system.

This is where genetic predisposition comes into focus, particularly with Tom, who has a family history of it. **Cancer is not inherited, but our metabolic patterns are**—that is, how we digest, absorb and use substances like fat, sugar, protein, vitamins and minerals from the food we eat. This is why, on precisely the same diet, some persons put on weight and some don't.

Tom, who was fair complexioned, was a keen sportsman, always out in the sun and, for the years before the first appearance of melanoma, usually unprotected by ultraviolet light screening creams. After the first operations, he was more aware and more careful. He took the anti-cancer slogans seriously for a time. 'Slip on a shirt! Slop on a sunscreen! Slap on a hat!' is the advice our Queensland Cancer Fund advertises so widely.

Over the years, however, the anxiety faded and anyway, both

doctors had said they had 'got it all'. He had been lazy about the 'Slip, Slop, Slap' for some time. But other factors were operating too:

- Tom was a keen cameraman. He had a proper darkroom in which he developed and printed his own films, often using chemicals such as sodium hyposulphite, with no protective gloves to avoid absorption of these products through the skin.
- Tom had always been a picky eater, a short but athletic man who disliked fruit and salads but loved meat and sugary foods. A 'real sweet tooth', he called himself. He was also a heavy coffee drinker. These, as I have said previously, upset some vitamin and mineral use.
- Tom had an itchy rash in the groin which, on examination under the microscope, proved to be *Candida* (monilia or thrush), a yeast-fungus organism. This rash had been a nuisance several times before. The itching and redness almost disappeared from time to time, only to recur, particularly when the weather was hot and Tom was perspiring.

On asking about Helen, his wife, it was not surprising to find that she had suffered from vaginal thrush intermittently for the last two years. Helen did not come to the course as a helper because someone had to stay home to look after the three children and the animals.

It was absolutely necessary, for reasons to be discussed shortly, for *both* Tom and Helen to use an aggressive anti-fungal program for several months to bring the Candida under control. The success of Tom's recovery from cancer depended on it, as did the success of the treatment he was taking for asthma. An overload of this organism in the alimentary tract, skin, respiratory system or any of the other places where it can reside will cause a breakdown of the immunity to it and possibly to cancer too.

Candida

Candida has at least two forms that we can recognise, yeast and fungal. In a slightly acidic body climate, the yeast form prevails.

Say: *Rainbows are made from rain and sunshine.*

The problem arises when the acid-base balance (pH) of the affected part becomes slightly alkaline. Then the yeast form, called the 'blastopore', starts to grow long mycelial threads and changes into the fungal form, which is invasive. The mycelia can enter the lining cells of any hollow organ such as the bowel, vagina, bladder or sinus, and there set up an inflammatory reaction with its attending symptoms. New colonies so embedded are difficult to eradicate unless the pH of the area can be made more acidic again.

In the vagina three or four days treatment with a cream or suppository is usually not enough. It simply clears the surface inflammation. The deeper layers of tissue can still harbour the yeast form which can start growing again when conditions are favourable.

Plan of action to control Candida

- **Eliminate from your diet altogether:**
  Sugar and all sweets, cakes, honey, syrup, and sugary fruits such as melons, dates, figs, dried fruits, grapes and custard apples. Refined and processed foods; e.g. white flour and foods containing it (these change to sugars, on which candida thrives).

- **Eliminate for 30 days:**
  Yeast containing substances; e.g. bread, vinegar, beverages made by fermentation, sauces, pickles.

- **Put foods back in rotation**
  Put foods back one at a time, every 12 hours, and watch for any allergy reactions. If a food makes you react, use it again only after seven days, and then in a tiny amount, increasing each week till you desensitise yourself to it (that is, rotate it every seven days).

- **Take antifungal compounds by prescription:**
  e.g. Nystatin tablets or Powder by mouth for 2 to 6 months as directed, usually $1/8$ teaspoon of powder with water 3 times daily *between* meals (Nizoral, Ketoconazole and Amphoteracin only in exceptional cases).

- **For local lesions:**
  Nystatin Cream, 'Anusol', 'Pevaryl' or other Ketaconazole creams for inflamed areas of skin, nails, anus or vagina.

- **Homemade Lotion:**
  Mix 1 tablespoon natural yoghurt with 1/16 teaspoon Vitamin C powder until dissolved and apply to affected area as often as necessary to control soreness, redness and itching in areas of skin, vagina, anus or mouth. Use an applicator for the vagina.

- **Use Tea-Tree Oil:**
  I teaspoon to 3 cups of tepid water as a douche, mouth wash or skin lotion.

- **Take regularly foods that inhibit candida:**
  Lactobacillus acidophilus as powder—1/8 teaspoon 3 times a day with cold food or drinks or as a capsule or tablet or as yoghurt, 1 tablespoon with each meal.
  Garlic (cooked or raw) or in capsules or tablets 3 times daily.
  Eat a salad every day containing at least 5 raw vegetables.
  Eat 3 pieces of non-sugary fruit aily.
  Use cold-pressed linseed oil—1 tablespoon daily in the butter, in cold food, off the spoon with food or in salad dressing.
  Turnip, cabbage and other of that family inhibit bowel yeasts.

- **Take supplements:**
  Multivitamin and mineral—1 daily (use a comprehensive one) containing the B group and many others.
  Vitamin C 1000 with bioflavinoids—1 three times a day.
  MaxEPA—1 three times a day or other essential fatty acid capsules.
  A and D Capsules—1 twice daily.
  For those severely affected:
  Digestive enzymes (D.E.F.)—1 with each meal.
  Thymus extract—1 twice a day.
  Biotin, 300 mcgm—1 three times a day.

Say: *Tolerance and love go hand in hand.*

Lysine 400 mgm—1 twice daily for cold sores.
Butter Mixture: Beat 500 g (½ lb) softened butter with ¾ cup cold-pressed linseed oil or cold-pressed safflower oil.

- **Use the dietary guidelines below:** The mycelial form of candida is contagious. Avoid sexual intercourse when vagina is affected. Shower rather than bath. Use cotton underclothes and wash separately.

Candida control diet—Guidelines for life
Note: Cancer patients should delete all foods prohibited for them from this diet.

- **Do eat:**

  Protein foods, unrefined grains, vegetables, raw fruits (low in sugar), as below:

  Lean meats of all types, fish of all types, poultry, eggs, milk, natural sugar-free yoghurt, dairy products

  All unprocessed nuts (watch for mould), seeds, fats and oils

  Products from unrefined grain flours such as wheat, rye, oats, barley, rice, corn; e.g. wholemeal pancakes, scones, taco, unleavened bread, burghul, unsweetened biscuits, porridges, polenta, buckwheat

  All salad vegetables, all root vegetables, all leafy green vegetables, especially of the cabbage family, all red, yellow and orange fruits and vegetables

  Cold-pressed linseed oil and other cold-pressed oils.

- **Do not eat:**

  Sugar, honey, glucose, glucodin, malt, molasses, chocolate, jams, sweets, biscuits, cakes, packaged cereals, white pasta, ice-cream, jelly, puddings and all foods containing sugars and/or white flour

  Fermented foods containing vinegar (pickles, chutneys, sauces), aged cheese

  Dried or canned fruit, canned beetroot, soft drinks, processed

> fruit juices, fruits high in sugar such as grapes, watermelon, dates, figs and custard apples
> - Those with *allergic* symptoms from yeasts *other* than candida should eliminate the following as well:
> Baker's yeast products such as bread, buns, doughnuts, etc.
> Brewer's yeast products such as alcohols of any variety including fermented drinks, vinegar, beer and wines
> Mushrooms
> Any processed food containing or prepared from the above
> Tea, coffee, herb teas (These usually contain mould spores, unless made of fresh herbs).

How to take nystatin oral powder

Nystatin powder is not soluble in water, but if you swill the dose around in a little water until it is evenly suspended, it may be drunk and washed down with more water. The pure powder contains no preservatives, colouring, flour agents, lactose or other fillers. It is very light so it may settle in the bottle and should be shaken up before measuring.

Nystatin is not much absorbed from the bowel and does its work in killing candida by contact with the bowel mucosa. Thus it is best to take it without food so that it will come into contact with the wall of the bowel more easily.

It may be necessary to work up to the full adult dose, of ¼ teaspoon three times a day between meals, slowly over four or five days, starting with ½ the usual dose twice a day. For an adult 1/8 teaspoon or 200 mg twice daily is the usual long-term maintenance dose, though in some people with longstanding candida infections such as some diabetics, ¼ teaspoon three times a day may be necessary for a long time. The amount is not critical.

There should be a change for the better within six weeks. If there

Say: | *Every day and every way I get happier and more contented.*

is not and the dietary and other guidelines have been adhered to strictly, it is no use continuing with nystatin. Contact your doctor to arrange new measures.

When the candida yeast fungus is being destroyed quickly by the nystatin antifungal, many toxins are released from the dying candida. These may sometimes give symptoms such as wind, bloating, stuffy nose, itching and nausea. This does not happen with many people and the symptoms quickly subside. However, if you don't know about this '**healing reaction**', you may think it is the flu and rush off to the doctor for antibiotics. This would, of course, allow the candida to grow again and cancel out your treatment.

If symptoms are very severe, take plenty of fluids to wash toxins out of the body. You may even have to stop the nystatin for two days and start again with a smaller dose, then work up more slowly.

See hints on helping the immune system in the appendix and read the miscellaneous instructions in the book, *The Yeast Connection*, by William Crook.

More importantly, there is some evidence* that fungal forms make an exotoxin that upsets the immune system cells' ability to manufacture antibodies against candida. The ongoing process, if not checked, has repercussions on the cancer organism, hastening the changes in its life cycle to form substances injurious to its human host.

But back to Tom and his need for knowledge. He was precipitated into taking the two-week course at Kelvin Grove because he was sitting in my waiting room this time, with a man who was the disastrous example of other treatments for the same type of cancer as his own. This young man looked ghastly and was dying of widely metastatic melanoma. He had undertaken the interferon and chemotherapy treatment that was being funded at one of the big hospitals at that time. He had gone to the hospital when the melanoma was at the same stage as Tom's, and had been offered either extensive surgery or this guinea pig treatment. (See Megan's case history, page 319.)

---

* C. Orion Truss, *The Missing Diagnosis*, and William D. Crook, *The Yeast Connection*.

Since I have seen both of these choices deplete the beleaguered immune system still further and allow melanoma to ravage on unhalted, I wonder why they are still used. (On the other hand, it has been reported in some studies that the interferon without the chemotherapy has been more successful.)

Luckily for Tom, a course at Kelvin Grove was starting in three days time. In his group were several older and much sicker people. Tom had such an unpleasant introduction into what cancer can do to thoroughly nice, clean-living people like the young man in the waiting room that he was eager to learn how to stop it going any further in himself.

Some people still half believe the old superstition that cancer only attacks reprobates who need to be punished. It was a shock for Tom to see this top athlete of impeccable reputation, hairless from chemotherapy, now deathly pale and cadaverously thin, covered in blackish lumps and so weak he could hardly stand.

Urged on by the staff and other participants, he took most of the juices in the Survival Plan diet without demur, but reneged for the first week on the liver juice. He had his first healing reaction of detoxification in the first week and then felt much better. By the time he went home, he was taking everything—all the supplements too.

On his return home, he had trouble describing the program to Helen, who phoned me several times with lists of questions about diet. She was amazed that he had given up so many of his favourites like sweets, desserts, coffee and beer because, since he was a picky eater, she had previously been pandering to his whims in this regard. We discussed making meals that would suit the whole family rather than cooking his food separately as she had always done.

Since there are others in the family with moles, I suggested that when he went for a check-up with his surgeon, the rest of the family should be examined for skin type too, and a watch kept on any suspicious areas. The family history is so strong for melanoma that all should be warned to take the precautions advertised in the 'Slip! Slop! Slap!' campaign and also to take up careers that do not mean

Say: *I will find the answer to my problem in prayer.*

constant exposure to the dangerous spectrum of ultraviolet light. Any suspicious moles should be removed.

Tom was able to get fresh, young, unfrozen calf liver once a week where he lived, so once he had become used to taking the liver juice, it was no problem. His blood tests for haemoglobin and iron were low at first, but after taking liver three times a week they soon picked up to normal.

He was also taking asthma and headache medication which it was not my ethical responsibility to stop, since they had been prescribed by another doctor. However I advised him, at his request, on the method of cutting down his medication safely without side effects. *It is dangerous to stop taking prednisone suddenly.* He had to make his decision to do this by himself.

The only medication that I gave him which was not a natural supplement was nystatin—an antifungal for the candida. The antifungal program, fits in well with the Survival Plan diet. Helen also had to take nystatin but, apart from the powder between meals they both took, she also had vaginal suppositories, whereas Tom had the skin preparations for his groin rash. These cleared the thrush in both at the same time. An added bonus was that Tom's dandruff disappeared.

Extra benefits of the survival plan

When Tom returned for his visit on 18 August 1986, his chest X-ray was clear, his asthma had gone and he was off all medication for it. His headaches had reduced to practically nil, also without medication, and he was controlling stress and tension with meditation. He had found meditation difficult at first, but now it was becoming part of his life.

At first Tom lost weight with his change of diet. This is not part of the program but it often happens if there has been an overload of sweet and fatty foods in the previous eating style. His weight dropped from 67 to 60 kilos, so I encouraged him to eat more calorific foods. There is plenty of everything in the grains, legumes, root vegetables and fruit—especially rice, beans, potatoes and bananas, all of which he liked.

Tom had always been keen on cricket which he took up enthusiastically now, using suitable sunscreens. He also liked music

Case 11: Tom—Melanoma 349

and was an expert guitarist, which gave him the scope to join a band and enjoy life more than before.

He was well and all his tests were normal when a close friend in the same district died of cancer. This man had a differnt type of cancer and a completely different lifestyle and personality from Tom's. But he had been on the Survival Plan diet. Tom was so upset and despondent that he lost faith in himself, in me and in the program. I lost touch with him for fourteen months while he was going through this bad patch. Possibly he would not have returned at all, but after he had been off the program altogether for a while, he contracted a severe viral infection which Helen and others in the area also had. In retrospect, and from the results of blood tests we did on 2 October 1987, it could well have been glandular fever or a similar virus.

Tom developed nasty secondary infections in the ears and persistent sore throats that finally cleared up with antibiotics from his local doctor. However, these brought on thrush again. Helen had it even more severely than Tom. Knowing that it was not a situation to leave unchecked, they very wisely returned to re-establish some balance in health again.

All tests have returned to normal through the six-monthly consultations in 1988 and 1990. Tom has been designing computer programs for his work. He has continued to set goals and reach them. He is using meditation and relaxation techniques as part of his regular routine. He is aware of and listening to his inner messages. Helen and the children are also doing well. Although this does not mean 'they lived happily ever after', it does suggest that Tom will be unlikely to have a recurrence of his cancer and even if the thrush does come back from time to time, he now knows how to treat it.

Say: *After a stormy night may come a beautiful day.*

37   CASE 12: PHILIP LINDSAY—BOWEL CANCER

My first contact with Philip was through his wife, Hilarie, by phone on 20 March 1985. She told me that Philip was in hospital following a bowel operation in which the surgeon had removed a malignant polyp and all of the sigmoid colon. I sent her a Survival Plan diet sheet for the meanwhile and asked her to keep in touch, as I thought something more would be necessary after he had recovered from the operation, given his history and type of cancer.

Philip was 67 years old at the time. He had been complaining of discomfort when sitting for about a year before. The doctor he went to in May, 1984, had a barium enema done, and explained that the x-ray showed a minute non-malignant polyp. Philip has a hearing deficiency so Hilarie usually went with him. She said that the doctor had been 'offhand' and would not explain how big the polyp was or how he knew it was not malignant. So the next month she took him to another doctor who looked into the bowel with a short instrument, a sigmoidoscope, and said he could not see any abnormality.

Philip was still very unwell. Within six weeks he was passing blood in his motions, so he went to another local doctor who gave him some ointment for haemorrhoids and, in spite of the past history, told him just to keep the bowels open.

In November 1984, when on a trip to Ballina, Philip became extremely tired and depressed. He had diarrhoea and was passing blood and mucus in his stools.

In frustration with their doctors, Hilarie treated him with juices, yoghurt and vitamin C, but though his condition improved (the bleeding stopped) the other symptoms persisted.

In February 1985, Philip went to another Veterans Affairs doctor who pronounced him to be 'quite healthy' and suggested he was overemphasising his symptoms and malingering. However, this time

Hilarie insisted on a colonoscopy and the polypoid mass was found and proved by biopsy to be cancerous—about a year after his first symptoms had occurred!

On 18 March 1985 a fifth doctor operated, took out the sigmoid colon and joined the bowel up so that Philip did not need a colostomy bag.

The doctor said that the cancer had not spread right through the wall of the bowel and that there was no obvious involvement of tissues in the rest of the abdomen.

Two weeks later Philip was back in the office at the family business which he and his wife run. She phoned me soon after from Sydney to arrange for the course, which they started in May 1985. They both came to the two-week briefing course.

Hilarie threw herself into the program with gusto. She is a very active, vibrant woman who lives life to the full with her husband and family, the business and her own creative talents. Philip is a keen tennis player and a most inventive, astute and dedicated businessman, but he is quieter and takes his time to consider each step. They are a happy and complementary couple.

Philip was still tired and thin and his blood pressure was always low, though pulse and temperature were in the mid-normal range. Of course, the doctor had said, 'I got it all'. Even though he had no metastatic spread of his cancer, we decided that the Gerson program would be the best way to get Philip's antibodies working again.

Immunoglobulins

Philip's tuberculin test was negative, showing that his immune system was still depressed. For this reason I gave him human immunoglobulins for several months as a means to afford passive immunity against cancer spread at this rather crucial period of recovery.

As I have mentioned elsewhere, all of us who do not have cancer are making antibodies against it. These are in the blood serum. Giving serum by intramuscular injection is well known as a short-term prevention against diptheria, tetanus and hepatitis. The donor's serum is broken down more or less quickly by the recipient, within

Say: *I live and thrive in a world of change.*

one to three weeks. But in the meantime the recipient is protected by the many antibodies it contains against every viral or bacterial illness those donors of the serum have overcome—including cancer in its formative stages. Immune serum is not so useful, in my experience, once the cancer is established somewhere with its own blood supply. However, used just after surgery it is theoretically and practically a prevention of colonisation from the primary site to the distant parts of the body. The doctor must watch for any problems of sensitisation to the serum by monitoring the immune system function with the weekly tuberculin PPD test.

Tuberculin, PPD or Mantoux test

In the Western world every adult should have developed an antibody reaction against the Tubercle bacillus (TB) now called *Mycobacterium tuberculosis*. Because the germ is not as virulent as it once was and may not have been encountered at all, Australia and most other countries have a testing program for children in the early teen years. This test is completely harmless and does not use the bacillus itself. It uses a minute (0.1 ml) quantity of the toxin (tuberculin) made by the bacillus—the germ itself is contagious but the toxin is not.

This is injected just under the skin, usually on the inner side of the forearm. Within twenty-four to seventy-two hours, immune antibody-making cells will recognise this toxin and attempt to destroy it, making an area of inflammation at the site of the injection. By measuring the size, colour, character and type of this reaction experienced immunologists can gauge the activity of the different manufacturing cells of the immune system.

If there is no reaction to the PPD—that is, no redness—then a vaccination is given to actively immunise the person against TB. This is done with an 'attenuated' (that is, devitalised) form of the live organism called 'Bacillus Calmette Guérin' (BCG), named after two clever French researchers who developed this useful germ by long and careful experiments.

When the person is tested six months after the vaccination, the PPD is positive and resistance to TB has developed.

The cancer organism is also a mycobacterium—one of the same family as leprosy, scleroderma and tuberculosis (see page 225).

When people lose immunity to TB they very often lose immunity to the cancer organism too. This is why the PPD test is a good monitor of the way the body defences are progressing with treatment.

Some people never get their immunity back. Those who do have a better chance of fighting the cancer with their own natural defences, improved by nutrition, supplements and stress control. Once the PPD is positive, there is also likely to be a good result from *autogenous vaccine*.

Philip had a negative PPD on 15 May 1985 so immunoglobulins were indicated. He also told me that he had suffered from 'sinus trouble' (see page 229). He could not breathe through both sides of the nose and had a poor sense of smell. Herpes and mouth ulcers were an on-going problem with him too. They are discussed at the end of this chapter. He was prone to bronchitis and had coughed up blood when he had pneumonia some years previously. (A chest x-ray showed no abnormality in May, 1985.) Because Philip was a mild but regular social drinker of beer, wine and spirits, Hilarie had made sure he took vitamin supplements daily for years. However, his preference was for sweet foods, and he still took coffee, tea, preserved and red meat.

Sweet tooth

The combination of sweet foods, coffee, tea and preserved and red meats causes trouble for people predisposed to bowel problems, not only by upsetting the vitamin B group uptake but by making carcinogens in the lower bowel. The sodium nitrite in any preserved food, but especially in meat such as ham, sausage, salami, mince (not made before your eyes), bacon, pickled and corned meat, can change during digestion to nitrosamine, which is carcinogenic, if there is not enough vitamin C and fibre to detoxify it in the diet. Fibre helps to pass them out of the bowel quickly, but for those who are even partly constipated, nitrosamines can sit in the sigmoid and rectum, causing trouble.

Philip and Hilarie enjoyed the course and on returning to Sydney continued with the Gerson program and my stress control tapes

Say: *I see the beauty in the world.*

most meticulously. We monitored progress mostly by telephone and blood tests sent from his local doctor. One of the cancer markers called 'Carcino Embrionic Antigen (CEA)' and others called 'CA 19-9' and 'CA 125' are very useful in monitoring for colon cancer.

The tests carried out before each return appointment are of the utmost importance for those who come to the surgery and also for those who cannot attend personally and must keep in contact by phone.

The Multiple Biochemicals Analysis or SMA 24, as it is called in the USA, shows the electrolyte balance, serum glucose (for the pancreas), kidney function, liver function, calcium and phosphate levels, protein levels, iron, cholesterol, triglycerides and others. It is an excellent monitor—so much can be learned from it about the general state of the body. The full blood count is also very useful since the state of the red cells, white cells and platelets monitor the very life blood of the person.

For about a year all went very well with Philip. The tests were all becoming normal and we were bringing the number of juices down and adding more allowable foods gradually.

On 5 August 1985, Philip wrote to the Livingston-Wheeler Medical Clinic in San Diego to enquire about having an autogenous vaccine made from the organisms in his own urine to help him build up antibodies against his cancer.

The letter of reply stated that this was possible only if he went to the Clinic personally and took the rest of the program too, including diet, vitamins and other immuno-stimulating boosters. He was referred to a doctor in Brisbane who had just started sending urine over to the Clinic by express courier. However, it would be necessary for Philip to become this doctor's patient and follow his program too. Since our methods did not entirely coincide, Philip decided not to get the vaccine. He was healthy and fit on my program however, and on 10 January 1986 we stopped the immunoglobulin injections.

Although Philip was a dedicated tennis player, he had started Tai Chi as a form of exercise and as meditation also—it is known as 'meditation in movement'. He found it helped him hold his enema longer.

In May 1986 he had an excellent report from his surgeon.

By June 1986, when he was down to six juices a day, I advised him to go back to the Cilento Survival Plan diet, which cut out the thyroid, potassium salts and niacin and all but one of the enemas. He was keen to have lamb and rabbit in his protein foods, so against my better judgment, I relented.

Then, on 1 August 1986, he phoned to say he had had blood in his motions again for the last three weeks and was losing weight, having gone from 64 kilograms to 62.5. There had been trouble with the business that had caused him a great deal of stress. His surgeon said it was nothing to worry about, that his CEA was still normal, but we decided to cut out meat again and go back to the Gerson Therapy to be on the safe side. We also arranged for him to have another colonoscopy.

Using wheatgrass juice implants of 60 grams twice daily into the rectum, the bleeding stopped within two days but, sure enough, there was another polyp which the surgeon removed on 15 August 1986. It was benign, but it was a warning that he could not let down his guard by falling into lax eating habits again.

Controlling familial polyposis

Some people inherit the tendency to make benign lumps (polyps) in the lining of the bowel. Some develop the type of polyps in the bowel that can change easily from benign to malignant. The tendency to turn like this is stronger if the genetic inheritance is present in both parents.

The myriad reactions going on in the body all the time depend on the absorption, use and excretion of our food. This is accomplished by enzymes that direct these processes. Sometimes one of these many and varied enzymes is missing or present only in a small quantity, so some processes in the body are imperfectly performed.

One important process in the bowel is the conversion of cancer-causing chemicals in our food to harmless substances that can be easily excreted. Not only enzymes are needed for this but also vitamins—vitamin C especially.

It is generally supposed that people who make polyps have a lack of enzymes in the bowel. If they also have a deficiency of vitamin C the risk of developing cancer in one or more of the bowel polyps is very great.

Say: | *What I see is what I get.* |

Polyposis is not a rare condition. People who have a known tendency to make polyps, and this is gauged from the family history, should take these precautions:

- Take plenty of vitamin C in ascorbate, non-acid form always. Sustained release 1000 milligram tablets or capsules are the only ones that reach the lower bowel (the usual site of these cancers) without being absorbed higher up. Take one twice a day to protect benign polyps from turning malignant.
- Do not eat any food preserved with sodium nitrate or nitrite. Without sufficient vitamin C these change to the carcinogenic substance called nitrosamide.
- Eat daily food containing fibre such as vegetables, unrefined grains and fruit. For those people who have trouble in the bowel from partial obstructions and adhesions the fibre can be flaked, made into a puree or cut very small.
- If cancer has already occurred but been healed by operation, the surgeon will usually suggest a follow-up colonoscopy every year to make sure that any further polyps that develop can be cauterised or otherwise removed before they become malignant.

Herpes and mouth ulcers

In his original questionnaire Philip had reported that he had had a severe herpes simplex (cold-sore, fever blister) infection on the top lip following a kick in the mouth at a football match in 1941, when he was a World War 2 serviceman. The lesion was inflamed and very painful and it took nine months to resolve. After many different treatments, it was finally cured with silver nitrate. The cold sore broke out every winter for years and only ceased to recur in 1982—three years before the cancer appeared. He felt strongly that his allergy to dogs sometimes precipitated an attack of herpes. I thought it could also be a combination of this allergy with cold weather, stress and nutrient imbalance.

Philip and his brother had also suffered since childhood from recurrent mouth ulcers. They were slow to heal and made eating miserable. These persisted into the time that Philip was using the Gerson Therapy. It became evident from tests then that his acid-base electrolyte balance was easily disturbed. Until this therapy started, he had been taking antacids off and on when stressed. Now his sodium and chloride were frequently low when he had the ulcers. He found that rubbing them with salt as soon as they started, although painful, would stop them forming. He had also used vinegar to this effect. I thought they may be caused by the herpes virus, but if this were so, they would have resolved with lysine. We tried this and the situation did not improve.

Not wanting to disturb the program too much, we put 1/8 teaspoon of salt into his otherwise saltless diet and added 300 mg of biotin twice daily to stabilise the salivary pH.

Scrapings from ulcers taken on 23 January 1987 showed no growth of pathogenic organisms. They are only occasionally troublesome now. On 16 January 1987 his weight was still at 62 kilos. His surgeon and his GP both pronounced him 'astonishingly well'. He was up to level six in his Tai Chi, giving a good account of himself at tennis twice weekly, and enjoying life with Hilarie and the business.

When Hilarie had some health problems Philip's CEA test increased immediately and his weight dropped a little, but this was simply a stress-related hiccup which he resolved by meditation.

In January 1989 he went back to the Cilento Survival Plan again. The change-over was a gradual one anyway, since his Gerson juices had reduced to six.

At last contact, in January 1992, Philip was fit and well and his CEA and CA 125 were entirely normal. He is still playing tennis with vigour, swimming regularly and running his business. He is resigned to having the regular supplements and healthy diet for life and has never had a recurrence of herpes on the lip.

The herpes family

This is an appropriate place to discuss the herpes family of viruses since herpes simplex was a coexistent factor in Philip's cancer. There are over sixty viruses in the Epstein-Barr family, occurring in more than thirty different species of animals. At least four of them can infect humans: in cold sores: herpes simplex of six different strains

Say: | *I make enjoyable plans and goals.*

so far known; chickenpox: herpes zoster, now believed to be the virus also causing shingles in later life; glandular fever (mononucleosis): Epstein-Barr virus, cytomegalovirus and hepatitis B virus. This is a very widespread and debilitating group and can be the cause of serious infections. The following are the notes I give to patients coming with herpes simplex infection. They also apply in some ways to other members of the family.

Herpes simplex

Herpes Simplex virus, HSV, has been known since ancient times and is now sweeping the world in epidemic proportions. Type 1, which comes mainly as cold sores or fever blisters round the mouth, nose and eyes, and Type 2, which occurs mainly in the genital regions, are no longer confined to above the waist and below the waist, since four other types are now known. It is claimed that one in ten people in America have herpes. It can occur on any margins or within mucous (wet) surfaces on the lips, nose, eyes, genitalia and anus but also on the skin surfaces.

Herpes is highly contagious. You catch it by coming into contact with an infected person's sores (lesions). The virus, which is smaller than a germ, multiplies enormously at the site where it enters the body and causes redness, then a cluster of blisters which break down, making raw areas that may be very painful. The toxins or poisons from them often drain to the nearest lymph glands, making them swollen and painful too. On the lips, throat or nose the glands that become swollen and painful are under the jaw. Those in the groin may be affected if the lesions are on or near the genitals. There are other causes of swollen glands which can be distinguished by your doctor—for instance, tonsillitis can cause swollen glands under the jaw and syphilis can cause a painless ulcer and swollen glands in the groin.

On the skin surfaces the broken blisters soon form crusts and then scabs which separate after about a week. On the moist surfaces such as inside the mouth and the lips of the female genitals, the blister stage is not so pronounced. The blisters may be tiny, like sand, breaking down quickly to form raw areas that are red, stinging, burning or very painful, especially when urinating. These mucous areas, being moist, never form scabs and can go on causing discomfort for months or years. Once the virus has become established it will stay in the body after the white cells of the defence system have brought the attack under control. Some immunity is built up but the virus lies dormant until the resistance is lowered and some trigger starts it growing again.

More than 30 million people in America are said to have annual recurrences of cold sores on the mouth, each lasting four to twenty-one days. More than 5 million Americans suffer from genital herpes. The trigger that sets off an attack can be sunburn, ultraviolet light, damage to tissue by trauma such as rubbing, a fever or sudden change in body temperature, protein imbalance in food, emotional stress and sex.

The attacks may be very close together at first, becoming less and less frequent as immunity is established. With Philip it was originally a trauma to the lip at football and the fact that the condition persisted meant that his immune system was very sluggish. Anything that helps the body to fight will be of great importance because, although the virus is still in the body, it can be controlled to the extent of never causing another attack. When poor nutrition, stressful situations and trauma continue, the virus may become a constant attacker and illness can go on throughout life.

The incidence of babies born with herpes contracted from lesions in the mother's birth canal is increasing. Herpes can cause very serious multiple lesions throughout the baby's body and brain. Since the death rate is at present 50 per cent in the newborn with herpes, doctors often do a Caesarian operation to save the baby from infection. Some doctors induce labour during a time when the mother has no lesions in the birth canal for the same reason.

Everybody has come in contact with HSV by the time adulthood is reached, but some people carry the virus in the body and it never causes any lesions at all. These people have high immunity to the virus. The immune responses of their bodies are strong so that the virions (virus particles) are never active enough to grow and reproduce. These are asymptomatic carriers who can pass on the virus without having illness themselves. Immunity rating can be tested

Say: *I love laughter and I laugh a lot.*

by a pathologist from a blood sample, but a positive test shows only that you have had the virus at some time in your life. Herpes simplex virus (HSV) can be cultured from the fluid of lesions and that fluid also contains 'giant cells' that can be recognised under the microscope. This method is most often used to prove the diagnosis of herpes in genital lesions of both men and women.

Genital herpes

In diagnosis in women the examination of the cervix and vaginal mucous surfaces by a doctor is particularly important. Lesions in this position may not be seen or felt by the infected persons, but they may infect the sexual partner. Another very important point is that cancer of the cervix more often occurs in women who have herpes there. It is easy to detect in the regular check-up that responsible women have yearly to make sure there is no cancer of the cervix. In this check-up, *'the Pap smear'*, the doctor slips a speculum into the vagina and scrapes some of the moisture from the cervix and vaginal wall onto a slide. Staining the cells on the slide 'the Papanicolaou smear' will not only show up any cancer cells present but also the giant cells of herpes.

There are other causes of rashes, sores, urethritis, vaginal discharge, itching, stinging and soreness of the genital area; syphilis, gonorrhoea, thrush, bacterial vaginitis and cystitis are some of them. The diagnosis may be obvious to you if there has been contact with an infected person. It is wise to always inspect your sexual partner to make sure there are no problems. Examination of your own genitalia may reveal the typical lesions. If there is any doubt, go to your doctor and have a test. There may be other diseases present.

What to do about it yourself

1 *Prevent infection of others and protect yourself*
Don't have sexual intercourse while you have lesions around the genitalia. If you have sex anyway, urinate immediately after and shower, washing the genitals and anal area thoroughly. Women should not douche as it spreads the infection. Do not have oral sex.

The virus is always around us, on used cups, cutlery, lipstick, glasses, toothbrushes, towels, drinking fountains, toilets, cosmetics, lips, saliva, and the clothes of people with lesions—even on your own hands. Wash your hands thoroughly and often with soap. Don't forget that 10 per cent of herpes infections of Type 2, which is supposed to be the genital one, are contracted this way. Use your own toiletries and utensils and wash up properly with hot water. Keep towels separate and launder clothes separately.

Herpes on the lips can be spread to other parts of the body by hands and tissues infected by picking and dabbing lesions. The eyes are particularly vulnerable. Do not rub your eyes. Herpes in the eye can be dangerous to the sight because the ulcers can scar the clear part of the cornea, giving permanently blurred vision.

Protect yourself from sunlight. Use a heavy ultraviolet screen such as zinc oxide and a broad-brimmed hat if you are prone to cold sores.

Avoid stress, both physical and emotional. Relief of stress makes the treatment more effective, as it is one of the main factors in keeping the immunity of the body high and the virus dormant. Techniques of relaxation such as are used in going to alpha brain-wave levels in yoga, Silva, biofeedback and other mind-control systems are very beneficial in keeping the body defence mechanisms in best shape.

If you cannot be in touch with any of these groups, books are available for do-it-yourself instructions on the best technique (see below and see also 'Relax for Health' on page 89).

Exercise can be relaxing so long as it is not frustrating and exhausting. Competitive exercise may be too stressful, as is overheating from any cause. Women are more prone to stress of all types at menstruation time or just before menstruation.

Laughter is one of the best forms of exercise and oxygenation.

2 Treat the lesions at home
For lesions inside the mouth and throat, use half a teaspoon of bicarbonate of soda and/or salt in one cup of warm water as a gargle. Do not swallow. Follow the gargle by sodium ascorbate

Say: *The atoms that vibrate in me pulse with the universe.*

(a non-acid form of vitamin C). Use half a level teaspoon of sodium ascorbate in half a cup of water. Do swallow this one, and follow it by a mouthful or two of natural yoghurt. After the whitish debris has been washed off the lesions by the gargle the acidophilus bacillus in yoghurt has an inhibiting effect on this virus as well as on thrush.

For lesions round the lips, skin, genitalia and anus, keep the lesions as dry as possible. As soon as lesions arise, apply one of the following:

- Idoxuridine (Stoxyl).
- Iodine (Betadine) or Acyclovir (Zovirax).
- A paste made of 'PC 1P', which is potassium chloride and iron phosphate in buffered soluble form.

If you are showering, wash carefully and pat the area dry with disposable tissues. Then apply one of the above. Towels may be infected by one use and should be laundered separately. Underclothes should be changed and washed daily.

For lesions that are in the vesicle or blister stage, apply Stoxyl (idoxuridine) or Acyclovir (or the lotions and ointments). Dry off thoroughly. Methylated spirit is too painful to use on the burst vesicles or ulcers, on these use only the lotions or ointments above or the non-acidic vitamin C and yoghurt paste. These may all be applied as many times daily as required.

When lesions on the skin are drying, methylated spirit should be applied after washing. Talcum powder (unscented) may be all that is necessary to keep the area dry.

Lesions on the uretha in women can make urinating excruciatingly painful. Take an alkalinising agent such as Citravescent, available from the chemist without a prescription, to make the urine less acid so that it will be less likely to sting as it passes over the lesions. Apply the Stoxyl as a lotion or ointment. Use disposable tissues for washing and drying genital and anal lesions.

Both men and women should wear cotton underwear, not synthetic fibre or mixed fibre, and tight trousers, underpants, girdles, pantyhose, jeans and bikinis will only make the condition worse. Whenever possible, long skirts and no panties are best for women and loose cotton boxer shorts for men. Whatever stops the lesions from drying will keep the virus active, so don't wear airtight underclothes.

Prevent constipation, if anal lesions are present, by taking a cereal, unprocessed bran, or a herbal laxative every morning and plenty of water daily and eat two or three fresh fruits and five raw fresh vegetables daily.

Diet for herpes control

Foods high in L-lysine (Foods to eat)	Foods high in Arginine (Foods to avoid)
Proportion of lysine in one average serving	*Proportion or arginine in one average serving*
fresh fish — HIGHEST	*hazel nuts
*canned fish	macadamia nuts
*chicken	*brazil nuts
*beef	*peanuts
goat's milk	*walnuts
cow's milk and milk foods	almonds
	cocoa
*lamb	*chocolate
*pork	sesame seeds
cheese of all types	*cashews
beans, cooked	carob
sprouts	*gelatine and jelly
brewers yeast	coconut
crustaceans	buckwheat
soybeans, cooked	chick peas
eggs	rice
figs	pecans
peaches	onions
tomatoes	cabbage
turnips	raisins
dates	sunflower seeds
asparagus	wholewheat bread
spinach — LOWEST	oatmeal

* People with cancer should not eat the asterisked foods on these lists (see page 66 for foods to avoid) and may have other supplements to take.

3 Build up your immune response

L-Lysine is an amino-acid building block of the body—one type of many that the body needs; arginine is another. L-lysine inhibits the growth of the herpes virus—arginine makes herpes grow better and often triggers an attack of the virus.

The reason for taking L-lysine is to put the lysine-arginine ratio of amino acids in your diet in favour of stopping the virus from becoming active.

If you eat foods that contain arginine make sure you also take a generous portion of high lysine food at the same meal. For instance, if there are onions in the stew, there should also be plenty of beef and turnips. It is best to avoid altogether the foods at the top of the arginine list, that is the nuts and seeds, if you are very prone to attacks.

The thymus gland controls your immunity. To make T-lymphocytes for combating the virus your immune system needs certain vitamins and minerals in plentiful supply. So take:*

- *Vitaminn C 500 mg* four daily until lesions have gone, then two daily as maintenance. Or use vitamin C powder. 2000 mg are needed, which equals half a heaped teaspoonful of ascorbate powder. Start with a little.

- *Zinc, magnesium and vitamin B6* together stimulate the immune response. Take two tablets twice daily for one week until lesions have disappeared. From then on take one tablet daily as maintenance.

- I use a *multivitamin and mineral tablet* containing all these, plus the rest of the B group, vitamin A and others in balanced proportion, one daily.

- *L-lysine 500 mg*—take four daily until the lesions have gone, then two daily to prevent recurrence.

- *Thymus extract*—take one tablet three times a day. White cells need it.

The regime described is a good one for keeping the herpes virus under control. If a severe stress weakens the immune system again

---

* People following the Cilento Survival Plan for Cancer should not take the substances marked with an asterisk.

and another flare-up occurs, resume the original number of tablets immediately. You may find a health food shop near you that has them. You may make up a potion that you can use for recurrent lesions by crushing up one zinc compound tablet and mixing it with a tablespoon of yoghurt. Keep this lotion covered in the refrigerator. You may also find a vitamin C tablet or half a teaspoon of sodium ascorbate (the salt of vitamin C) dissolved in a little water gives relief to lesions—but if you mix the two lotions together, although effective, it will stain clothing red.

Above all, be responsible. Don't pass the virus on by careless hygiene.

Most people develop immunity to the flare-ups within the first six months of contracting the lesions. Attacks become less and less frequent and shorter in duration. If stress levels remain high, however, the process of control takes longer. The supplements should be taken for at least six months, but don't forget that infected cells take two and a half to three *years* to replace completely.

I have described the Epstein-Barr family of viruses more fully than others because it is particularly heinous in the instigation of cancer. Members of the family are suspected of causing oncogenes (see page 195) which carry the damaged DNA material susceptible to the abnormal growth-stimulating factor that triggers cancerous change.

Intensive study is progressing on the following relationships:

- *Glandular fever* as a precursor of leukaemias and lymphomas.
- *Herpes* as a precursor of cervical, bowel and postnasal space cancer.
- *Hepatitis B* as a precursor of primary liver cancer or hepatoma.

The best safeguard for people who have had these illnesses is to consistently take 2000 mg of Vitamin C daily, for ever. If that is not available, take fresh, raw fruits and vegetables and the natural herbal compounds that can be used as infusions or extracts.

Among many others that are currently researching the effects of new anti-viral drugs on herpes are the following:

Dr Arthur Norins, Director, Dermatology Department, Indiana University School of Medicine;

Dr Richard Griffith, Research Director, Lilly Pharmaceuticals; and

Dr Christopher Kagan, Radiologist, California.

NOTE: If you have had these illnesses it does **NOT** mean that you will get cancer!

Appendixes

1 WHAT FORM OF VITAMIN C WILL I TAKE?

There need be no controversy over the merits of various forms of Viamin C (ascorbic acid). By clinical experience in treating thousands of patients with this substance in all its available forms I know there is some way available for each person.

Ascorbic acid

This is the first form of choice as it is a normal form for body use of the substance. It is especially good for people who are not making enough hydrochloric acid in the stomach. These are usually people past middle age who feel a little nauseated and burpy straight after eating. Most people can take ascorbic acid with water and after food. For a few it is too acidic and even small amounts cause looseness of motions and bladder discomfort which stop as soon as it is ceased.

Ascorbate

The non-acidic salt of vitamin C, ascorbate, is usually better for people who cannot tolerate ascorbic acid. Whether it is given as calcium or sodium ascorbate depends on the problem being treated and the type of metabolism the patient has. For instance *calcium* ascorbate is the form of choice for women after menopause since they are prone to lose calcium when oestrogen levels decrease. If taking any calcium salts, make sure that *magnesium* is also in the daily food intake.

I give a pinch of epsom salts (magnesium sulphate) or magnesium orotate to those having calcium ascorbate, and also encourage the use of salads and green vegetables, which should contain magnesium.

Those women who have the type of breast cancer in which microcalcification in the breast has been apparent on the mammogram, have a basic calcium/magnesium/ oestrogen imbalance and should take *sodium* ascorbate since they may not always hold enough magnesium to balance their calcium.

Calcium ascorbate is also contraindicated in people with some types of cancer in which the calcium metabolism can be deranged. These include sarcomas such as osteogenic sarcoma, bone secondaries from breast and prostate cancer and some types of lung and kidney cancer in which calcium excretion is disturbed and serum calcium rises.

For people who have *congestive heart disease*, staight ascorbic acid or magnesium ascorbate would be best for the same reason, especially if they are also taking calcium antagonist tablets for the heart. Sodium ascorbate may not be suitable for people taking *steroids* such as cortisone and prednisone. They usually need calcium ascorbate to make up for the loss of calcium that this medication causes.

Sodium can cause fluid retention so sodium ascorbate should be monitored carefully in some types of anxiety and depression and in women who have menstrual disturbances with fluid retention, since it can increase the bloating.

Conclusion

Confused? I could go on with more examples. You can see that broad simplistic generalisations make no sense. Thousands of my patients have used calcium ascorbate over the years with excellent results and no side effects. I advise sodium ascorbate for the few who can't take calcium or who hate the bitter taste of it.

Vitamin C is a very useful substance in so many ways that we should each seek out the form that is most palatable for us. Personally I take one teaspoon daily of calcium ascorbate because I had osteoporosis some years ago and I found it the easiest and best way to take calcium—but I eat my greens for magnesium too. My mother always took sodium ascorbate, on the other hand.

There are some people who have become hyper-sensitive to *all* commercial forms of vitamin C, even Ester C, which is usually well tolerated. They need to eat the foods that contain it naturally in abundance, such as fresh raw fruits and vegetables.

2 CILENTO SURVIVAL PLAN SHOPPING GUIDE, MENUS AND RECIPES

All amounts are based on medium-sized fruit and vegetables. If small fruit is all that is available then increase the quantity. Three medium carrots and one Granny Smith apple give 8-9 ounces of juice.

Ten to twelve people require thirty carrots and six apples, approximately, for morning juice.

Afternoon juice

Large bunch celery, 2 large chokos, 4 apples *or* 1 cabbage, 1 bunch celery, 3 carrots, 3 apples *or* 1 bunch celery, 1 lettuce, 4 apples.

Lunch shopping

Check:

Lemons	Millet or Dr	Capsicum
Mint	Bronner bread	Cabbage
Parsley	(wholemeal)	Chokos
Sultanas	Carrots	Zucchini
Brown Rice	Granny Smith Apples	Yoghurt
Barley	Celery	Oranges
Lentils	Potatoes	Bananas
Split Peas	Lettuce	Grapes
Kelp powder	Swede or turnip	Melons
Arrowroot Powder	Beetroot	Mandarins
Garlic	Corn	Apples
Bernard Jensen seasoning mix	Broccoli	Other fruit in season, but *not* berries or pineapple
	Cauliflower	

Menu 1 for nutrition and stress control centre

10 a.m. Morning juice

For each person: 8 oz of carrot and granny smith apple. Wash everything well in clean water and put through juicer and into pouring container.

12.30 Lunch

Soup (see suggestions below). Baked potatoes (dry) in jackets (one per person). Cooked vegetable dish, hot or cold*. Dish of brown rice with sultanas. Salad of 5 raw vegetables include carrot and lettuce. Vegetables to be grated or torn into bite-size pieces. Yoghurt in separate jug. Linseed oil, with orange and lemon juice as dressing. Bread (wholemeal, Pritikin). Fruit salad (made of fresh fruit in season). Garlic, cloves and crusher on table.

3 p.m. Afternoon juice

Green juice—vary from the combinations given below.

Three soup suggestions for rotation

Vegetable soup

¼ cabbage (1 cup chopped)
6 onions (1 cup chopped)
½ celery and some tops (1-2 cups)
¼ pumpkin puree (1-2 cups)
kelp powder (1 teaspoon)
Bernard Jensen or Dr Bonner seasoning mix (1 teaspoon)
Water (pure) or vegetable water (2 litres)

Simmer till vegetables are tender. The soup can be thickened with arrowroot powder, 1 tablespoon mixed with a little water. Add when off the heat source and stir until thickened. This may also be used as a creamed soup by blending until smooth in a blender with no thickening.

---

* Vegetable dishes and soup may be chosen from my cook book (*Anti-Cancer Cookbook*) and varied.

Appendix

Pea soup

1 lb split peas	several medium chopped onions
ginger	2 stalks chopped celery

Cover all ingredients with 2 litres of water in a large pan (pressure cooker) and cook till the peas have made a puree. If preferred, put through a sieve and also stir in 2 tablespoons of cold-pressed linseed or safflower oil per serve when cooling.

Barley soup

1 cup washed barley	1 cup diced swede turnip
1 large chopped onion	1 cup green peas and pods
1 teaspoon kelp powder	1 teasp. Bernard Jensen seasoning

Simmer all in 2 litres of water until barley is tender—may be served directly or put through a sieve or blender to puree.

Vegetable dishes

Bean and vegetable pot

2 cups diced potato	¼ teaspoon each oregano and rosemary
2 cups green beans	
2 cups cooked red kidney beans (soak beans overnight then cook in tomato juice)	¼ cup chopped parsley
	1 cup sliced carrot
	1 or 2 sliced onions

Place all ingredients except parsley in saucepan, including bean liquid. Bring to the boil and simmer 20 minutes, adding extra water if necessary. Stir in parsley before serving.

Vegetable casserole

1 thinly sliced potato	1 cup any other finely chopped or sliced vegetables
1 thinly sliced tomato	
juice of ½ lemon	½ thinly sliced onion
½ small sweet potato, thinly sliced	1 cup chopped silverbeet
	pinch mixed herbs

Layer ingredients in casserole dish, finishing with tomato. Sprinkle with lemon juice and herbs, cover tightly and bake at 375⁰-400⁰ for 1 hour or until food is soft.

Lentil shepherd's pie

1 cup dry brown lentils
1 cup chopped carrots
1 or 2 tomatoes, chopped
crushed garlic to taste
herbs (perhaps ¼ teaspoon each sage, rosemary and oregano)
2 cups potatoes mashed with a little of the lentil stock
1 chopped onion
1 cup diced celery
1 small capsicum, chopped
chopped parsley

Cook lentils and vegetables and herbs in water to cover, adding more liquid (water or maybe fresh tomato juice) if needed. When lentils are cooked, place mixture in baking dish and cover with potato mixed with parsley. Bake at 350⁰F for 30 minutes.

Potato cakes

3 cups diced potato
handful of grated carrot
¼ teaspoon each sage and basil
1 chopped onion
¼ cup chopped parsley

Steam potato and onion. Mix in other ingredients after mashing the cooked vegetables. Form into patties and bake on a tray lightly oiled with olive oil. Bake at 350⁰F for 30 minutes. Turn up heat a little to brown tops if needed. Any leftover vegetables may be added for variation.

Menu 2 for Nutrition & Stress control centre

10 a.m. Morning juice

8 oz or 200 ml of carrot and Granny Smith apple each. Only sound fruit and vegetables to be used, wash everything well in clean water (no detergent) before use.

3 p.m. Afternoon juice

Each 200 ml to contain three of the following in combination, depending on what is in season, freshest and most available:

Celery, carrot, parsley, parsnip, radish, capsicum (red or green), potato, choko, spinach, silverbeet, beetroot and tops, sorrel, cos or romaine lettuce, other lettuce, kale, artichoke, garlic, fennel, endive, dandelion, cabbage, sprouts, cauliflower, broccoli, asparagus, turnip and tops.

(*NO* tomato or cucumber on Gerson and Herbal programs.)

Fruit may be added in combination. Choose one or more from the following:

Apple, peach, pear, apricot, orange, mandarin, grapefruit, papaw, passionfruit, melon, guava.

Blueberries, strawberries, currants, grapes, bananas (these do not juice well), coconut, pea pod, onion.

(Pineapple, babaca, kiwifruit, gooseberries, mulberries, raspberries should be used only under doctor's instructions, *not* if on Gerson or herbal programs.)

Popular combinations (plus apple or grape):

Carrot, celery, lettuce,
Celery, beetroot, carrot
Spinach, celery, lettuce
Cabbage, beetroot, choko
Capsicum, parsley, spinach
Cabbage, celery, carrot and apple

Lunch

Daily, soup
Salad of five or more raw vegetables.
Dry baked potato in jacket
Cooked vegetable dish, cold or hot
Dressings and sauces, as allowed
Dish of brown rice (with sultanas or mint)
Bread and butter with cold-pressed linseed oil
Fruit salad
Yoghurt, natural, unsweetened

Some juice favourites

(All ingredients should be carefully washed.)

1 part carrot, 1 part apple (green type).
3 parts carrot, 1 part celery.

3 parts carrot, 1 part cabbage (green).
1 part tomato, 1 part carrot.
2 parts cucumber, 1 part beetroot, 1 part apple.
2 parts grape, 1 part choko, 1 part cucumber or zucchini.
all watermelon (with rind too).
1 part carrot, 2 parts apple, 1 or 2 whole limes.
3 parts orange, ½ part lettuce greens, ½ part broccoli.
2 parts pineapple, 1½ part cabbage, ½ part comfrey.
2 parts pear, 1 part cabbage, 1 part choko or zucchini.
2 parts apple, 1 part guava, 1 part zucchini.
2 parts apple, 1 part pear, 1 part guava.
2 parts grape, 2 parts choko.
2 parts carrot, 2 parts beetroot.
1 part celery, 1 part beans, 1 part zucchini, 1 part apple.
1 part cucumber, 1 part capsicum, 1 part silverbeet, 1 part apple.
2 parts apple, 1 part celery, 1 part beetroot.
1 part grape, 1 part celery, 1 part choko, 1 part apple.
2 parts grape, 1 part carrot, 1 part apple.

Liver dishes

Liver and onion

1 lamb's liver, young and fresh
1 large onion, chopped finely
3 tablespoons fresh parsley
1 tablespoon wholemeal flour seasoned with herbs to taste
1 large tomato, chopped
fresh or dried Oregano leaves
water

Put 3 tablespoons of water into a wok or stainless steel pan. Simmer the onion, herbs and tomato in it until onion starts to soften. Slice liver thinly. Dredge with seasoned flour. Cook gently on top of vegetables, turning often until colour changes. Add oregano, stir in and simmer briefly. Add more water if it is too thick. Serve covered with parsley.

Lamb's liver paté

1 lamb's liver
1 cup buttermilk
1 teaspoon dried or finely chopped fresh mixed herbs
1 teaspon Bernard Jensens vegetable seasoning powder
2 eggs
1 clove garlic, crushed

Peel liver. Cut into slices. Dredge both sides of each slice with seasoning powder. With a little water in pan, sear quickly on a wok or coated pan. Watch it change colour, then cool. Mince the liver. Beat in buttermilk, eggs, garlic and herbs. Fill a small deep casserole dish with mixture, cover top with lid or foil, stand in a pan of hot water. Cook one hour in moderate oven. Remove and press with heavy weight until quite cold. Turn out whole or serve in a crock. Spread on wholemeal toast. Keep well refrigerated. Lasts no more than 3 days.

Tangy citrus liver

1 calf's liver, peeled and diced
2 onions, chopped
2 cloves garlic, chopped
juices of 3 oranges plus a little grated rind
2 tablespoons wholemeal flour or 1 tablespoon of arrowroot

Seal and cook the liver and onions gently in a little water in a wok or stainless steel pan. Add garlic, citrus juices and peel. Thicken with wholemeal flour or arrowroot.

Liver loaf

1 large lamb's fry
¼ cup diced celery
2 tablespoons minced parsley
¼ teaspoon paprika
1 tablespoon celery leaves, minced
4 tablespoons finely chopped green pepper
1 teaspoon mixed herbs, dry or chopped fresh
½ cup minced onion
1½ cups grated carrots
3 tablespoons fresh wheatgerm
2 free-range eggs, beaten

Put liver through finest mincing blade, followed by the vegetables. Combine all ingredients and mix thoroughly. Put mixture in a large casserole dish and distribute evenly. Cover and bake in moderate oven (325–350°F). Uncover for 15 minutes for browning. This mixture is delicious if used for pies and pasties or as potato pie. The vegetables can be what is left from the juicer.

3 WHY WE NEED VITAMIN SUPPLEMENTS
by Lady Phyllis Cilento

Everyone, even the most conservative, now concedes that vitamins are essential to health, but there is much confusion about the amounts that give the best results.

The most heated arguments I have about nutrition are with doctors and dietitians who assert that we can obtain all the vitamins we need from a good, mixed ordinary Australian diet.

In the first place, what is a good mixed Australian diet?

Everyone differs. For years I have recorded a detailed daily diet from every patient I see, and most do not contain even the Recommended Daily Allowance of vitamins and minerals, let alone those needed to combat the stress and pollution of modern life.

Some few who are nutrition conscious suspect deficiencies, but do not know how to overcome them with ordinary food.

If we lived in a quiet country area, unpolluted by traffic exhaust fumes and industrial waste, grew our vegetables and fruits organically and obtained our dairy products and meat, fish and poultry from paddocks and rivers unpolluted by pesticides—then it would be possible, with careful food preparation, to obtain sufficient vitamins and minerals in our daily meals to maintain abundant health and energy.

The actual lifestyle and food of most Australians, however, is far otherwise. Over 60 per cent live in cities, a further proportion in country towns, where the food supplies are still obtained from supermarkets, and eggs and poultry from battery hens. The usual run of food storage, preparation and cooking tends to destroy most of the vitamins and minerals originally present in the best of food.

All in all, Australian food is pretty good—and wonderful compared with that in the crowded countries around us.

What happens to much of its value before ever it reaches our dinner table or is bought prepared as a fast food from the local takeaway?

Researchers in the United States Department of Agriculture have shown (and their findings would apply to Australia also) that meat today does not deliver the amount of iron shown in the food tables— pork only a quarter of its supposed iron; beef 20 per cent less; the fat in chickens has doubled or trebled over the last 15 years— and the more fat the less muscle meat, including iron.

Still considering meat, which is rich in the B vitamins, it is not always realised that when your liver or steak is browned one-third to two-thirds of its vitamin B_1 (thiamine) and one-third of the B_2 (riboflavine) are destroyed.

In thawing out frozen meat for cooking, one-third of another important B vitamin—pantothenic acid—is lost in the drip; while of vitamin B_6 (pyridoxine)—so important to women— 70 per cent is destroyed in the cooking process.

We also depend on the germ of wheat and cereals for B vitamins but most Australians, from Hobart to Darwin, live on white bread and white flour products from which practically all vitamins (as well as valuable fibre) is stripped in the milling—and sold to pig farmers and health food stores—where we buy wheat germ and bran as supplements. Silly, isn't it?

Vitamin C is recognised by the 'newer knowledge of nutrition' as invaluable in resistance to all infections; as a universal detoxifier to fight poisons and pollution and as a nontoxic chemotherapy in the control of cancer. It could well be called 'the Vanishing Vitamin'.

Surely there is enough in fresh fruits and vegetables to keep us healthy?

Actually, as soon as you remove the skin of C-rich fruits and start juicing them or cutting them up, a large percentage of the vitamin C is lost. Cutting greens like lettuce, cabbage and beans causes bruising that destroys C, while keeping them in the 'fridge till next day accounts for further loss—30–40 per cent.

Commercial 'orange juice' bought in plastic or waxed containers has lost so much available C that it cannot be relied on to supply adequate vitamins. A pleasant drink certainly, and better than sugar-laden soft drinks and cordials, which are laced with artifical flavourings and colourings and iron-destroying pesticides.

Potatoes may not be high in C, but because Australians eat so much of them they are an excellent source of the vitamin, that is if it is not all soaked and cooked out of them and thrown away in the vegetable water, or if potatoes are not eaten as an 'instant mix' or as fried chips. Strangely enough, the thin potato flakes (crisps), analysed by a scientist recently, were found to retain much of their C.

Long boiling of vegetables—specially when soda is added or the water contains chlorine—is well know to destroy vitamin C, while much of what is left and their B vitamins plus their valuable potassium and other minerals usually go down the sink when straining them for the table. Vegetable water—which should be low in salt—should not be discarded but used in soups or gravies or drunk as an adjunct to meals.

An unsuspected example of C loss was recently found by Israeli scientists. When mashed banana pulp was mixed with orange juice—such as is often given to babies—75 to 80 per cent of the vitamin C was lost.

Drying fruits and vegetables destroys all their vitamin C; canning some of it, depending on the canning process, but much of the vitamin remains in the fluid rather than the vegetable or fruit itself.

Freezing is the best means of preserving the vitamins in vegetables, but it is known that minerals such as zinc are lost from the surface of frozen greens.

Recently a Melbourne pathologist took the trouble to test the vitamin C content of a good day's meals with restaurant dinner. He found only 5 mg of vitamin C, and that was in the prawn cocktail. Even the restaurant fruit salad contained none.

Vitamin deficiencies in most takeaway-restaurant and institutional meals have been surveyed by several scientific groups and they are well documented.

It is so easy and time-saving, especially for the growing number of working mothers, flatting students and those living alone, to buy most meals prepared, processed or packaged and to let white bread, biscuits and refined carbohydrates dominate the diet, that they simply do not realise how depleted in vitamins and minerals their nutrition has become.

Vitamin A, for example, is essential not only for normal growth in children, but for insuring clear sight and maintaining a healthy condition of the skin, hair and nails, and also of all the lining and covering membranes in the body—nose, throat, respiratory tract, digestive, urinary and reproductive passages.

Vitamin A is obtainable in butter, well-fortified margarine, egg yolk, liver, fish liver oils, dairy products, and its precursor, beta carotene, in red, orange, green and yellow fruits and vegetables.

The present vogue of cutting down fats and dairy products and eggs in the diet, through fear of cholesterol, depletes much vitamin A in the diet of many normal people and prevents its absorption, while very few take sufficient greens and coloured vegetables in their daily diet to supply adequate A. More than half of them turn up their noses at the mention of liver and would never think of including fish liver oils (the best source) in their own or their children's daily intake.

Hence we have such universal hypersensitivity to sun glare that dark glasses are the vogue. Strong sunlight and fluorescent lights on white paper so use up the vitamin A-dependent visual purple in the retina of the eyes that our ordinary diet does not supply sufficient A to replace it.

Widespread A deficiency is also obvious in the prevalence of adolescent acne, chronic sinusitis, respiratory tract infections, cystitis in the bladder, dry scaly skin and premature wrinkles. Deficiency in vitamin A allows heaping up of dead cells on these areas, creating an invitation for the growth of bacteria and viruses which could never flourish in normal, A-nourished tissues.

The proof of the pudding is in the eating. When adequate supplements of vitamin A (specially when coupled with E) are given these infections can be practically eliminated and a healthy condition and resistance restored to the areas.

Before the discovery of antibiotics, ear, nose and throat specialists used concentrated vitamin A to combat infections. The practice ceased when an antibiotic would quickly destroy the invading bacteria. It is now realised, however, that unless A, C and some B supplements are added to the usual diet, the trouble recurs soon after the antibiotics have fulfilled their immediate function and been discontinued.

This is why so many people, young and old, are only kept infection-free by continuing courses of various antibiotics.

There is, however, a widespread fear of vitamin A supplements as it is (with vitamin D) the only vitamin in which symptoms of 'hypervitaminoses' have occurred and it has been misnamed 'toxic'. Strangely enough they are much the same symptoms as in a deficiency.

However, many times the RDA is needed to maintain healthy skin and mucous membranes in our polluted environment on the ordinary Australian diet as consumed by the ordinary Australian.

So prevalent is vitamin A deficiency in the United States that the Health Department has now forbidden the term 'toxic' to be used in relation to it.

Vitamin E

Now that most of our wheaten and cereal products are denatured before ever we get them, it is well nigh impossible to get enough vitamin E to maintain healthy heart, blood vessels and normal fertility and prevent premature ageing without supplements of this vitamin.

Few people include enough wheat germ, whole grain cereals, nuts and seeds, wheat-germ oil or cold-pressed vegetable oils in their daily diet to obtain even the RDA of 15 mgs of E. But much more is needed in our stressful and polluted environment.

E is so versatile in its benefits as an anti-coagulant, anti-oxidant and preserver of vitamin A, that supplements included in the daily regime from infancy to old age would prevent many of the common disabilities to which we have become prone.

I refer particularly to the health of heart and arteries. Overwhelming clinical evidence has shown that vitamin E supplements are effective in preventing angina and coronary thrombosis and curing cases that have already occurred—if taken in sufficient amounts.

I believe that if every man over thirty and every woman over forty were to take 400 to 1000 mgs. of vitamin E (d alpha tocopherol) daily, increasing with age and stress, and add wheatgerm, cold-pressed oils and whole grain bread and cereals to their daily diet, the incidence of coronary thrombosis, angina and poor leg circulation would be a thing of the past. Many sudden deaths of men in their prime of life would be prevented.

It should be taken regularly and in sufficient dosage. Vitamin E may be expensive, but worth the cost in added efficiency and longevity.

4 CORRECT BREATHING FOR PHYSICAL AND MENTAL HEALTH

Most of us breathe incorrectly. We breathe superficially, using only a small part of the capacity of our lungs. Our breathing is not rhythmical or in harmony. The sad result is that our whole body and brain is literally starved of nourishment, and this is completely unnecessary in view of the plentiful supply of oxygen in the air that surrounds us. By shallow respiration we also tend to encourage the build-up of stagnant air in the lower regions of the lungs for long periods of time. This is conducive to the onset of various diseases that inflict modern people, such as tuberculosis. Wearing tight clothing around the waist impedes deep breathing. Remember, without breathing we cannot live; with half breathing we only half live.

The process of breathing can be divided into two parts: abdominal and thoracic breathing.

Abdominal breathing

This is also known as diaphragmatic respiration. Sit or lie flat on the back and place one hand on the naval. Inhale deeply and you will see the hand rise as the abdomen expands outwards. The more the abdomen expands outwards, the lower down the diaphragm moves. This is the strong muscle membrane that separates the lungs from the abdominal organs. The lower it moves during inhalation the more air is taken into the lungs.

Exhale deeply and your hand moves inwards towards the spine as the abdomen contracts. The diaphragm will move higher if the contraction of the abdomen is accentuated with maximum expulsion of air from the lungs. During this practice do not move the chest or the shoulders.

Thoracic or chest breathing

Maintain the same position as in the abdominal breathing exercise, sitting or lying flat on the back. Inhale while expanding the chest or rib cage. You will find that the ribs move outwards and upwards.

Exhale and you will find that the ribs move inwards and downwards. Try not to move the abdomen at all in thoracic breathing.

Do each of these five times daily, separately, then five times together, from diaphragm first to chest breathing. This aerates the lungs and gives you oxygen.

5 DESCRIPTION OF THE CANCER ORGANISM—GASTON NAESSENS

Here is Gaston Naessen's description of the cancer organism he calls 'the somatid', quoted from *Aids, Cancer and the Medical Establishment* by Raymond Keith Brown, MD

> The standard microscope permits a maximal enlargement to 1800X with a maximal resolution (index of clarity) of 0.1 micron. The electron microscope can achieve an enlargement into the millions with a resolution of 30 to 50 angstroms but the object of study must be dried and fixed so that only its skeletal outlines can be seen.
>
> Using a combination of laser and ultraviolet technology, we have developed an instrument which we call the 'Somatoscope' that permits the observation of living organisms up to a magnification of 30 000 with a resolution of 150 angstroms. Because of the infinite time and intricacies of working at the higher magnifications, most of our work has been done at the lower ranges.
>
> With this instrument, we have observed in all biologic liquids, and particularly in the blood, an elementary particle endowed with movement and possessing a variable life cycle of many forms. We have called this particle a 'somatid' and in the proper media, it can be isolated and cultured. Its dimensions vary from a few angstroms to 0.1 of a micron and it is present in the blood of all individuals. It is the diversity of forms emerging in many disease states that distinguishes their possessors from healthy individuals.
>
> We postulate and have evidence that the normal life cycle of this organism consists of somatids, spores and double spores and that these produce a hormone-like substance (which we have

termed 'trefons' after the usage of Alexis Carrel), that initiate cell division within the body. In healthy individuals, the somatid cycle is regulated and controlled by blood inhibitors (usually certain trace minerals and organic substances).

If, due to stress or other biologic disturbances, these inhibitors within the blood are diminished, the relatively simple cycle of somatids, spores and double spores is diverted into another and more elaborate cycle; one then sees with the tissues, and particularly within the blood, the diverse forms of bacteria known as 'Syphonospora Polymorpha' that were so well demonstrated by the German scientist von Brehmer in the 1930s. Within this group can be placed the wide range of mutable organisms that have been variously described as 'Pleomorphic Organisms', 'L' forms, or 'Cell Wall Deficient Organisms' (see page 173).

Little is known of bacterial evolution and there is no really adequately comprehensive classification for many microbial forms but it appears that the infinite variations of pleomorphic bacteria that are present in many disease states can be aligned within the expanded somatid cycle. They can be aerobic, anaerobic, motile or non-motile, with varying staining capacity (especially for Gram and acid-fast stains). The diagrams on pages 174-5 demonstrate their forms which can range from coccal (ie. Streptococcus and Staphylococcus) to bacillary, from the rod-like forms of Mycobacteria to the curves of spirochetes). The pathogenically prominent Mycobacteria evolve and burst (Eclatment), releasing yeast-like 'levurids' at a level which can be termed 'fungal' although this term applies more to the appearance than the physical characteristics of the organisms. The 'Levurids' evolve through 'ascospores' to 'asci' which are indistinguishable by ordinary laboratory means from small lymphocytes. Forming cytoplasm, the 'asci' in an adequately nutritious environment develop as 'thalli' whose walls burst and liberate an enormous quantity of new somatid that initiate another complete cycle. The fibrous thallus, emptied of its cytoplasm and contents, is often observed on stained smears and catalogued and dismissed as being an artifact. (Except to call them 'fibrin formations' no one has ever explained the wide prevalence of these 'artifacts' in carefully prepared and usually sterile slides!!).

In our laboratory we can show that derivatives of the somatid cycle, and other substances that react with these organisms, are capable of effects that pertain to many current problems and challenges of medicine. They are relevant to cancer, organ transplantation and many aspects of degenerative diseases.

Bacteriological classification of the cancer microbe

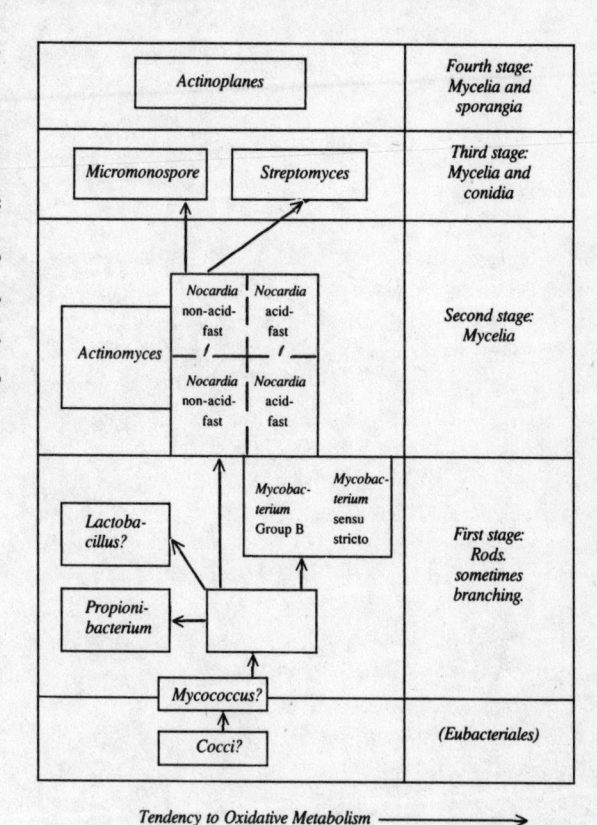

Degree of Morphological Differentiation →

	Actinoplanes		Fourth stage: Mycelia and sporangia
	Micromonospore *Streptomyces*		Third stage: Mycelia and conidia
Actinomyces	*Nocardia* non-acid-fast / *Nocardia* acid-fast / *Nocardia* non-acid-fast *Nocardia* acid-fast		Second stage: Mycelia
Lactoba-cillus? *Propioni-bacterium*	*Mycobac-terium* Group B *Mycobac-terium* sensu stricto		First stage: Rods, sometimes branching.
Mycococcus? *Cocci?*			(Eubacteriales)

Tendency to Oxidative Metabolism →

Tentative philogenic scheme of the Actinomyretales.
Chart by H.L. Jensen, International Congress of Microbiology, Rome 1953.
Progenitor cryptocides Pluripotential Actinomycete has all the above forms.

Appendix

Schematic representation of filaments from spores in the blood, after Dr Von Brehmer

1	Red blood cells with sporanges of syphonospora
2 & 3	The sporanges discharging their mature spores into the haematin
4	The red cell becomes deformed by the sporanges within it
5	The sporanges stretch the red cell membrane
6, 7, 8, 9	The red cell membrane is drawn out by the sporanges which are still attached to it
10	The sporanges free themselves from the red cell and begin to move, carrying red cell membrane material around them
11	Free forms

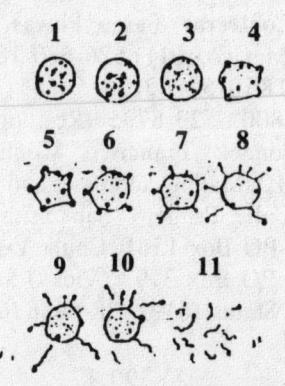

HEALING INSTITUTIONS

Burzynski Research Institute, Outpatient Clinic, 6221 Corporate Drive, Houston, Texas 77036, United States (713) 777-8233; Research Institute, 12707 Trinity Drive, Stafford, Texas 77477 United States, (713) 240-5227 (713) 777-8241 (Lee Trombetta); Primary personnel: Stanislau R. Burzynski, MD PhD.

Bio-medical Center (Hoxsey), PO Box 727, General Ferreira #616, Col. Juarez, Tijuana BC Mexico, (706) 684-9011 (706) 684-9081 (706) 684-9082 (706) 684-9376; Primary personnel: Fernando Arriola, MD, Mildred Nelson RN; Information: (619) 228655 Leona Rogers.

Yolanda Fraire, MD, Calle 8 1941 (Entre Revolution and Madero) 4th floor, Tijuana, B.C. Mexico, (706) 685-4664 (706) 685-4665.

Gerson Therapy: Hospital de Baja, California Gerson Institute, P.O. Box 430, Bonita, California 92992 United States, (619) 267-1150; Hospital: Playas, Tijuana, B.C. Mexico; Information: Charlotte Gerson, Gar Hildebrand, Norman Fritz at the Institute.

Hospital Ernesto Contreras, Paseo Playas de Tijuana, No 19, Tijuana, B.C. Mexico, (011) 526-680-1850/51/52/53/54/55, (706) 680-1850/51/52/53/54/55, (800) 262-0212 (California), (800) 523-8795 (Rest of the United States); Primary personnel: Francisco Contreras, MD Ernesto Contreras Sr MD; Mailing addresses and U.S. Contact: Patricia Prince, 190 Calle Primero, San Ysidro, California 92073 United States, PO Box 1561, Chula Vista, California 92912 United States, PO Box 3793 (Vicky) San Ysidro, California 92073, United States, (619) 428-6438 (619) 428-4486.

Immuno-Augmentative Therapy Centre (IAT Centre) Primary personnel: Lawrence Burton, PhD, John Clements MD, P.O. Box F-2689, Freeport, Grand Bahama Island, Bahamas (809) 352-7455/6; IAT Patients' Association Inc. Box 10, Otho, Iowa 50569-0010, United States (515) 972-4444; IAT West Mailing Address, 416 West San Ysidro Boulevard, San Ysidro, California 92073, United States (619) 428-2211 (706) 680-6830; IAT West Clinic: Baja region of Mexico.

Livingston-Wheeler Medical Clinic, 3232 Duke Street, San Diego, California 92110, United States, (619) 224-3515.

Lukas Klinik, CH-4144 Arlesheim, Switzerland; Primary Personnel: Rita Leroi, MD, (011) 41-61-72-3333 for Iscador etc.

Electro-Chemical and Cancer Institute, Hasumi, Ken-ichiro, KH MD, 5-45-6, Kokuryo-cho, Chofu-shi 182 Tokyo, Japan, 0424-82-2037/0424-88-3437, telefax 0424-86-6452.

Institute of Applied Biology, 164 East 91st Street, New York 10128, United States, (212) 876-9669; Primary personnel: Emanuel Revici MD; Contact person: Elena Avram.

Bristol Cancer Help Centre, Grove House, Cornwallis Grove, Clifton, Bristol Bs8 4PG, England, United Kingdom; 011-44-0272-743216 (from Australia), (0272) 743216 (England).

E.D. Danopoulos, MD, Rigillis Str. 26 (Private Practice: 12 Rigillis Str) 106-74 Athens, Greece, 011-301-721-1332 011-301-721-5318; Primary personnel: Prof E.D. Danopoulos, MD

Hans A. Nieper MD, Outpatient Office: Sedan Strasse 21, 3000 Hannover 1, West Germany, 011-49-511-348-08-08; Inpatient Clinic: Paracelsus Klinik at Silbersee, Oertzweg 24, 3012 Langenhagen, West Germany, 011-49-511-733031.

The Australian Cancer Patients' Foundation Inc., The Melbourne Living Center, 360 Mont Albert Road, Mont Albert, Victoria 3127, Australia (03) 8902209.

The Yarra Valley Living Centre, P.O. Box 77, Yarra Junction, 3797, Australia (059) 671730.

BIBLIOGRAPHY

Achterberg, J., *Imagery in Healing*, New Science Library, Shambhala, Boston & London, 1985.

Bechamp, A., *The Blood*, Veritas Press, Bundaberg, Australia, 1988.

Berkley, G., *Cancer, How to Prevent It and How to Help Your Doctor Fight It*, Spectrum, Prentice Hall Inc, Inglewood Cliffs, New Jersey, USA, 1978.

Beyers, M., Durburg, S., Werner, J., *Complete Guide to Cancer Nursing*, Medical Economics Company, New Jersey, USA, 1984.

Bishop, B., *A Time To Heal*, Severn House Publishers, London, 1985.

Bradford, R., *Now That You Have Cancer*, Choice Publishers, Los Altos, USA, 1977.

Brown, R.K., *Aids, Cancer & the Medical Establishment*, Robert Speller Publishers, New York, 1986.

Buckman, R., *I Don't Know What to Say*, Paper Mac, MacMillan Publishers, London, 1988.

Cameron, E. and Pauling, L., *Cancer and Vitamin C*, Warner Books, New York, 1979.

Cantwell, A., Jr, *The Cancer Microbe*, Aries Rising Press, Los Angeles, USA, 1990.

Carter, S.K., Glatstein, E., Livingston, R.B., *Principles of Cancer Treatment*, McGraw Hill Book Co. Inc, New York, 1982.

Cassileth, B., *The Cancer Patient*, Lea Febiger, Philadelphia, USA, 1979.

Chaitow, L., *An End to Cancer*, Thorsons Publishing Group, Wellingborough, UK, 1983.

Chopra, D., *Quantum Healing*, Bantam Books, New York, 1989.

Cilento, P., *Better Health*, Veritas Press, Perth, Australia, 1991.

Clinkard, C.E., *The Uses of Juices*, Pitman Publishing, London, 1988.

Clyne, R., *Coping With Cancer—Making Sense of it All*, Thorsons Publishing Group, New York, 1986.

Cohen, A., *The Dragon Doesn't Live Here Anymore*, Alan Cohen Publications, Kula, Hawaii, 1981.

Cousins, N., *Anatomy of an Illness*, Bantam Books, New York, 1979.

Creasey, W.A., *Cancer—An Introduction*, Oxford University Press, New York, 1981.

Davison, J., *Cancer Winner*, Midwest Press, Pierce City, USA, 1977.

de Vore, S., White, T., *The Appetites of Man*, Anchor Press, Double Bay, New York, 1978.

Dewar, D., *Breast Cancer—A Woman's Handbook*, And Books, South Bend, USA, 1983.

Dude, D., *A Guide to Dying at Home*, John Muir Publications, Sante Fe, Mexico, 1982.

Eisen, H.N., *Immunology*, Harper & Row Publishers, Philadelphia, USA, 1980.

Erasmus, U., *Fats and Oils*, Alive Books, Vancouver, Canada, 1986.

Eyre, R.B., *I Fought Leukaemia and Won*, Hawkes Publishing Inc, Salt Lake City, USA, 1982.

Fredericks, C., *Breast Cancer—A Nutritional Approach*, Hill of Content, Melbourne, Australia, 1978.

Friedberg, E., 'Cancer Biology' in *Scientific American*, W.H. Freeman & Co., New York, 1986.

Gawler, I., *You Can Conquer Cancer*, Hill of Content, Melbourne, Australia, 1984.

Gerson, M., *A Cancer Therapy—Results of Fifty Cases*, Totality Books, Del Mar, USA, 1977.

Gilshenan, P., *Where There's Hope*, (available from 8 Sycamore Street, Redland Bay, Queensland, Australia) 1990.

Griffin, G.E., *World Without Cancer (The Story of Vitamin B17, Part 1)*, American Media, Thousand Oaks, USA, 1974.

Halpern, S., *Clinical Nutrition*, 2nd Edition, J B Luppincott Co, Philadelphia, USA, 1987.

Hanawalt, P.C., 'Molecules to Living Cells', in *Scientific American*, W.H. Freeman & Co, New York, 1980.

Harris, T., *I'm OK, You're OK*, Pan Books, London 1979.

Hasumi, K., *Cancer Has Been Conquered*, Maruzen Co Ltd, Tokyo, 1980.

Hay, L., *Heal Your Body*, Specialist Publications, Concord, Australia, 1988.

Heinerman, J., *The Treatment of Cancer with Herbs*, Biworld Publishers, Orem, USA, 1980.

Henderson, C., Raymond, A., *Cancer Help*, Simon & Schuster, Sydney, Australia, 1988.

Hersey, P., ed., *Biological Agents in the Treatment of Cancer*, Proceedings of the International Conference at Newcastle, September 1990.

Hicks, R., *Understanding Cancer*, University of Queensland Press, Brisbane, 1980.

Hoxsey, H.M., *You Don't Have to Die*, Milestone Books Inc, New York, 1956.

Hsu, H-Y., *Treating Cancer with Chinese Herbs*, Oriental Healing Arts Institute, Los Angeles, USA, 1982.

Hunsberger, E.M., *Edyie Mae's Natural Recipes*, Avery Publications Group, Wayne, NJ, USA, 1978.

Hunter Trum, B., *Be Kitchen Wise*, Unwin paperbacks, Sydney 1986.

Hunter Trum, B., *Consumer beware*, Touchstone, 1972.

Issels, J., *Cancer: A Second Option*, Hodder & Stoughton, London, 1975.

Jacka, J., *Cancer—A Physical and Psychic Profile*, Judy Jacka, Sydney Australia, 1977.

Jung, C.G., *Memories, Dreams, Reflections*, Collins, Fontana Library, London, 1975.

Kelley, W.D., *One Answer to Cancer*, International Association for Cancer Victims and Friends, The Kelley Foundation, Playa del Rey, USA, 1974.

Kidman, B., *A Gentle Way With Cancer*, Century Publishing, London, 1983.

Kittler, G.D., *Laetrile—Nutritional Control for Cancer with B17*, Royal Publications Inc, Denver, USA, 1982.

Koch, W., *The Survival Factor in Neoplastic and Viral Diseases*, Natural Immunity Series, Portuguese Edition, 1960.

Kormondy, E.J. and Essenfeld, B.E., *Biology: Addison—Wesley*, 2nd edition, Reading, Massachusetts, USA, 1984.

Kyokai, B.D., *The Teaching of Buddha*, Buddhist Promoting Foundation, Tokyo, Japan, 1966.

Lewis, J., *Positive Thoughts for Successful Living*, Unity Church, Denver, 1979.

Livingston-Wheeler, V. and Addeo, E.G., *The Conquest of Cancer—Vaccines and Diet*, Franklin Watts, New York, 1984.

Livingston-Wheeler, V. and Webster Wheeler, O., *Food Alive*, Livingston-Wheeler Medical Clinic, San Diego, USA, 1977.

The Microbiology of Cancer Compendium, A Livingston-Wheeler Medical Clinic Publication, San Diego, USA, 1977.

Lynch, H.T. and Fusaro, R.M., eds., *Cancer-Associated Genodermatoses*, Van Nostrand Reinhold Co, New York, 1982.

Mae, E., and Loeffler, C., *How I Conquered Cancer Naturally*, Production House, San Diego, USA, 1975.

Manning, M., *A Guide to Self Healing*, Thorsons Publishing Group, Wellingborough, UK, 1989.

Marks, J., *A Guide to the Vitamins: Their Role in Health and Disease*, Medical and Technical Publishing Co, Lancaster, UK, 1975.

McKhann, C.F., *The Facts About Cancer*, Spectrum, Prentice Hall Inc, New Jersey, USA, 1981.

Meares, A., *The Wealth Within*, Hill of Content, Melbourne, Australia, 1978.

Mervyn, L., *Complete Guide to Vitamins and Minerals*, Thorsons Publishing Group, London, 1989.

Morris, N., *The Cancer Blackout*, Regent House, Los Angeles, USA, 1977.

Moss, R., *The Cancer Syndrome*, Grove Press, New York, USA, 1980.

Nieper, H., *Dr Nieper's Revolution in Technology, Medicine and Society*, MTI Verlag, Oldenburg, Germany, 1985.

Nordenstrom, B.E.W., *Biologically Closed Electric Circuits*, Nordic Medical Publications, Stockholm, Sweden, 1983.

Ostander, S. and Schroeder, L., *Psychic Discoveries Behind the Iron Curtain*, Prentice Hall Inc, New Jersey, USA, 1970.

Ott, J.N., *Health and Light*, Pocket Books, Simon & Schuster, New York, 1973.

Parker, M. and Mauger, D., *Children with Cancer*, Cassell Ltd, London, 1979.

Parker, M., *Why Me—Commonsense About Cancer*, ANZ Book Co. Auckland, New Zealand, 1981.

Passwater, R., *Cancer and Its Nutritional Therapies*, Keats Publishing Inc, New Canaan, USA, 1978.

Porth, C.M., ed., with eleven contributors, *Pathophysiology; concepts of altered health states*, J B Lippincott, 1986.

Pottinger, F.M., *Pottinger's Cats: A Study in Nutrition*, Price-Pottinger Nutrition Foundation Inc, New Jersey, USA, 1983.

Reading, C. and Meillor, R., *Your Family Tree Connection*, Keats Publishing Inc, New Canaan, USA, 1988.

Richards, D., *The Topic of Cancer*, Pergamon Press, New York, USA, 1982.

Riddle Wright, J., *Diagnosis: Cancer, Prognosis: Life*, Allbright & Co, Huntsville, Alabama, USA, 1985.

Roger, J. and McWilliams, P., *You Can't Afford the Luxury of a Negative Thought: A book for people with life-threatening illness, including life!* Thorsons, Harper Collins, London, 1991.

Russ, P. and Tanner, L., *The Politics of Pollution*, Visa, Widescope International Publishers Pty Ltd, Melbourne, Australia, 1978.

Sattilaro, A., Monte, T., *Recalled By Life*, Houghton Mifflin, Boston, USA, 1982.

Schwartz, D.J., *The Magic of Thinking Big*, Wilshire Book Co, California, USA, 1990.

Schwartz, L.M., *Compendium of Immunology*, Van Nostrand Reinhold Co, New York, 1980.

Scott Peck, M., *The Road Less Travelled*, Hutchinson, London, 1983.

Shealy, C.N., Myss, C.M., *The Creation of Health*, Stillpoint Publishing, Walpole, USA, 1988.

Siegal, B.S., *Love, Medicine and Miracles*, Harper & Row Publishers, New York, 1986.

Siegal, B., *Peace, Love and Healing*, Rider, London, 1990.

Simonton, S., *The Healing Family*, Bantam Books, New York, 1984.

Silva, J. and Miele, P., *The Silva Mind Control Method*, Pocket Books, New York, 1977.

Silva, J. and Stone, R.B., *You the Healer*, H.J. Kramer Inc, Tiburon, USA, 1989.

Suzuki, D., *Inventing the Future*, Allen & Unwin, Sydney, Wellington, London, 1990.

Thomas, L., *The Lives of a Cell*, Bantam New Age Books, New York, 1975.

Thompson, R.F., ed., 'Progress in Neuro Science', in *Scientific American*, W.H. Freeman & Co, New York, 1986.

Tropp, J., *Cancer: The Whole Body Approach to Cancer Therapy*, Cancer Resource Centre, Los Angeles, 1980.

Twycross, R.G. and Lack, S.A., *Therapeutics in Terminal Cancer*, Churchill Livingstone, New York, 1990.

Waerland, E., *Cancer, A Disease of Civilisation*, The Provoker Press, St Catherines, Canada, 1976.

Whelan, E., *Preventing Cancer*, Sphere Books, London, 1979.

Wilner, B.I., *A Classification of the Major Groups of Human and Other Animal Viruses*, Burgess Publishing Co, Minneapolis, USA, 4th edition, 1969.

INDEX

Aborigines, 141, 271, 314
abscisic acid, 50, 61-2, 67-8
acidophilus, Lactobacillus, 53-4, 137
adenosine triphosphate (ATP), 50
adjuvants, 141
adrenal glands, 89, 165-6
aerobic metabolism, 42
affirmations, 94-5
age and healing, 166
Agens, 180
AIDS, 176
air-conditioning, 42
alcohol, 42, 78, 242
Alexander-Jackson, Eleanor, 222-4
allergy
    eosinophils, 138
    grains, 52, 56-7
    yeast, 342, 345
aloe vera, 310
alpha rhythms, 89-90, 95
amino acids, 323-4, 364
amygdalin, 111, 306
anaemia, 210
anger, 337-8
animal cancers, 207, 209, 223-4
antibiotics, 136, 145, 241, 346, 349
antiblocking agents, 125-6, 137
antibody (Ab), 128-32, 137-9, 351-2
anticancer serum, 179, 351-2
antigen (Ag), 128-32, 282
antineoplastons, 189-90, 324
antivin, 230
appetite stimulation, 48
arginine, 363-4
ascorbate, 369-70
ascorbic acid, 369
asparagus, 61
asthma, 317, 348

attitudes
    family, 84-8
    healing, 88, 325
    positive, 24-7
Australian Cancer Patients' Foundation, 391
Australian Medical Association (AMA), 32-4, 82
auto-immune reaction, 132
B cells, 128-32, 138, 195-6
Bacillus Calmitte-Guerin (BCG), 172, 208, 323, 352
bacteria, 44, 53-4
Barley Green, 253
basal cell carcinoma, 270-1, 327-8
Béchamp, Antoine, 169
benzaldehyde, 111
beta carotene, 62-3
Bhagwan Maharishi Rajneesh, 311-12
bifidis, Lactobacillus, 53-4
biological product therapy, 139-50, 215-19, 301
bladder cancer, 61, 247-54
blood
    acid and alkaline, 180
    cancer organism, 177
    serum, 351-2
    spread of cancer, 327
    stem cells, 126, 129-30
    tests, 23, 138, 233-4, 266-7, 353-4
    see also Progenitor cryptocides, white cells
bone cancer, 215
bone marrow, 126, 129-30, 137
Bonifacio, A., 221
bougie, 48
bowel, 345, 353
bowel cancer, 54, 215, 255-63, 327, 349-56

brain
    cancer, 36-7, 102, 320, 326-7, 329
    left and right sides, 89
    physiology, 81-2
bread, 57, 73
breakfast, 51-7, 68-9
breast cancer, 78-9, 177, 215, 222, 274-318, 327, 369-70
breathing exercises, 74, 90, 383-4
Brehmer, Wilhelm von, 179-80, 386-8
brewer's yeast, 53
Bristol Cancer Help Centre, 391
Budwig, Johanna, 162-4
bulgaricus, Lactobacillus, 54
Burzynski, Stanislau R., 189-90, 390
butter, 72
BX and BY virus, 227
caffeine, 46
calcium ascorbate, 369-70
calcium metabolism, 369-70
cancer
    causes, 78-80, 289, 340
    formation, 326-7
    indolent, 40
    prognosis, 29-30, 32-3, 36-40
    spread, 326-7
    stages, 8-9
    types, 36
    see also animals; cell; survival
Cancer Care Program, 33
Cancer Control Society (CCS), 109-13
Cancer Facts and Fallacies seminar, 31-4
cancer markers, 125, 281-2, 354
cancer organism, 135-6, 141-2, 168-77, 221-35, 385-7
cancer virus, 159, 168-72, 206-10, 225-30
cancer weed, 270
Candida, 23, 53, 148, ,232, 275-7, 333, 341-9
Cantwell, Alan, *vii*, 176
carotanaemia, 63
carotinoids, 62-3
cell
    cycles, 159
    growth, 61-2
    membrane, 158-60, 184-5, 191-2
    physiology, 155-96
    stages in cancer development, 191-6
    stress, 155-96

cell-wall-deficient organism (CWDO), 173, 195, 227
Centro Medico del Mar, 305-8
cervical cancer, 116, 360
chemicals
    household use, 43
    photography, 341
    see also food
chemotherapy, 8, 136-7, 149-50, 166-7, 215, 268-9, 274, 320, 346-7
children, 135-6, 284-5
chlorine, 46
cholesterol, 333-5
chymotrypsin, 230
Cilento, Phyllis, 14-15, 108-9, 162, 295-8, 305-6, 378
Cilento Survival Plan, 15, 141, 164, 371-7
Cilento Way, 15
coffee enemas, 244
cold-pressed oils, 54-6, 164
cold sores, 356-62
Coley, William B., 230-1
colon therapy, 300
colony stimulating factors (CSF), 126
colostomy, 332-3, 336
colour meditation, 96-7
computers, 241, 246
confidence, 98-103
contact inhibition, 159
contraceptive pill, 275, 278, 319, 322
Contreras, Ernesto, 305-9, 390
cookbooks, 47, 77
Coryne-bacterium, 180
cosmetics, 67
Crofton, William Mervyn, 178, 221
Culver-Evans, Celia, 227
Curaderm, 272
Danopoulos, E. D. and I., 328-9, 391
Deaken, Thomas, 221
death, *see* dying
dehydration, 44
denial, 86-7
dentistry, 118, 120, 250-2
depression, 335-6
detergents, 43
Devil's Apple, 272-3
diet, 15, 378-82
    bowel problems, 353
    Candida control, 342-5
    dying, 293

eating habits, 51
fat-free, 55
food plan, 66-74, 308
herpes, 363-5
modern, 162-3, 242
tribal, 190-1
see also food; meals; nutrition; supplements
digestive enzymes, 142
Diller, Irene Corey, 223-3
dinner, 71-2
Dique, John C. A., 107
doctors, 12-14, 29-30
dolomite, 53
dormin, 50
drawings, interpretation, 96-7
drug manufacturing firms, 75-6, 111-12, 184, 187, 224, 329, 331
Dubos, Rene, 171-2
ductless glands, 140-5
Durovic, Stevan and Marco, 221
dying, 289-99
economics of treatment, 330-1
egg flip, 49
electrical charge, cell membrane, 158-60, 184-5, 194
electrolytes, 44, 63, 185, 354
electron microscope, 204-7, 210
emotions
immune system, 130
negative, 24, 83-4, 91-3, 336-8
endocrine system, 140-2
endoscopy, 39-40
enemas, 244, 300
energy and physiology, 155-7
eosinophils, 138, 252
Epsom salts, 50, 67, 369
Epstein-Barr viruses, 357-8, 365
Erasmus, Udo, 161-2
erysipelas, 230
Escherichia coli, 139
essential fatty acids (EFA), 55, 157-8, 160-4, 184-6
Ester C, 370
Euphorbia peplus, 270-1
exercise, 74, 79, 312, 335-6, 361
faith, 98-101, 261-2, 325
family
as helpers, 22-4
attitudes to cancer, 84-8
stress, 258-60, 283-7, 334-7
see also genetics

fats, dietary, 41, 46, 78, 156-7, 160-4
Feez, Kharmine, 85
fibre, 356
fibrin, 111
film
pathology of the blood, 107-9, 120-2, 232
flatulence, 60, 65
flaxseed oil, 163-4
flour, 42-3, 379
fluid retention, 370
fluids, 49-50
fluorescent light, 381
Fonti, Clara, 177
food
additives, 42-3
availability, 330
combining, 59-60
immune system, 41-3
mould, 54, 65
plan, 47-74
preserved, 353, 356
raw, 15
refined, 42
vitamins and minerals, 133-4, 378-82
see also diet; meals; nutrition
Fraire, Yolande, 148, 390
free radicals, 157, 166, 187
fruits, 54, 58, 371-6, 379-80, *see also* juices
fucose, 160
fungus
cancer organism, 222-3, 228
gastrointestinal tract, 54
infections, 44
gastrointestinal tract, 48, 53-4, 61
Gawler, Ian, 82
genetics, 26, 78-9, 240-1, 340, 355-6
genital herpes, 358-65
Gerlach, Franz, 228
German measles, 135, 319-20
Gerson, Max and Charlotte, 112-14, 143, 390
Gerson Therapy, 59, 243-5, 248-53, 256-7, 262-3
glandular fever, 279, 365
Glover, Thomas J., 179, 221
glutamine, 44
grains, 42-3, 52-3
gregomycin, 230
Gregory, John E., 230
grooming, 67

growth hormone, 192-3, 195, 228
gum diseases, 118
Gye, Dr, 206
Haemaview, 233
haemopoietic system, 149
haptens, 132
Hartman, Phillipina, 226-7
Hasumi, Kiichiro and Ken-ichiro, 182, 199, 203-15, 226, 391
headaches, 348
healing
  attitudes to, 88, 325
  nature, 313-14
  reaction, 244, 312, 346
Healthy Revolution diet, 55
heart disease, 370, 382
helplessness, 286
hepatitis B, 365
herbs, 8, 49, 72, 145-8
herpes simplex virus (HSV), 357-65
herpes viruses, 355-65
hip sarcoma, 240-5
Hoekstra, Phillip, 232-3
homeopathy, 142
honey, 44
hormone imbalance, 322
Hoxsey Biomedical Clinic, 146-8, 390
human chorionic gonadotrophin (HCG), 193, 195, 228
hydroxyurea, 329
hyperalimentation, 37
immune system, 127-38, 149
  foods, 41-3
  interferon, 139-40
  tests, 23, 29, 205, 208
  vitamins, 12
immunity, cellular and humoral, 128
Immuno-Augmentative Therapy (IAT), 125, 391
immuno-suppressive drugs, 37-8
immunoglobulins, 351-2
interferon, 126, 139-40, 229, 268-9, 347
interleukin, 127, 140, 229
International Union Against Cancer (UICC), 219-20
iron, 379
iscador, 301-3, 391
Issels, Joseph, 117-18, 180, 226
Ivy, Andrew C., 221
Japan, cancer vaccination trial, 182, 210-11
juices, 15, 49-50, 57-65, 68, 371-6

apple and carrot, 72
liver, 72, 142-4
orange, 379-80
pawpaw leaf, 244-5
wheatgrass, 72
juicing machines, 57-8, 143
Kaposi's sarcoma, 176
kidney transplant, 37-8
Koch, William, 186-8
Krebs virus, 180
L forms, 135-6, 173
L-lysine, 363-4
lactobacillus, 53-4
laetrile, 110-11, 306
lecithin, 164
leukaemia, 136-7, 227, 275
leukotriene, 140
life force, 88-9, 315
lifestyle, 41-6, 119-20, 322
light and physiology, 121-2, 241-2, 245-6, 322, 338, 341, 381 *see also* sunlight
Lincoln, Robert E., 229
linoleic acid, 162-3
linolenic acid, 163
linseed oil, 55-6
lip cancer, 272-3
lipids, 185-6, 233-4
liver (human)
  biological products, 139-40
  cancer, 215, 327
  cancer formation, 195-6
  functions, 45-6
  macro 2 globulin, 126
  nutrition, 41-2
liver (meat), 72, 140-4, 334, 376-7
Livingston, Virginia Wuerthele Caspe, 107-8, 115-21, 180-1, 199-200, 222-6, 232-3, 321-2, 391
low-density lipid (LDL), 333-4
lunch, 70
lung cancer, 36-7, 61, 86-8, 101-3, 138
lymph nodes, 320, 327, 339, 358
lymphocytes, 128-32, 137-8, 229
lymphoma, 166
lysine, 48
macro 2 globulin, 126, 139
macrophages, 131, 196
magnesium, 50, 67, 369-70
magnetic resonance imaging, 159
mammogram, 281
Manion, Helen and Gerard, 32-3

Mantoux test, 205, 208, 323, 352-3
margarine, 162-3
Maruyama, Chisato, 226
mash, 52-6
mastitis, chronic, 278
Mattmann, Lida, 173, 232
meals, 68-74, 371-7
Meares, Ainslie, 82
meat, 42, 45, 73, 141-2, 323-4, 379
meditation, 96-7, 261-2, 333-4
melanoma, 264-71, 319-31, 339-41, 347-9
memory cell, 131
mesothelioma, 215
metabolism
 aerobic and anaerobic, 42
 cell, 125-36, 191-6
 different types, 51, 59-60
 stressed cells, 155-96
microbacillus, 180
microbiology, 168-72
micromyces blastogenes, 228
microzyma, 169, 180
milk, skim, 49, 163
milkweed, 270
mind, 46-8, 81-97, 130
minerals, 378-82
 food sources, 133-4
 herpes, 364-5
 immune system, 12
 radiation therapy, 150
 see also supplements
mistletoe, 301
Mixed Bacterial Toxins (MBT), 230
monilia, see Candida
monocytes, 138, 279
Morales, Betty Lee, 109-12
Mortal Oscillary Rate (MOR), 227
motile rod, 135-6
Mountford, Caroline, 160
mouth ulcers, 356-7
muesli, 52-6
Multiple Biochemicals Analysis, 354
mycobacterium, 180, 352
Naessens, Gaston, 227-8, 385
natural therapists, 151-2, 331
Nauts, Helen Coley, 230-1
neutrophils, 138
Nieper, Hans A., 180, 391
nitrosamine, 353, 356
Norwalk juicer, 57-8, 143
nursing care, 28-9, 291-4

nutrition, 37, 41, 75, 129-30, 292-3, see also diet; food; supplements
Nutrition and Stress Control Centre, 10, 21-4
nuts, 54
nystatin powder, 345-6
oat bran, 57
oesophagus cancer, 206
oestradiol, 279
oestrogen, 278-9
oils, dietary, 41, 54-6, 160-4
oncogene, 168, 195, 365
orange juice, 379-80
Ott, John, 121-2, 241, 245-6
ovaries
 cancer, 102-3
 cysts, 322
oxidation, 157,-67, 186-8
pain, 74, 185, 291-2
Papanicolaou (Pap) smear, 360
para amino benzoic acid (PABA), 269-70
parotid cancer, 251
Pasteur, Louis, 170
pawpaw leaf juice, 244-5
Pennsylvania Quality of Life Inventory, 116-17
peptides, 127, 140, 189-90, 324
peritoneal metastases, 215
pesticides, 45-6
petty spurge, 270-3
phenylalanine, 323
plants, Australian, 148
plasma cell, 131
pleomorphic organisms, 135, 173-6, 386
pleuro-pneumonia-like organism (PPLO), 173
polyposis, 355-6
potassium, 42, 44-5, 50, 67, 157, 185
potatoes, 380
pregnancy, 257
Pressor K, 67
Pritikin diet, 55
Progenitor cryptocides, 107-8, 115-16, 118, 122, 180, 225-6, 232-3, 321
prostate cancer, 108, 118
protamide, 144
protein, 45, 141-2, 160-1, 189-91
psychotherapy, 82-3
Purified Protein Derivative (PPD), 205, 208, 215, 225, 323, 352-3
Quality of Life Inventory, 116-17

Quality of Life Support Group, 32, 101-3
radiation, *see* light
radiation therapy, 8, 48, 150-1, 166-7, 215, 248, 309-10
radium plant, 270
rebirthing, 313-14
rectal cancer, 332-8
relaxation techniques, 74, 89-91
research, 34-5, 182-3, 231-2
retinol, 63
retrovirus, 168-9
Revici, Emanuel, 183-6, 391
Rife, Royal, 227
Rous, Francis Peyton, 169, 206
Rous sarcoma, 169, 224
rubella, 135, 319-20
Russell, William, 179
saliva, 48
salt, dietary, 42, 44-5
sarcomas, 242, 370
scarring, 48
Scott, M. James, 179, 221
seafood, 73
Seibert, Florence, 225
selenium, 184-5
self-awareness courses, 312-13
self-esteem, 85, 98-103, 277-8, 286-8
Selye, Hans, 170
Shukokai Institute, 204-5, 212-13
Simonton, Carl and Stephanie, 82-3
skin
    cancer, 61, 271-3, 326-7, 339
    sunscreens, 269-70
    tests, 229
SMA 24, 354
smoking, 42, 242
sodium, 42, 44-5, 157
sodium ascorbate, 369-70
solasadine, 273
somatid, 180, 385-8
Somatoscope, 227, 385
soups, 372-3
spirit, 9, 47-8, 98-103, 261-2
sports injuries, 242
sprouts, grain, 57
spurge, 270-3
squamous cell carcinoma, 327
Staphage Lysate (SPL), 144, 148, 229
stem cells, 126, 129-30
steroids, 139, 370
sterols, 184

stomach cancer, 38-40, 48-9
stress, 78, 92, 165, 258-60, 277-80, 334-8, 361 *see also* cell; family
sugars, 42, 44, 73, 160
sunglasses, 242, 322
sunlight, 156, 338, 340, 381
sunscreen, 269-70
supplements, dietary, 67-8, 75-7, 167, 330-1, 334, 378-84 *see also* minerals; vitamins
support group, 32, 101-3
surgery, 8, 88, 268, 327-8, 339-40
survival
    factors, 36-8
    rates, 16-17, 35-40, 113
Survival Plan, *see* Cilento Survival Plan
Synthetic Survival Reagent (SSR), 187
syphonospora polymorpha, 180, 389
T cells, 128-32, 138, 195-6, 229, 364
tamoxifen, 308-9
teeth, 118, 120, 180, 250-1
tender trap, 285-7
therapies
    economic factors, 330-1
    history, 8
    natural, 151-2, 331
thrush, *see* Candida
thymosin, 130-1
thymus, 131, 140, 364
thyroid gland, 142, 333-4
thyroxine, 142, 333-4
Tozinal, 180
triglycerides, 160
trophoblasts, 111
trypsin, 111, 308
Tswett, Mikhail S., 207
tuberculosis (TB), 172, 323, 352-3
tumour necrosing factor (TNF), 126, 140, 143
TV sets, 246
ultraviolet (UV) light, 246, 320
urea, 328-9
urine filtration, 210
uterine cancer, 94
vaccines, 117-18, 126, 137-8, 178-81, 199-235, 323, 330, 352
    autogenous, 24, 115-16, 137-8
vegetables, 58, 371-6, 379-80, *see also* juices
victimisation, 78-80, 91
Villequez, E., 178, 199

virus, 44, 138
    cancer, 159, 168-72, 206-10, 225-30
visual display terminal (VDT), 241, 246
visualisation, 83, 93-7, 309-10
vitamins, 41-2, 75-6, 378-82
    A, 63, 308, 380-2
    administration, 322
    antibiotics, 136-7
    antioxidant, 164, 167
    B group, 48-9, 111, 149-50, 379
    C, 329, 355-6, 362, 364, 369-70, 379-80
    E, 48, 273, 310, 382
    food sources, 133-4
    herpes, 364-5
    immune system, 12
    radiation therapy, 150
    see also supplements
von Brehmer, Wilhelm, 179-80, 386-8
Warburg, Otto, 186
water, drinking, 46, 49, 74
weight gain and loss, 47, 333, 348
wheatgerm, 57
wheatgrass, 253, 355
white cells, 41, 55, 136, 246, 252, *see also* lymphocytes
wobe mugos, 142, 146, 148
worms, 249
Yarra Valley Living Centre, 391
yeast, 53, 341-6
yoghurt, 53, 362